SPRINGHOUSE NOTES

Anatomy and Physiology

Cecelia Gatson Grindel, RN, PhD
Assistant Professor, College of Nursing
Northeastern University
Boston

Leonard V. Crowley, MSc, MD
Professor
Century College
St. Paul, Minnesota
Clinical Assistant Professor
University of Minnesota Medical School
Minneapolis

Charlotte A. Johnston, PhD
Chairman, Department of Health Information Management
Medical College of Georgia
Augusta

Springhouse Corporation
Springhouse, Pennsylvania

Staff

Executive Director
Matthew Cahill

Editorial Director
June Norris

Art Director
John Hubbard

Managing Editor
David Moreau

Acquisitions Editors
Patricia Kardish Fischer, RN, BSN; Louise Quinn

Clinical Consultants
Maryann Foley, RN, BSN; Collette Bishop Hendler, RN, CCRN

Senior Project Editor
Nancy Priff

Editors
Naina Chohan, Karen Diamond, Michael Shaw

Copy Editors
Cynthia C. Breuninger (manager), Christine Cunniffe, Brenna Mayer

Designers
Arlene Putterman (associate art director), Lesley Weissman-Cook (book designer), Joseph Clark, Elaine Ezrow, Jacalyn Facciolo, Donald G. Knauss, Matie Patterson, Mary Stangl

Production Coordinator
Margaret A. Rastiello

Editorial Assistants
Beverly Lane, Mary Madden, Jeanne Napier

Manufacturing
Deborah Meiris (director), Pat Dorshaw (manager), T.A. Landis

---

The clinical procedures described and recommended in this publication are based on research and consultation with nursing, medical, and legal authorities. To the best of our knowledge, these procedures reflect currently accepted practice; nevertheless, they can't be considered absolute and universal recommendations. For individual application, all recommendations must be considered in light of the patient's clinical condition and, before administration of new or infrequently used drugs, in light of the latest package-insert information. The author and the publisher disclaim responsibility for any adverse effects resulting directly or indirectly from any suggested procedures herein, from any undetected errors, or from the reader's misunderstanding of the text.

Printed in the United States of America.

SNAP- D N
03 10 9 8 7

Library of Congress Cataloging-in-Publication Data
Grindel, Cecelia Gatson
Anatomy and physiology/ Grindel, Cecelia Gatson, Leonard V. Crowley, Charlotte A. Johnston
p. cm. — (Springhouse notes)
Includes bibliographical references and index.
1. Human anatomy and physiology. I. Crowley, Leonard V. II. Johnston, Charlotte A. III. Title. IV. Series.
DNLM: 1. Human anatomy and physiology—outlines. 2. Nursing—Outlines.
DNLM/DLC 97-65156
ISBN 0-87434-901-X (alk. paper) CIP

Contents

Advisory Board

How to Use Springhouse Notes

Springhouse Notes is a multivolume study guide series developed especially for nursing students. Each volume provides essential course material in an outline format, enabling the student to review information efficiently.

Special features appear in every chapter to make information accessible and easy to remember. **Learning objectives** encourage the student to evaluate knowledge before and after study. **Chapter overview** highlights the chapter's major concepts. Within the outlined text, key points appear in color to facilitate a quick review of critical information. Key points may include pivotal structures, critical steps in physiological processes, current theories, and cardinal signs and symptoms. **Points to remember** summarize each chapter's major themes. **Study questions** then offer another opportunity to review material and assess knowledge gained before moving on to new information. **Critical thinking and application exercises** conclude each chapter, challenging students to expand on knowledge gained.

Other features appear throughout the book to facilitate learning: **Teaching tips** highlight key areas to address with patient teaching. **Alerts** point out health concerns that may stem from a structural problem or the breakdown of a normal physiologic process. **Physiologic processes** graphically illustrate the steps that normally maintain homeostasis in the body. Difficult, frequently used, or sometimes misunderstood terms are indicated by SMALL CAPITAL LETTERS in the outline and defined in the glossary, Appendix A; answers to the study questions appear in Appendix B. Finally, a brand-new Windows-based software program (see diskette on inside back cover) poses 100 multiple-choice questions in random or sequential order to assess your knowledge.

The Springhouse Notes volumes are designed as learning tools, not as primary information sources. When read conscientiously as a supplement to class attendance and textbook reading, Springhouse Notes can enhance understanding and help improve test scores and final grades.

CHAPTER 1

Overview of Anatomy and Physiology

Learning objectives

After studying this chapter, you should be able to:

- Define anatomy and physiology.
- Describe common terms used in anatomy and physiology.
- List the 10 directional terms used to describe the locations of body structures.
- Identify and describe the body reference planes.
- Name the major body cavities and list the organs found in each.
- Identify the nine subdivisions of the abdominal region.
- Describe how the human body achieves homeostasis.

Chapter overview

Every health care professional needs a basic understanding of anatomy and physiology. This includes knowledge of how the body is organized, how its parts function together, and how its structures and functions may be affected by disease and other factors. To build this understanding, the health care professional must be familiar with basic anatomy and physiology terms, body reference planes, the contents of body cavities and body regions, and the principles of homeostasis.

♦ I. Introduction to anatomy and physiology

A. Definitions

1. *Anatomy* is the study of the structure of the body and the relationship of its parts
2. *Physiology* is the study of how body parts function, including their chemical and physical processes
3. The functions of a body part reflect its structure; this is called the complementarity of structure and function
    a. An example of complementarity is the direction of blood flow through the heart, which is controlled by the structure of the heart valves
    b. Another example is the relationship of blood pressure to the anatomic and physiologic status of structures in the kidney
4. Anatomy has several subdivisions, each addressing a specific aspect of structure
    a. *Gross anatomy* (macroscopic anatomy) is the study of anatomic structures visible to the unaided eye
    b. *Regional anatomy* is the study of limited portions or regions of the body, such as the head and neck
    c. *Developmental anatomy* is the study of structural changes from conception through old age
    d. *Microanatomy* (microscopic anatomy) is the study of anatomic structures using a microscope
    e. *Applied anatomy* is the application of anatomic findings to the diagnosis and treatment of medical disorders
    f. *Pathologic anatomy* (morbid anatomy) is the study of abnormal, diseased, or injured tissue
5. Physiology has several subdivisions, each addressing a specific aspect of function
    a. *Cell physiology* is the study of cell functions
    b. *Systems physiology* is the study of organ system operation
    c. *Pathophysiology* is the study of functional changes caused by disease and aging
    d. *Exercise physiology* is the study of cell and organ functions during skeletal muscle activity
    e. *Neurophysiology* is the study of nerve cell functions
    f. *Endocrinology* is the study of the effects of hormones on body functions

   g. *Immunology* is the study of the body's defense mechanisms
   h. Other subdivisions of physiology address the function of the specific structures, such as the heart and blood vessels (cardiovascular physiology), air passageways and lungs (respiratory physiology), kidneys (renal physiology), and reproductive structures (reproductive physiology)

B. Structural organization
1. Structural organization is characteristic of the body and all of its parts
2. The body is composed of increasingly complex levels of structural organization
   a. The *chemical level* includes the atoms and molecules that are needed to maintain life
   b. The *cellular level* consists of cells — the body's basic structural and functional units
   c. The *tissue level* combines similar cells and surrounding substances into groups that work together
   d. The *organ level* organizes different kinds of tissues — usually in recognizable shapes — to perform a special function
   e. The *systems level* consists of different kinds of organs arranged to perform complex functions
   f. The *organismic level,* which is the highest level, brings together all lower level structures into one functioning, living being
3. Body structures change gradually
   a. Usually, body structures grow and develop until young adulthood
   b. After young adulthood, body structures typically age and atrophy

C. Anatomical position
1. To describe regions or parts of the body accurately, health care professionals assume that the body is in the *anatomical position*
2. In the anatomical position, the body is erect and facing forward, with arms at the sides and palms turned forward
3. Use of this position makes directional terms clear

D. Directional terms
1. *Directional terms* are terms used to describe the exact location of a body structure
2. Derived mainly from Greek or Latin words, directional terms are standard throughout the various health science fields
   a. When used as a directional term, SUPERIOR (CRANIAL) means toward the head
   b. INFERIOR (CAUDAL) means toward the tail or lower part of the body
   c. ANTERIOR (VENTRAL) means toward the front of the body
   d. POSTERIOR (DORSAL) means toward the back of the body
   e. MEDIAL means toward the midline of the body

f. LATERAL means away from the midline of the body
g. PROXIMAL means closest to the trunk, point of origin of a part, or center of the body
h. DISTAL means farthest from the trunk, point of origin of a part, or center of the body
i. SUPERFICIAL means toward or at the body surface
j. DEEP means farthest from the body surface

3. Anatomical features are demarcated by dividing the body into planes, cavities, and regions

♦ II. Body reference planes

A. General information
1. In the study of anatomy, the body and its organs are sectioned (cut) along imaginary lines called planes
2. Planes are used to describe the structural plan of the body and the anatomic relationship of one part to another
3. The three major body reference planes are the sagittal, frontal, and transverse; the three planes lie at right angles to one another (see *Body reference planes*)

B. Reference planes
1. A SAGITTAL PLANE runs longitudinally (lengthwise) and divides the body into right and left regions
   a. When exactly midline, it is called a median sagittal plane or a midsagittal plane
   b. When not exactly midline, it is called a parasagittal plane
2. A *frontal plane* (coronal plane) also runs longitudinally but at a right angle to a sagittal plane; it divides the body into anterior and posterior regions
3. A *transverse plane* runs horizontally at a right angle to the vertical axis; it divides the structure into superior and inferior regions
4. An *oblique plane* is a slanted plane that lies between a horizontal plane and a longitudinal plane

♦ III. Body cavities

A. General information
1. *Body cavities* are spaces within the body that house the internal organs; the dorsal and ventral cavities are the two major closed cavities containing internal organs (see *Body cavities,* page 6)
2. Other cavities include the oral, nasal, orbital, tympanic, and synovial

B. Dorsal cavity
1. The *dorsal cavity* is located in the posterior region of the body
2. It is divided into the cranial and vertebral cavities
   a. The *cranial cavity* (skull) encases the brain

Body reference planes

Body reference planes are directional terms used to locate body structures. The illustration below shows the median sagittal, frontal, and transverse planes, which lie at right angles to one another.

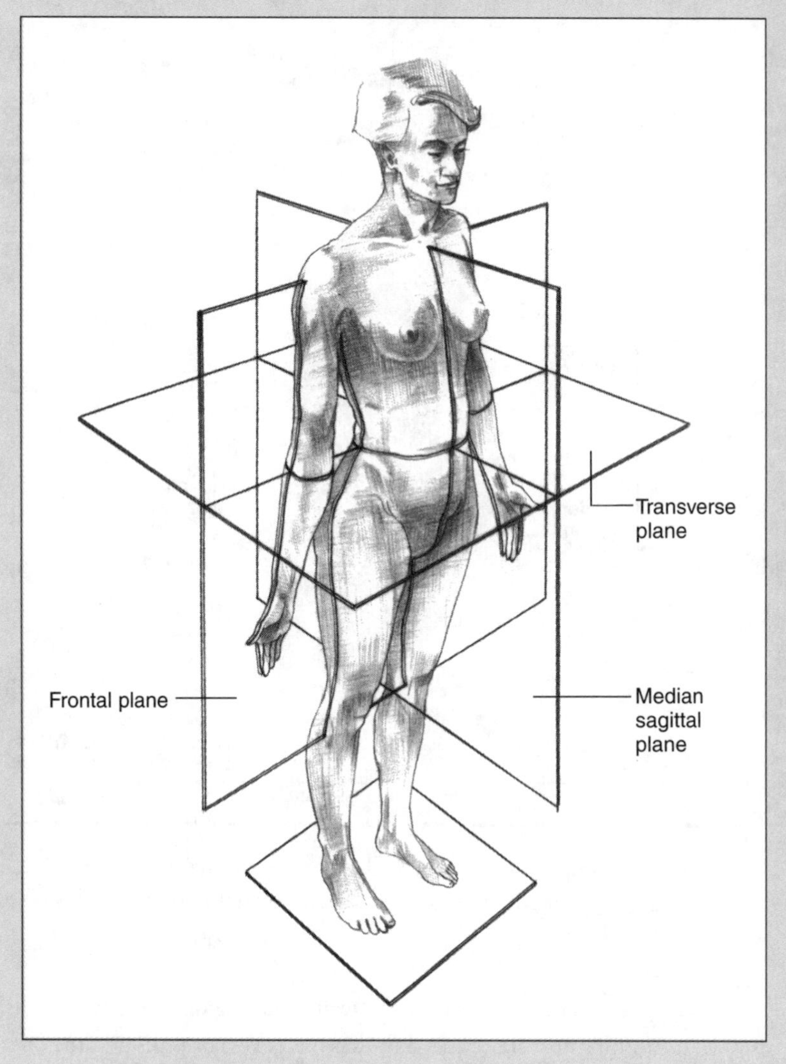

Body cavities

The body has two major cavities—dorsal and ventral. The dorsal cavity, located posteriorly, is subdivided into the cranial and vertebral cavities. The ventral cavity, located anteriorly, is subdivided into the thoracic and abdominopelvic cavities.

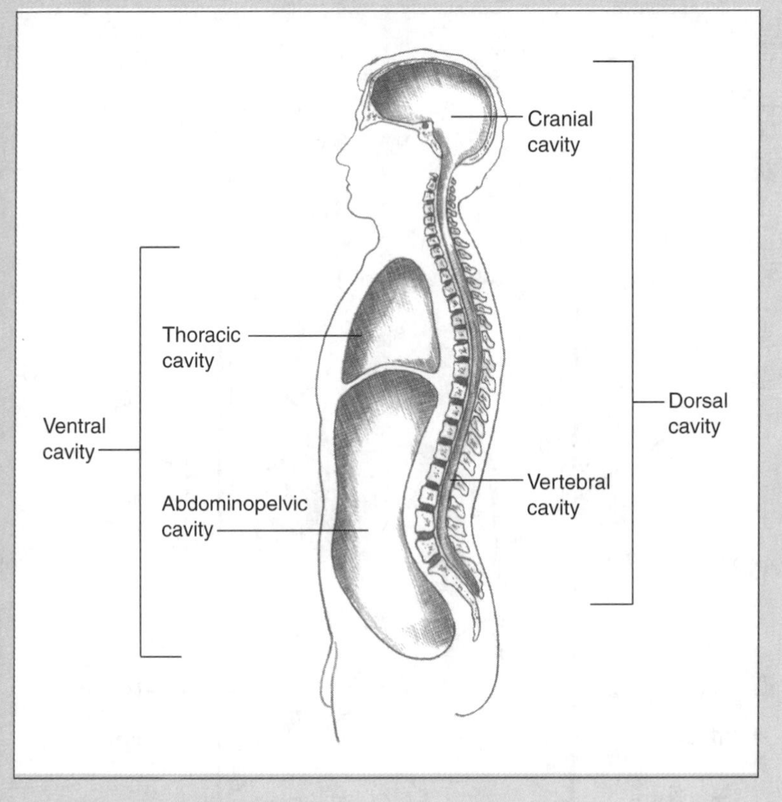

   b. The *vertebral cavity,* also called the spinal cavity or vertebral canal, is formed by the series of bones (vertebrae) that enclose the spinal cord

C. Ventral cavity
   1. The *ventral cavity* is located in the anterior region of the trunk
      a. A thin membrane called the SEROSA covers its walls and the outer surface of its organs
      b. The portion of the membrane that lines the cavity wall is called the *parietal serosa;* the portion that covers the organs is called the *visceral serosa*
   2. The ventral cavity is divided into the thoracic and abdominopelvic cavities

3. The thoracic cavity is superior to the abdominopelvic cavity; it is surrounded by the ribs and chest muscles
   a. It is subdivided into the pleural cavities and the mediastinum
      (1) The two lateral pleural cavities each contain a lung; the serosa in these cavities is called the *pleura*
      (2) The mediastinum contains the heart (enclosed in a membranous serosal sac forming the pericardial cavity), the large vessels of the heart, the trachea, the esophagus, the thymus, lymph nodes, and portions of other vessels and nerves
      (3) The serosa of the pericardial cavity is called the *pericardium*
   b. The thoracic cavity is separated from the abdominopelvic cavity by the *diaphragm,* a large dome-shaped muscle
4. The abdominopelvic cavity is subdivided into two parts (regions), which are not separated by muscle or membrane
   a. The two subdivisions are the abdominal cavity and pelvic cavity
      (1) The abdominal cavity — the superior portion of the abdominopelvic cavity — contains the stomach, spleen, liver, small intestine, most of the large intestine, and other organs
      (2) The pelvic cavity is inferior to the abdominal cavity and contains the bladder, some of the large intestine, some reproductive organs, and the rectum
   b. The serosa in the abdominal and pelvic cavities is called the *peritoneum*

D. Other cavities
1. The oral cavity (mouth) contains the teeth and tongue; it is continuous with other gastrointestinal structures
2. The nasal cavity, located in the nose, is divided medially; it is continuous with the respiratory tract
3. The two orbital cavities house the eyes
4. The tympanic cavities, etched into the temporal bone, contain the auditory ossicles (the small bones of the middle ear)
5. The synovial cavities are enclosed within fibrous capsules that surround freely movable joints

♦ IV. Body regions

A. General information
1. Body regions are universally accepted designations for specific areas of the human body having a special nerve or vascular supply or a special function
2. The terms applied to these regions help describe the anatomic locations of various body structures

Abdominal regions

The nine abdominal regions include the epigastric, right and left hypochondriac, umbilical, right and left lumbar, hypogastric, and right and left iliac regions.

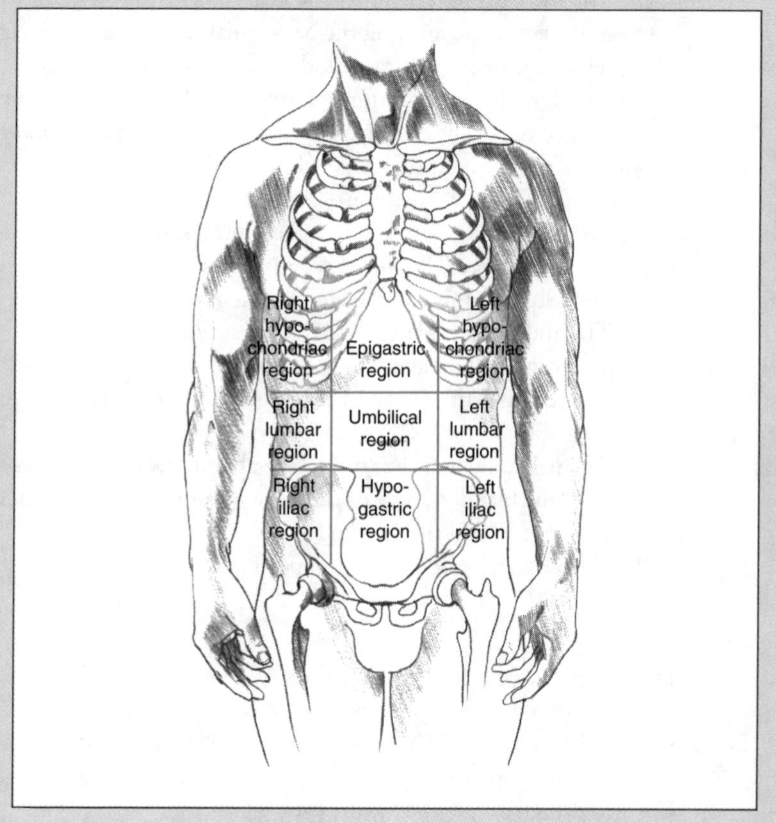

B. Abdominal regions

1. The abdomen commonly is subdivided into nine regions (see *Abdominal regions*)
2. The umbilical region (navel) is the area around the umbilicus; its most prominent structures are sections of the small and large intestines, inferior vena cava, and abdominal aorta
3. The epigastric region (stomach) is superior to the umbilical region; prominent structures are the pancreas and portions of the stomach, liver, inferior vena cava, abdominal aorta, and duodenum
4. The hypogastric region (pubic region) is inferior to the umbilical region; prominent structures include portions of the sigmoid colon, urinary bladder, ureters, and small intestine

5. The right and left inguinal regions (iliac regions) are lateral to the hypogastric region; they include portions of the small and large intestines
6. The right and left lumbar regions (loin regions) are lateral to the umbilical region; prominent structures include portions of the small and large intestines and portions of the right and left kidneys
7. The right and left hypochondriac regions are lateral to the epigastric region; both contain portions of the diaphragm and kidneys
   a. The right region also contains the right side of the liver
   b. The left region also contains the spleen and a portion of the pancreas

♦ V. Homeostasis

A. General information
1. HOMEOSTASIS is a condition of relative constancy in the body's internal environment
2. Homeostasis is present when the body's internal environment meets three requirements
   a. It has the proper concentration of water, gases, and ions
   b. It maintains a normal temperature
   c. It has sufficient volume to maintain cellular health

B. Regulation of homeostasis
1. The nervous system and endocrine system help maintain and restore homeostasis; their actions in this effort are called homeostatic mechanisms
2. Homeostatic mechanisms operate by negative feedback; a change in one direction feeds back in some way to cause a change in the *opposite* direction

POINTS TO REMEMBER

- Anatomy is the study of the body's structures; physiology is the study of the body's functions.
- The body is composed of increasingly complex levels of structural organization, from the chemical level to the organismic level.
- Anatomic features are demarcated by dividing the body into planes, cavities, and regions.
- Homeostasis requires a proper concentration of water, gases, and ions, temperature, and volume.

- Homeostatic mechanisms maintain or restore homeostasis by using negative feedback.

STUDY QUESTIONS

To evaluate your understanding of this chapter, answer the following questions in the space provided. Then compare your responses with the correct answers in Appendix B, page 328.

1. How is anatomy related to physiology?

____

____

2. What are the basic structural levels of the body?

____

____

3. How are anatomical features demarcated?

____

____

4. What organs are housed by the body's two major closed cavities?

____

____

CRITICAL THINKING AND APPLICATION EXERCISES

1. Draw a human body in the anatomical position.
2. On a model of the human body, indicate the sagittal, frontal, and transverse planes.
3. Ask a partner to name a body structure. Using the 10 directional terms, describe its location. Then you and your partner reverse roles.
4. On an illustration of the human body, draw and identify the nine abdominal regions.

CHAPTER

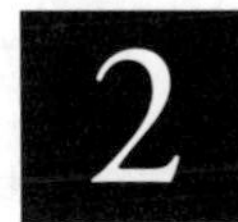

Chemical Organization

Learning objectives

After studying this chapter, you should be able to:

- Define matter and energy.
- Describe an atom and identify its subatomic particles.
- Differentiate between ionic and covalent bonds.
- Compare different types of chemical reactions.
- Discuss the roles of inorganic compounds in the body.
- Discuss the roles of organic compounds in the body.

Chapter overview

The chemical level is the simplest level of structural organization, yet it is the most important. Without the proper chemicals in the proper amounts, the cells — and eventually the body — will die. Not only is the body composed of chemicals, but all of its activities are chemical in nature. To comprehend the importance of chemicals in anatomy and physiology, the health care professional must be familiar with the basic principles of chemistry, such as atomic structure and chemical bonds and reactions. The health care professional also must understand the inorganic and organic compounds in the body.

♦ I. Principles of chemistry

A. Matter and energy
   1. Matter is anything that has mass and occupies space; it may be a solid, liquid, or gas
   2. Energy is the capacity to do work (put mass into motion); it may be potential energy (stored energy) or kinetic energy (energy of motion)
   3. Forms of energy include chemical, electrical, and radiant energy
   4. Matter and energy cannot be created or destroyed; however, matter can be converted to energy

B. Chemical elements
   1. An ELEMENT is a form of matter that cannot be broken down into simpler substances by normal chemical reactions
      a. All forms of matter are composed of chemical elements
      b. The periodic table of elements lists 109 chemical elements; each element has a chemical symbol, such as Fe (the chemical symbol for iron)
   2. Carbon, hydrogen, nitrogen, and oxygen comprise 96% of total body weight
   3. Calcium and phosphorus comprise another 2.5% of total body weight

C. Atomic structure
   1. An ATOM is the smallest unit of matter that can take part in a chemical reaction; an element is composed of atoms of a single type, such as carbon
   2. Each atom has a nucleus (dense central core) and one or more electron shells (surrounding energy layers)
   3. Atoms contain three basic subatomic particles: protons, neutrons, and electrons
   4. PROTONS (p+) are positively charged particles in the atom's nucleus
      a. The number of protons is unique for each element
         (1) The number of protons determines the element's *atomic number;* for example, sodium's atomic number is 11 because its nucleus contains 11 protons
         (2) Each element has a different atomic number
      b. A nucleus's positive charge equals the number of its protons; for example, the nucleus of a carbon atom has positive charge of 6 (6p+) because it contains 6 protons
      c. One proton weighs the same as 1 neutron, which is equal to 1,836 times the weight of 1 electron
      d. An atom's *atomic weight* (atomic mass) equals the total mass of its protons, neutrons, and electrons (p + n + e)

    e. An atom's *mass number* is the sum of its protons and neutrons (p + n); because electrons have little mass, an atom's mass number may nearly equal its atomic mass
5. NEUTRONS are uncharged (neutral) particles in the atom's nucleus
    a. All atoms of an element do not necessarily have the same number of neutrons
    b. *Isotopes* are atoms that have a different number of neutrons from most atoms of an element
6. ELECTRONS are negatively charged particles that orbit around the nucleus in different electron shells
    a. The number of electrons in an atom equals the number of protons in its nucleus
        (1) The electrons' negative charges cancel out the protons' positive charges
        (2) Because of this cancellation, atoms are electrically neutral
    b. Each electron shell surrounding the nucleus can accommodate a maximum number of electrons
        (1) The innermost shell can hold no more than two electrons
        (2) The outermost shells can hold many more
7. Electrons play a key role in chemical bonds and reactions
    a. An atom with single (unpaired) electrons in its outer electron shell can participate in chemical reactions
    b. An atom's *valence* (combining capacity) equals the number of unpaired electrons in its outer shell; for example, sodium ($Na+$) has a plus-one valence because it has an unpaired electron in its outer shell
        (1) A chemical reaction occurs when one atom combines with or breaks apart from another atom
        (2) A molecule is a substance composed of two or more atoms
        (3) A compound is a substance composed of two or more elements

D. Chemical bonds
1. Chemical bonds are forces of attraction that hold together the atoms of a molecule
2. Chemical bond formation usually requires energy; chemical bond breakage usually releases energy
3. Several types of chemical bonds exist
    a. An *ionic bond* forms when valence electrons are transferred from one atom to another
    b. A *covalent bond* forms when atoms share pairs of valence electrons
    c. A *hydrogen bond* forms when two atoms associate with a hydrogen atom; oxygen and nitrogen commonly form hydrogen bonds

Summary of chemical reactions

The four types of chemical reactions can be expressed with the following formulas.

Synthesis reaction

$A + B \longrightarrow AB$

Exchange reaction

$AB + CD \longrightarrow AD + BC$

Decomposition reaction

$AB \longrightarrow A + B$

Reversible reaction

$A + B \longleftrightarrow AB$

E. Chemical reactions
   1. The occurrence of a chemical reaction depends on energy as well as particle concentration, speed, and orientation
   2. Four basic types of chemical reactions exist (see *Summary of chemical reactions*)
      a. *Synthesis reactions* involve the combination of two or more substances (reactants) to form a new, more complex substance (product)
         (1) In these reactions, chemical bonds are formed
         (2) Collectively, synthesis reactions in the body are called ANABOLISM
      b. *Decomposition reactions* involve the breakdown of a substance into two or more simpler substances
         (1) In these reactions, chemical bonds are broken
         (2) Collectively, decomposition reactions in the body are called CATABOLISM
      c. *Exchange reactions* combine decomposition and synthesis reactions
         (1) Two complex substances undergo decomposition into simpler substances
         (2) Through synthesis, the simple substances combine with different simple substances to form new complex substances
      d. *Reversible reactions* allow the product to revert to its original reactants and vice versa; these reactions may require special conditions, such as heat or light, to take place

♦ II. Inorganic compounds

A. General information
   1. Some biomolecules form *inorganic compounds;* these compounds usually lack carbon and are small

2. Most biomolecules form *organic compounds;* these compounds contain carbon and hydrogen, and use covalent bonds
3. Inorganic compounds include water and inorganic acids, bases, and salts

B. Water
1. Water is the body's most abundant substance
2. This versatile substance serves many vital functions
   a. Water is an excellent solvent and suspension medium; it easily forms polar covalent bonds
   b. It acts as a lubricant in mucus and other body fluids
   c. It enters into chemical reactions, such as nutrient break down during digestion
   d. It absorbs and releases heat slowly, which helps the body maintain homeostasis
   e. It needs a great deal of heat to convert from liquid to gas; this function keeps the body cool through perspiration

C. Inorganic acids, bases, and salts
1. In water, molecules of inorganic acids, bases, and salts undergo *ionization* (separation into ions)
   a. ACIDS ionize into hydrogen ions (H^+) and anions (negatively charged ions); for example, HCl dissociates into H^+ and the anion Cl^-
   b. BASES ionize into hydroxide ions (OH^-) and cations (positively charged ions); for example, KOH dissociates into OH^- and the cation K^+
   c. SALTS ionize into cations and anions, but not H^+ or OH^- ions; for example, KCl dissociates into the cation K^+ and the anion Cl^-
2. When acids and bases react together, they form salts
3. To maintain homeostasis, body fluids must achieve ACID-BASE BALANCE
   a. The greater the number of hydrogen ions in a solution, the more acidic it is
   b. The greater the number of hydroxide ions in a solution, the more basic (alkaline) it is
   c. The pH scale measures the acidity or alkalinity of body fluids
      (1) A neutral solution has a pH of 7; it contains equal amounts of H^+ and OH^-
      (2) An acidic solution has a pH below 7; it contains more H^+ than OH^-
      (3) A basic (alkaline) solution has a pH above 7; it contains more OH^- than H^+

4. In the body, pH is maintained by various BUFFER SYSTEMS (see Chapter 16, Fluid, Electrolyte, and Acid-Base Balance)

♦ III. Organic compounds

A. General information
   1. Organic compounds include CARBOHYDRATES, LIPIDS, PROTEINS, and NUCLEIC ACIDS
   2. Carbohydrates include sugars and starches, as well as glycogen and cellulose
   3. Lipids are a diverse group of water-insoluble biomolecules
   4. Proteins are polypeptides composed of amino acids
   5. Nucleic acids include deoxyribonucleic acid (DNA) and ribonucleic acid (RNA)

B. Carbohydrates
   1. Based on size, carbohydrates are grouped as monosaccharides, disaccharides, and polysaccharides
      a. Monosaccharides have three to seven carbon atoms
      b. Disaccharides are a combination of two monosaccharides; examples include sucrose (table sugar) and lactose (milk sugar)
      c. Polysaccharides are large carbohydrates made from many monosaccharides; glycogen is the major polysaccharide
   2. Monosaccharides are combined to form disaccharides or polysaccharides through dehydration synthesis; this process yields the more complex saccharide and water
   3. Disaccharides and polysaccharides are broken down into monosaccharides by hydrolysis; by adding water to larger molecules, this process yields smaller molecules
   4. The main functions of carbohydrates are energy release and energy storage

C. Lipids
   1. The major lipids include triglycerides, phospholipids, steroids, lipoproteins, and eicosanoids
   2. Triglycerides (neutral fats) are the most plentiful lipids in the diet and the body
      a. They protect, insulate, provide energy, and store energy
      b. They have three molecules of a fatty acid and one molecule of glycerol
   3. Phospholipids function as the major component of cell membranes
      a. Phospholipids have one molecule of glycerol, two molecules of a fatty acid, and a phosphate group
      b. Phosphatidylcholine (lecithin) is a common phospholipid

4. Steroids, which come in four main types, have different functions
   a. Cholesterol is a part of animal cell membranes and is required for the formation of all other steroids
   b. Bile salts emulsify fats during digestion and promote the absorption of vitamins A, D, E, and K
   c. Male and female sex hormones are responsible for reproduction function and sexual characteristics
   d. Vitamin D helps regulate the body's calcium concentration
5. Lipoproteins helps transport lipids to various parts of the body
6. Eicosanoids include prostaglandins and leukotrienes
   a. Prostaglandins serve diverse functions, such as modifying hormone responses, promoting the inflammatory response, and opening airways
   b. Leukotrienes function in inflammatory and allergic responses

D. Proteins
1. *Amino acids* are the building blocks of proteins; the sequence of amino acids in a protein's polypeptide chain determines its conformation (shape), which determines its functions
2. Typical protein functions include providing structure and protection, regulating processes, promoting muscle contraction, transporting substances, and serving as enzymes
3. *Enzymes,* the largest group of proteins, act as catalysts for vital chemical reactions

E. Nucleic acids
1. DNA and RNA are nucleic acids composed of nitrogenous bases, sugars, and phosphate groups
2. DNA has a double-helix shape; it is the primary hereditary molecule
   a. In DNA, two long chains of deoxyribonucleotides coil into double-helix shape
      (1) Deoxyribose and phosphate units alternate in the backbone of the chains
      (2) Base pairs of adenine-thymine and guanine-cytosine hold the two chains together
   b. Each human DNA molecule contains a specific sequence of more than 100 million base pairs; this sequence is the same in all the DNA in one individual and different from the DNA of all other individuals
3. Unlike DNA, RNA has a single-chain structure, contains ribose instead of deoxyribose, and substitutes uracil for the base thymine; RNA guides protein synthesis from amino acids

POINTS TO REMEMBER

- Every atom contains protons and neutrons in its nucleus. Electrons orbit around the nucleus.
- A chemical reaction occurs when one atom combines with or breaks apart from another atom. It may create a molecule or a compound.
- Chemical bonds include ionic, covalent, and hydrogen bonds.
- Types of chemical reactions include synthesis, decomposition, exchange, and reversible reactions.
- Inorganic compounds usually lack carbon. They include water and inorganic acids, bases, and salts.
- Organic compounds contain carbon and hydrogen. They include carbohydrates, lipids, proteins, and nucleic acids.

STUDY QUESTIONS

To evaluate your understanding of this chapter, answer the following questions in the space provided. Then compare your responses with the correct answers in Appendix B, page 328.

1. Which chemical elements make up most of the human body? __________

____

____

2. What role do electron shells play in chemical reactions? __________

____

____

3. What is the difference between ionic and covalent bonds? __________

____

____

4. What is water's role in the body? __________

____

____

5. How is dehydration synthesis different from hydrolysis? ______________

____

____

6. How does DNA's structure differ from that of RNA?______________

____

____

CRITICAL THINKING AND APPLICATION EXERCISES

1. Choose one element on the periodic table. Identify its atomic number, mass number, atomic mass, and valence.
2. Express the synthesis reaction that occurs when you add H_2 and Cl_2.
3. Using a reagent strip, test and record the pH of three different solutions. Determine which are neutral, acidic, or alkaline.
4. Record your daily food intake for one day. Then highlight the carbohydrates in blue, lipids (fats) in yellow, and proteins in red.

CHAPTER

3

Cell Organization

Learning objectives

After studying this chapter, you should be able to:

- ♦ Describe the cell's main components and functions.
- ♦ Explain how mitochondria convert food nutrients into the energy in adenosine triphosphate (ATP) and how ATP is broken down and recycled to provide cellular energy.
- ♦ Describe the ways in which substances can pass through a cell membrane.
- ♦ Discuss the function of genes and the significance of heterozygous and homozygous gene pairs in dominant, recessive, codominant, and sex-linked genetic expression.
- ♦ Compare the roles of deoxyribonucleic acid and ribonucleic acid in cell division.
- ♦ Identify and discuss the phases of cell division.
- ♦ Contrast mitosis and meiosis.

Chapter overview

The cellular level is the second level of structural organization. Yet it is the first level for living matter. A knowledge of cell organization and function can help the health care professional better understand certain disease processes, drug actions, and laboratory tests. This chapter highlights cellular components, energy production, genetic material, and reproduction. It also explains substance movement across the cell membrane and the actions of ribonucleic acid (RNA).

♦ I. Cellular components

A. General information
   1. The cell is the structural and functional unit of all living matter; it is the smallest body structure that can perform all the fundamental activities of life, such as movement, ingestion, excretion, and reproduction
   2. Although most cells are specialized, they all have these four major components: *cell membrane, cytosol, organelles,* and *inclusions*

B. Cell membrane
   1. The cell is surrounded by a semipermeable cell (plasma) membrane that regulates the passage of certain materials in and out of the cell (see "Substance movement across the cell membrane," page 24, for more information)
   2. This membrane separates the cell's internal environment from its external one

C. Cytosol
   1. The term *cytoplasm* refers to all the cell's contents from the cell membrane to the nucleus
   2. Cytosol is the semifluid medium in the cytoplasm; it constitutes the intracellular fluid, which contains such material as proteins, enzymes, nutrients, and ions
   3. Organelles and inclusions are embedded in the cytosol

D. Nucleus and organelles
   1. The *nucleus* is the control center of the cell; it directs the activities of the cytoplasmic structures
      a. The nucleus contains the genetic material of the cell
      b. It also contains one or more *nucleoli,* spherical structures that synthesize RNA
      c. A nuclear membrane separates the nucleus from the cytoplasm; pores in this membrane allow certain substances to pass through
   2. Each organelle, or little organ, performs a specific function
   3. Not all organelles are used to the same degree, depending on the function of a particular cell; for example, cells that synthesize large amounts of lipids have an abundant smooth endoplasmic reticulum, whereas cells that synthesize protein have a rough endoplasmic reticulum

4. The major organelles are the mitochondria, ribosomes, endoplasmic reticulum, Golgi apparatus (or complex), lysosomes, and centrioles
   a. MITOCHONDRIA are the energy-producing cellular structures
      (1) They contain enzymes that oxidize food nutrients
      (2) This oxidation produces ADENOSINE TRIPHOSPHATE (ATP), which provides the energy for many cellular activities
   b. *Ribosomes* are nucleoprotein particles that are attached to the endoplasmic reticulum; protein synthesis takes place in these organelles
   c. *Endoplasmic reticulum* is a system of interconnecting tubular channels
      (1) Rough (granular) endoplasmic reticulum is covered with ribosomes
      (2) Smooth endoplasmic reticulum contains enzymes to synthesize lipids
      (3) Both types of endoplasmic reticula have fluid-filled channels that appear to connect all parts of the cytoplasm
   d. *Golgi apparatuses* synthesize carbohydrate molecules
      (1) These molecules combine with protein produced by rough endoplasmic reticulum
      (2) This combination forms secretory products, such as lipoproteins
   e. *Lysosomes* are digestive bodies that break down damaged or foreign material in the cells
      (1) Each lysosome is surrounded by a membrane separating its digestive enzymes from the rest of the cytoplasm; its enzymes digest materials brought into the cell by phagocytosis
      (2) The membrane of the lysosome fuses with that of the vacuoles, or cytoplasmic spaces, that have phagocytized material, allowing the lysosomal enzymes to digest the engulfed material
         (a) Digestion occurs in the phagocytic vacuole
         (b) Digestive enzymes do not escape into the cell cytoplasm
   f. *Centrioles* are short cylinders adjacent to the nucleus; during cell division, they move to opposite poles of the cell and form the mitotic spindle

E. Inclusions
   1. Cell inclusions are chemicals produced by the cell; they are not contained by a membrane, but some have particular shapes
   2. Melanin, glycogen, and triglycerides are examples of cell inclusions

Adenosine triphosphate structure

The illustration below shows the chemical structure of adenosine triphosphate.

Adenine

Ribose

Phosphate

1 2 3

$O-P(=O)(OH)-O\sim P(=O)(OH)-O\sim P(=O)(OH)-OH$

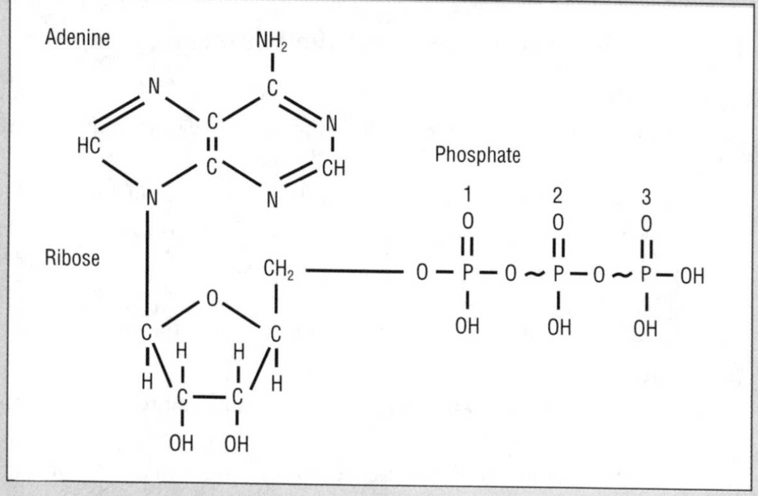

♦ II. Cellular energy generation

A. General information
   1. Cellular activities require energy
   2. Mitochondria are the cellular power stations
      a. They contain enzymes that oxidize food nutrients
      b. This oxidation produces ATP, a chemical fuel for cellular processes

B. Adenosine triphosphate
   1. ATP is composed of a nitrogen-containing compound (adenine) joined to a five-carbon sugar (ribose), forming adenosine; adenosine is joined to three phosphate groups (see *Adenosine triphosphate structure*)
   2. The chemical bonds between the first and second and the second and third phosphate groups contain a large amount of energy
      a. When the terminal high-energy phosphate bond ruptures, ATP is converted to adenosine diphosphate (ADP)
      b. Liberation of the third phosphate releases the energy stored in the chemical bond

3. Mitochondrial enzymes reconvert ADP and the liberated phosphate to ATP
   a. Mitochondria obtain the energy needed for this reattachment by oxidizing food nutrients
   b. The recycled ATP then is available again for energy production

♦ III. Substance movement across the cell membrane

A. General information
1. Each cell interacts with body fluids through the interchange of substances
2. Movement of substances between cells and body fluids is accomplished by several methods of transport: DIFFUSION, OSMOSIS, ACTIVE TRANSPORT, and *endocytosis*
3. Transfer of fluids and dissolved substances across capillaries into interstitial fluid is facilitated by filtration

B. Diffusion
1. This is a method of PASSIVE TRANSPORT; it does not require cellular energy
2. In diffusion, dissolved particles (solute) move from an area of higher concentration to one of lower concentration
3. Several factors influence the diffusion rate
   a. The CONCENTRATION GRADIENT (difference in the particle concentration on either side of the plasma membrane) affects diffusion: the greater the concentration gradient, the faster the diffusion
   b. The particle size affects diffusion; small particles diffuse faster than large ones
   c. Lipid solubility affects diffusion; lipid-soluble particles diffuse more rapidly through the lipid layers of the cell membrane
   d. The electrical charge of the diffusing particles also affects diffusion
      (1) Electrically charged particles (ions) on one side of the membrane diffuse more rapidly when ions on the other side of the membrane have the opposite electrical charge, because ions of unlike charges are attracted to each other
      (2) Ions with the same electrical charge repel each other, slowing diffusion
4. FACILITATED DIFFUSION is a special type of diffusion in which a carrier molecule in the cell membrane picks up the diffusing substance on one side of the membrane and deposits it on the other side

C. Osmosis

1. Like diffusion, osmosis is a passive transport method that involves molecule movement from a solution of higher molecular concentration to one of a lower concentration
2. Unlike diffusion, osmosis involves water (solvent) molecule movement across the cell membrane from a dilute solution (with a high concentration of water molecules) to a concentrated one (with a lower concentration of water molecules)
3. Osmosis depends on the OSMOTIC PRESSURE of a solution
   a. Osmotic pressure measures the "water-attracting" property of a solution; it is determined by the number of dissolved particles in a given volume of solution, not on their size or electrical charge
   b. For example, a calcium chloride molecule ($CaCl_2$) dissociates (ionizes) in solution into three particles, a calcium ion and two chloride ions; its osmotic pressure is higher than that of a larger glucose molecule, which does not dissociate into ions when dissolved in solution
4. Water movement in and out of cells by osmosis depends on the osmotic pressure differences between intracellular and extracellular fluids
   a. Normally, intracellular osmotic pressure equals the extracellular osmotic pressure; as a result, the water content of cells does not change
   b. Osmotic pressure changes in body fluids causes water to shift between cells and extracellular fluids, impairing or disrupting cell functions
      (1) When the osmotic pressure of extracellular fluid is lower than that of intracellular fluid, water enters the cells, causing them to swell and possibly rupture
      (2) Conversely, when the osmotic pressure of extracellular fluid is higher than that of intracellular fluid, water moves into extracellular fluid, causing the cells to shrink

D. Active transport

1. Active transport is a transport method in which a substance is moved across the cell membrane
   a. Usually, the transport mechanism moves a substance from an area of lower concentration to an area of higher concentration (against the concentration gradient)
   b. This mechanism also can move a substance from an area of higher concentration to one of lower concentration (with the concentration gradient)
2. In active transport, a carrier molecule in the cell membrane combines with the substance, transports it through the membrane, and deposits it on the other side of the membrane

3. Unlike facilitated diffusion, which also uses a carrier molecule, active transport requires energy from ATP breakdown to transport a substance across a cell membrane

E. Endocytosis
   1. In this active (energy-requiring) method of transport, a substance is engulfed by the cell rather than passing through the cell membrane
      a. The cell surrounds the substance with part of the cell membrane
      b. This part of the membrane separates, forming a vacuole that moves to the cell interior
   2. Endocytosis may be divided into phagocytosis and pinocytosis
      a. PHAGOCYTOSIS is the engulfment and ingestion of particles too large to pass through the cell membrane
      b. *Pinocytosis* is similar to phagocytosis, except that it is used only to engulf substances in solution or very small particles in suspension

F. Filtration
   1. Movement of fluid and dissolved substances across a cell membrane also can be accomplished by *filtration*
   2. In filtration, the application of pressure to a solution on one side of the cell membrane forces fluid and dissolved particles through the membrane; the filtration rate depends on the amount of pressure
   3. Filtration serves several purposes
      a. It promotes the transfer of fluids and dissolved materials from the blood across the capillaries into the *interstitial fluid* (fluid surrounding the cells); the pressure of capillary blood provides the filtration force
      b. Urine formation depends on fluid filtration from the blood flowing through capillaries in the kidneys (see Chapter 15, Urinary System, for more information)

♦ IV. Cellular genetic material

A. General information
   1. Chromosomes in the nucleus control cell activities
   2. Chromosomes contain the genetic material of the cell

B. Chromosomes
   1. *Chromosomes* control cellular activities; they direct protein synthesis by ribosomes in the cytoplasm
      a. Chromosomes are composed of deoxyribonucleic acid (DNA) and protein
      b. They appear as a network of granules (chromatin) in the nondividing cell
   2. Chromosomes exist in pairs, except in the GAMETES (male and female reproductive cells); one chromosome from each pair comes from the male parent, the other from the female parent

3. Normal cells contain 23 pairs of chromosomes
   a. In these cells, 22 pairs are sets of homologous chromosomes, or autosomes; they contain genetic information that controls the same characteristics or functions
   b. One pair is composed of sex chromosomes
      (1) The composition of these chromosomes (X and Y) determines sex
         (a) XX is genetic female
         (b) XY is genetic male
      (2) In the female, the genetic activity of both X chromosomes is essential only during the first few weeks of embryonic development
         (a) Later development requires only one functional X chromosome
         (b) The other X chromosome is inactivated and appears as a dense chromatin mass called a *Barr body* (or sex chromatin body), which is attached to the nuclear membrane in the cells of a normal female
      (3) The Barr body is absent in the cells of a normal male (who has only one functional X chromosome)

C. Genes
   1. *Genes* are segments of chromosomal DNA chains that determine a cellular property; they are arranged in a line on the chromosomes somewhat like beads on a string
   2. The *gene locus* refers to the location of a specific gene on a chromosome
      a. *Alleles* are alternate forms of a gene that can occupy a particular locus on a chromosome
      b. Only one allele can occupy a specific gene locus
   3. Because chromosomes are paired, genes also occur in pairs on homologous chromosomes, with one allele at its locus on both homologous chromosomes
      a. If the alleles for a particular gene are the same on both chromosomes, the individual is HOMOZYGOUS for that gene
      b. If the alleles are different, the individual is HETEROZYGOUS for the gene
   4. Genes are responsible for inherited traits; the effects they produce vary with the gene
   5. *Gene expression* refers to the effect of a gene on cell structure or function
      a. A *dominant gene* is expressed in the heterozygous state
         (1) A dominant gene is expressed even if only one parent transmits it to the offspring
         (2) The genes for dark hair and eyes are dominant

b. A *recessive gene* is expressed only in the homozygous state
   (1) A recessive gene is expressed only when both parents transmit it to the offspring
   (2) The genes for blond hair and blue eyes are recessive
c. *Codominant genes* allow expression of both alleles, as in the genes that direct specific types of hemoglobin synthesis in red blood cells
d. *Sex-linked genes* are carried on sex chromosomes
   (1) Almost all appear on the X chromosome and are recessive
   (2) In the male, sex-linked genes behave like dominant genes because there is no second X chromosome

D. DNA
1. *DNA,* a large nucleic acid molecule found in the chromosomes in the nucleus, is the carrier of genetic information in living cells
2. The basic structural unit of DNA is the *nucleotide;* it consists of a phosphate group linked to a five-carbon sugar, deoxyribose, joined to a nitrogen-containing compound called a base
   a. Deoxyribose is similar to ribose, except for the substitution of a hydrogen (H) atom for hydroxyl (OH) connected to a carbon (C) atom
   b. Four different DNA bases exist
      (1) Adenine and guanine are double-ring compounds classified as purines
      (2) Thymine and cytosine are single-ring compounds classified as pyrimidines
   c. Consequently, four different DNA nucleotides exist, differing only in the base joined to deoxyribose
3. Nucleotides are joined into long chains by chemical bonds between the phosphate group of the nucleotide and a carbon atom in the deoxyribose molecule of the adjacent nucleotide
4. The nitrogen bases project from the deoxyribose molecule at right angles to the long axis of the chain
5. DNA chains exist in pairs; they are held together by weak chemical attractions (hydrogen bonds) between the nitrogen bases on adjacent chains
   a. Because of the chemical configuration of the bases, adenine bonds only with thymine, and guanine bonds only with cytosine; bases that can link with each other are *complementary*
   b. Linked DNA chains form a spiral structure, or double helix, which resembles a spiral staircase
      (1) The deoxyribose and phosphate groups form the railings
      (2) The nitrogen base pairs form the steps
6. The sequence of nucleotide bases in DNA chains forms the *genetic code,* a series of coded messages

7. Each group of three bases, called a *codon,* specifies the synthesis of a specific amino acid by attracting a specific amino acid, which is carried to the ribosomes to synthesize protein

♦ V. RNA

A. General information
   1. *RNA* transfers genetic information from nuclear DNA to ribosomes in the cytoplasm where protein synthesis occurs; several types of RNA are involved in this process
   2. Like DNA, RNA consists of nucleotide chains; however, some of its components are different
      a. RNA contains the five-carbon sugar ribose rather than deoxyribose
      b. Uracil — not thymine — is the complementary base of adenine in RNA
      c. Guanine and cytosine are complementary bases in RNA

B. Types of RNA
   1. The nucleus produces three types of RNA, which pass into the cytoplasm: ribosomal RNA (rRNA), messenger RNA (mRNA), and transfer RNA (tRNA)
   2. *rRNA* is used to make ribosomes in the endoplasmic reticulum of the cytoplasm, where the cell produces proteins
   3. *mRNA* specifies how the amino acids are arranged to make proteins at the ribosomes
   4. *tRNA* carries specific amino acids during protein synthesis

C. Protein synthesis in the cytoplasm
   1. One or more ribosomes attach themselves to the mRNA strand that contains instructions for protein synthesis
   2. tRNA chains attach themselves to amino acids in the cytoplasm and transfer them to the ribosomes
   3. The ribosomes join the amino acids into a chain according to the sequence of bases on the mRNA strand to form a protein
   4. When the chain is complete, the new protein is released and the mRNA strand detaches from the ribosomes

♦ VI. Cell division

A. General information
   1. Each cell must replicate itself for life to continue
   2. Before a cell divides, its chromosomes are duplicated
   3. Duplication involves separation of the DNA chains
   4. Cells normally divide by MITOSIS or MEIOSIS (ALERT)
   5. When cell division is uncontrolled, excess tissue may form; it may develop into a tumor, growth, or neoplasm

6. Although cell division is continuous, it may be divided into four phases: prophase, metaphase, anaphase, and telophase

B. Chromosome and DNA duplication
1. During this process, the double helix separates into two DNA chains; each serves as a template for constructing a new chain
2. Individual DNA nucleotides are linked into new strands with bases complementary to those in the originals
3. In this manner, two identical double helices are formed, each containing one of the original strands and a newly formed complementary strand
4. These double helices are duplicates of the original DNA chain (see *DNA duplication*)

C. Mitosis
1. All cells except gametes undergo this form of cell division
   a. The parent cell, containing 46 chromosomes, undergoes division and gives rise to two daughter cells
   b. Both daughter cells are identical to each other and to the parent cell
2. During *prophase,* the first active phase of mitosis, the chromosomes (each consisting of two chromatids) thicken and shorten; the centrioles move to opposite sides of the cell and form the mitotic spindle, a network of protein microfibers; and the nuclear membrane breaks down
3. During *metaphase,* the chromosomes line up in the center of the cell; the two chromatids of each chromosome begin to separate but remain joined at the centromere, where spindle fibers are attached
4. During *anaphase,* the chromatids of each chromosome separate and are pulled to opposite poles of the cell by spindle fibers
5. During *telophase,* nuclear membranes form around both groups of chromosomes, and the cytoplasm divides, and forms two identical daughter cells

D. Meiosis
1. Only gametes (ova and spermatozoa) undergo this type of cell division
2. Meiosis is characterized by intermixing of genetic material between homologous chromosomes and a reduction by half in the number of chromosomes in the four daughter cells
3. Meiosis consists of two separate divisions
4. The first meiotic division involves four phases
   a. During prophase, homologous chromosomes align so that matching genes are side by side, a condition called *synapsis;* chromatid segments may break off and interchange, or CROSS OVER, mixing the genetic material

DNA duplication

The basic structural unit of deoxyribonucleic acid (DNA) is the nucleotide, which is composed of a phosphate group, deoxyribose, and a nitrogen base made of adenine (A), guanine (G), thymine (T), or cytosine (C). Many nucleotide strands become twisted to form a double helix of a DNA molecule. During duplication, linked DNA chains separate. Then new complementary chains form and link to the originals (parents). This results in two identical double helices, consisting of parent and daughter, as shown.

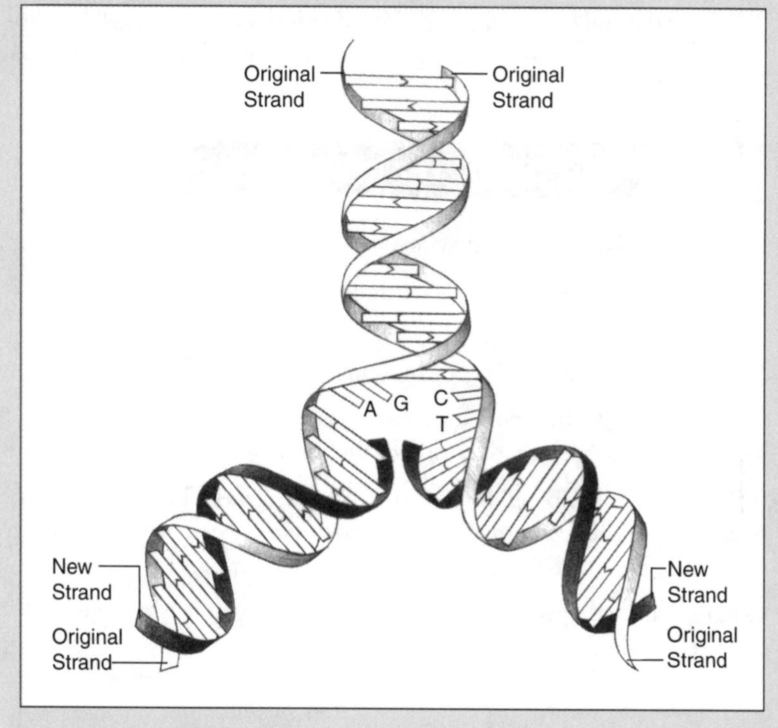

b. During metaphase, the chromosomes move to the center of the cell and the spindle fibers form
c. In anaphase, the homologous chromosomes — but not the chromatids — of each pair separate and move to opposite poles of the cell
d. During telophase, nuclear membranes form around the chromosomes, and the cytoplasm divides, forming two new daughter cells
   (1) Each cell has only 23 chromosomes

(2) Each contains genetic material from both parents because of cross over and because the chromosomes of each parent do not all move to one side of the cell during anaphase

5. The second meiotic division resembles the four phases of mitotic division
   a. In each cell, the two chromatids of each chromosome separate to form new daughter cells
   b. However, because each cell that enters the second meiotic division has only 23 chromosomes, each daughter cell formed during this division has only 23 chromosomes
6. At the end of the second meiotic division, each parent cell has produced four daughter cells genetically different from the parent cell

POINTS TO REMEMBER

- The cell is the basic unit of all living matter.
- The major components of the cell include the nucleus, cytoplasm, and organelles. All components are surrounded by the cell membrane.
- Mitochondria generate energy by breaking down ATP.
- Substances may be transported across the cell membrane by diffusion, osmosis, active transport, endocytosis, or filtration.
- Within the chromosomes, DNA carries the cell's genetic information. RNA transfers this genetic information to ribosomes in the cytoplasm, where protein synthesis occurs.
- Cells reproduce themselves by cell division. Gametes divide by meiosis; all other cells divide by mitosis.

STUDY QUESTIONS

To evaluate your understanding of this chapter, answer the following questions in the space provided. Then compare your responses with the correct answers in Appendix B, pages 328 and 329.

1. What are the major components of the cell? ______________________

____

____

2. How do mitochondria create energy for the cell?

3. How is active transport different from passive transport?

4. When is a dominant gene expressed? When is a recessive gene expressed?

5. What is the primary function of DNA?

6. What are the three types of RNA and what do they do?

7. What are the four phases of cell division?

CRITICAL THINKING AND APPLICATION EXERCISES

1. Draw a cell and identify its major components.
2. Prepare an oral presentation for your class on the actions of mitochondria in using ATP and recycling ADP.
3. Create of a model of a cell, and demonstrate a method of transporting substances across the cell membrane.
4. Summarize the functions of DNA and RNA in the cell.
5. Create a poster showing the phases of mitosis or meiosis.

CHAPTER

4

Tissue Organization

Learning objectives

After studying this chapter, you should be able to:

- ♦ State the relationship between tissues and cells.
- ♦ Identify the types of epithelial tissue.
- ♦ Describe the classifications of connective tissue.
- ♦ Name the distinguishing characteristics of muscle fibers.
- ♦ Identify the two main attributes of nervous tissue.

Chapter overview

The tissue level is the third level of structural organization. Tissues are groups of cells with the same general function. They include epithelial, connective, muscle, and nervous tissues. By knowing the location and function of each type of tissue, the health care professional can gain a better understanding of their roles in health, illness, and recovery.

♦ I. Epithelial tissue

A. General information
   1. *Epithelial tissue* (epithelium) is a continuous multicellular sheet with at least two types of epithelial cells; it covers the body's surface, lines body cavities, and forms certain glands
   2. Epithelial tissue is classified by the number of cell layers and the shape of the surface cells (see *Differentiating among epithelial tissues,* page 36)

B. Cell layer types
   1. Based on the number of cell layers, epithelial tissue is classified as simple, stratified, or pseudostratified
      a. Simple epithelial tissue has only one layer
      b. Stratified epithelial tissue has two or more layers
      c. Pseudostratified epithelial tissue has only one layer but appears to have more
   2. The cell layer depends on its location and function; for example, simple epithelium appears in areas with little wear and tear, whereas stratified epithelium appears in areas with much greater wear and tear

C. Surface cell shapes
   1. Based on the shape of its surface cells, epithelial tissue is classified as squamous, columnar, or cuboidal
      a. Squamous epithelial tissue has flat surface cells
      b. Columnar epithelial tissue has tall, cylindrical, prismatic surface cells
      c. Cuboidal epithelial tissue has cube-shaped surface cells
   2. Transitional tissue has cells that change shape easily
      a. Transitional tissue usually appears in the stratified epithelium
      b. It is located in areas that require ready distention (ability to stretch)

D. Characteristics of epithelium
   1. Some columnar epithelial cells have vertical striations (microvilli); these are called a striated, or brush, border
   2. Stereociliated epithelial cells have long piriform (pear-shaped) tufts; such cells line the epididymis
   3. Ciliated epithelial cells possess CILIA
      a. Cilia are fine hairlike protuberances on the free border
      b. Larger than microvilli, cilia propel fluid and particles through the lumen of an organ
   4. Typically, epithelium lacks blood vessels; in some epithelial tissues (such as the olfactory mucosa), branches of sensory nerves pierce the underlying layer (basement lamina) of the tissue

Differentiating among epithelial tissues

The number of cell layers and the shape of surface cells determine how epithelial tissue (epithelium) is classified. Thus, epithelium may be simple (one-layered), stratified (multilayered), or pseudostratified (one-layered but appearing to be multilayered). It also may be squamous (containing flat surface cells), columnar (containing tall cylindrical surface cells), or cuboidal (containing cube-shaped surface cells). The top left illustration shows how the basement membrane of simple squamous epithelium joins the epithelium to underlying connective tissues. The remaining illustrations show the five other types of epithelial tissue.

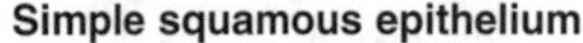

Simple squamous epithelium

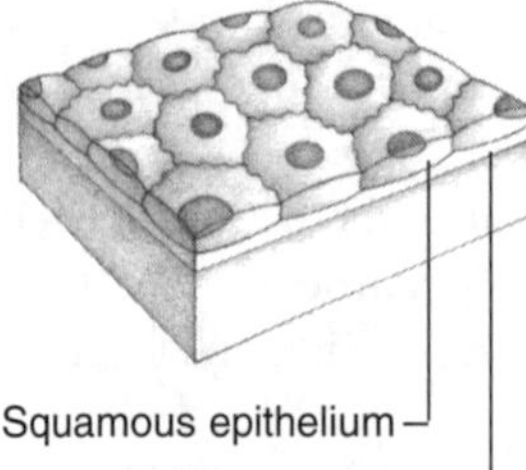

Stratified columnar epithelium

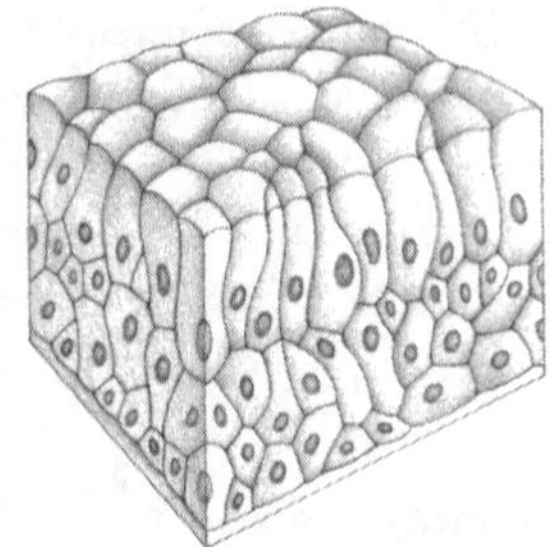

Simple cuboidal epithelium

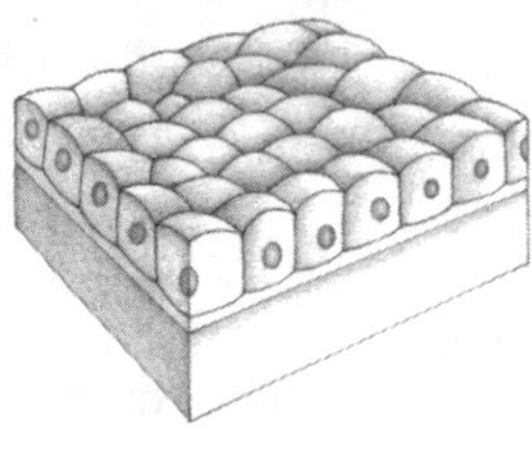

Stratified squamous epithelium

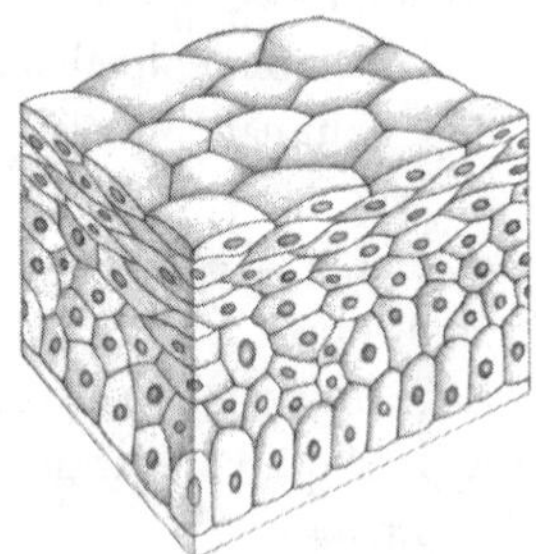

Simple columnar epithelium

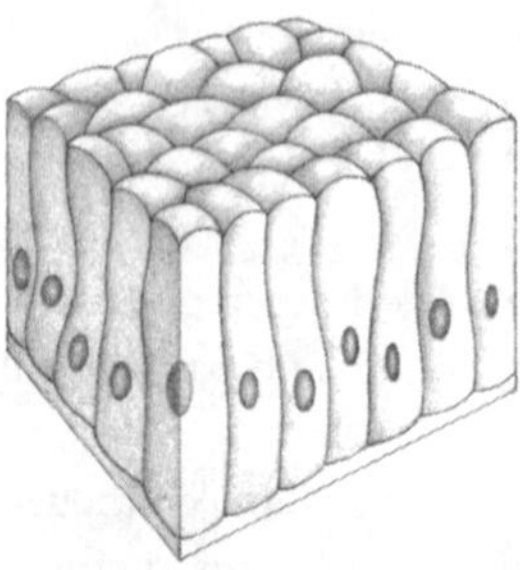

Pseudostratified columnar epithelium

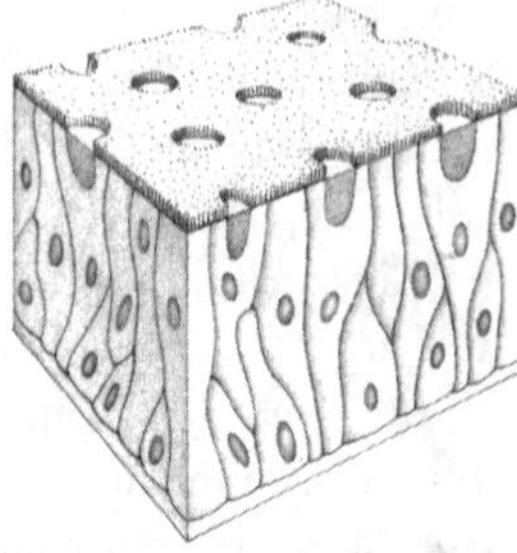

5. *Wandering cells* are macrophages (PHAGOCYTES) that enter the epithelium from connective tissue
6. Some types of epithelium are desquamated (shed) and regenerated continuously by transformation of cells from deeper layers
7. Epithelial tissue with a single layer of squamous cells attached to a basement membrane is called *endothelium;* it lines the heart, lymphatic vessels, and blood vessels

E. Glandular epithelium
   1. Glands — organs that produce secretions — are composed of a special type of epithelium called *glandular epithelium*
      a. Many glands are enclosed in a dense connective tissue capsule
      b. They are divided into lobes, then into smaller units called lobules
   2. Depending on its secretion mode, a gland is classified as exocrine or endocrine
      a. *Secretion* is the process of elaborating a specific product; it may involve separation of an element of the blood or elaboration of a totally new chemical substance (such as the urine secreted by the kidneys)
      b. *Excretion,* in contrast, refers to elimination of a product from the body; for instance, the urinary bladder excretes urine
      c. Endocrine glands release secretions into the blood or lymph; for example, the medulla of the adrenal gland secretes epinephrine and norepinephrine into the bloodstream
      d. Exocrine glands discharge secretions onto external or internal surfaces; for instance, sudoriferous (sweat) glands secrete sweat onto the surface of the skin
      e. Mixed glands contain endocrine and exocrine cells
         (1) The pancreas, for instance, contains alpha and beta cells (in the islets of Langerhans); these endocrine cells produce glucagon and insulin, respectively
         (2) The pancreas also contains acinar cells; these exocrine cells secrete digestive juices

♦ II. Connective tissue

A. General information
   1. Connective tissue binds together and supports body structures
   2. It is composed of cells, fibers, and ground substance
      a. Outside of the cells, the fibers and ground substance create the tissue MATRIX
      b. The matrix separates cells from each other; they do not touch like epithelial cells do

B. Tissue cells
   1. Connective tissue cells include fibroblasts, macrophages, plasma cells, mast cells, adipocytes, and white blood cells
   2. Each type of cell performs a distinct function
      a. Fibroblasts secrete substances that form matrix
      b. Macrophages perform as phagocytes
      c. Plasma cells secrete antibodies
      d. Mast cells produce histamine and contain heparin
      e. Adipocytes store fat
      f. White blood cells act as a defense mechanism
   3. Connective tissue cells may be fixed or wandering
      a. Fixed cells are typical cells that remain in place
      b. Wandering cells may move from one site to another

C. Tissue matrix
   1. The tissue matrix has two components — fibers and ground substance
   2. The fibers, which provide strength and support, come in three types — collagenous, reticular, and elastic
   3. The *ground substance* includes extracellular fluid chemicals as well as large molecules, such as hyaluronic acid and proteins

D. Classification
   1. Connective tissue is classified as loose, dense, cartilage, bone (osseous), and blood
   2. *Loose connective tissue* develops from the mesenchyme after other embryonic tissues have formed
      a. Large spaces separate its fibers and cells; it contains much intercellular fluid
      b. Types of loose connective tissue include areolar, adipose, and reticular
   3. *Dense connective tissue* has a greater concentration of fibers than does loose connective tissue
      a. It provides structural support
      b. Types of dense connective tissue include dense regular, dense irregular, and elastic connective tissue
         (1) Dense regular connective tissue consists of tightly packed fibers arranged in a consistent pattern; it includes TENDONS, ligaments, and APONEUROSES
         (2) Dense irregular connective tissue consists of tightly packed fibers arranged in an inconsistent pattern; it is found in the dermis, the submucosa of the gastrointestinal tract, fibrous capsules, and fascia

(3) Elastic connective tissue consists of freely branching elastic fibers; it is found in lung tissues, arterial walls, bronchial tubes, and other structures that must stretch

4. *Cartilage* and *bone tissues* are the connective tissue of the skeletal system (for details on them, see Chapter 6, Skeletal System)
5. *Blood (vascular tissue)* is an opaque, viscous fluid that circulates through the heart, arteries, capillaries, and veins
   a. Blood is connective tissue that uses plasma as the liquid matrix
   b. Formed elements (blood cells) are suspended in the plasma (for details on blood, see Chapter 11, Hematologic System)
6. Some types of connective tissue have special properties
   a. Mucous connective tissue (Wharton's jelly) of the umbilical cord is a temporary tissue that derives from the mesenchyme; it supports the umbilical cord
   b. Elastic connective tissue of the vocal cords permits speech
   c. Pigmented connective tissue of the sclera gives the eyeball its white color

E. Membranes

1. An *epithelial membrane* is the plane of contact between an epithelial layer and the connective tissue layer beneath it; the three main types of epithelial membranes are mucous, serous, and cutaneous membranes
2. A *synovial membrane* contains connective tissue only; it lines joint cavities, bursae, and tendons

♦ III. Muscle tissue

A. General information

1. Muscle tissue consists of well-vascularized muscle cells
   a. These cylindrical cells may measure several centimeters long; their elongated shape enhances their ability to contract (contractility)
   b. MYOFIBRILS (muscle fibers) of muscle tissue contain the contractile proteins ACTIN and MYOSIN
2. The three basic types of muscle tissue are STRIATED, cardiac, and smooth (for details on muscle tissue, see Chapter 7, Muscular System)

B. Striated muscle

1. *Striated muscle* tissue has a characteristic striped (striated) appearance
   a. Striated muscle fibers are multinucleated masses of protoplasm innervated by cerebrospinal nerves

b. These fibers contain specialized myofibrils — bundles of fine fibers made up of even finer fibers called thin and thick filaments
   (1) Thin filaments contain the contractile protein actin
   (2) Thick filaments contain the contractile protein myosin

2. *Skeletal muscle* includes all striated muscle tissue capable of voluntary contraction

C. Cardiac muscle

1. *Cardiac muscle* is the striated muscle of the heart
   a. Cardiac muscle fibers are separate cellular units; they are not multinucleated, as are other striated muscle fibers
   b. Some references classify cardiac muscle as striated muscle rather than as a separate category; however, unlike other striated muscle, it contracts involuntarily
2. Cardiac muscle fibers are connected to each other by interwoven discs

D. Smooth muscle

1. *Smooth-muscle* tissue is composed of long spindle-shaped cells; it lacks the characteristic striped pattern of striated muscle
2. Smooth-muscle tissue is innervated by the autonomic nervous system; thus, its activity is not under voluntary control
3. Smooth-muscle tissue lines the walls of many internal organs
   a. It lines the digestive tract from the middle of the esophagus to the internal anal sphincter, forming the contractile portion of the gastrointestinal tract
   b. It lines the walls of the respiratory passages from the trachea to the alveolar ducts
   c. It also lines the urinary and genital ducts, the walls of arteries and veins, and larger lymphatic trunks
   d. In the skin, smooth-muscle fibers form the ARRECTORES PILORUM, tiny muscles whose contraction causes the hair to stand erect
   e. In the mammary glands, smooth muscle causes the nipples to become erect; in the scrotum, it wrinkles the skin to help elevate the testes
   f. Smooth muscle in the ciliary body of the eye plays a role in accommodation; smooth-muscle contraction in the iris results in pupil dilation

♦ IV. Nervous tissue

A. General information

1. The main function of nervous tissue is communication (for details on nervous tissue, see Chapter 8, Nervous System)
2. Its two basic attributes are irritability and conductivity
   a. *Irritability* is the capacity to react to various physical and chemical agents
   b. *Conductivity* is the ability to transmit the resulting reaction from one point to another

B. Cell types

1. Nervous tissue includes two types of cells — neurons and neuroglia
2. *Neurons* are highly specialized cells that generate and conduct nerve impulses
   a. A typical neuron consists of a cell body with cytoplasmic extensions — numerous dendrites on one pole and a single insulated axon on the opposite pole
   b. These cytoplasmic extensions allow the neuron to conduct impulses over long distances
3. *Neuroglia* form the support structure of nervous tissue
   a. They insulate and protect neurons
   b. They are found only in the central nervous system

POINTS TO REMEMBER

- There are four main types of tissue: epithelial, connective, muscle, and nervous.
- Epithelial tissue covers the body's surface, lines body cavities, and forms certain glands. It is classified by the number of cell layers and the shape of the surface cells
- Connective tissue binds together and supports body structures. It is composed of cells and a matrix made of fibers and ground substance.
- Muscle tissue consists of well-vascularized muscle cells that contract. The basic types of muscle tissue are striated (skeletal), cardiac, and smooth.
- Nervous tissue communicates information throughout the body. It includes two types of cells: neurons and neuroglia.

STUDY QUESTIONS

To evaluate your understanding of this chapter, answer the following questions in the space provided. Then compare your responses with the correct answers in Appendix B, page 329.

1. What are the three layers of epithelial tissue? ______________________

____

____

2. Which fibers comprise the connective tissue matrix? ________________

____

____

3. What are the three types of muscle tissue and where are they located?_____

____

____

4. How are neurons different from neuroglia? ______________________

____

____

CRITICAL THINKING AND APPLICATION EXERCISES

1. Draw and identify the shapes of the three types of epithelial cells.
2. Look at several types of connective tissue under a microscope, and document the characteristics you see.
3. Develop a chart that compares the location, function, and characteristics of the three types of muscle tissue.

CHAPTER

5

Integumentary System

Learning objectives

After studying this chapter, you should be able to:

- ♦ Identify the components of the integumentary system.
- ♦ Name the six functions of the skin.
- ♦ Describe the five strata of the epidermis.
- ♦ Compare the appearance and functions of the two regions of the dermis.
- ♦ Name the skin derivatives and describe their functions.
- ♦ Explain the mechanisms involved in thermoregulation.

Chapter overview

The integumentary system consists of the skin, hair, nails, and certain glands. The integumentary system is one of the largest and most visible organs of the body, and it is commonly affected by changes in other systems. For these reasons, the health care professional who is familiar with its anatomy and physiology can quickly detect signs of disease — and recovery.

♦ I. Skin

A. General information

1. The integumentary system includes the skin and its derivatives — hair, nails, sudoriferous glands, sebaceous glands, and ceruminous glands
2. The skin (also called the INTEGUMENT) weighs about 9 lb (4.1 kg) and covers a surface area of roughly 15 to 20 ft^2 (1.4 to 1.9 m^2)
   a. Every square inch (6.5 cm^2) of skin contains approximately 15′ (4.6 m) of blood vessels, 12′ (3.7 m) of nerves, 650 sweat glands, 100 oil glands, 1,500 sensory receptors, and 3 million cells
   b. Skin cells die and are replaced continuously
3. Skin thickness varies from 1⁄32" to 1⁄8" (0.5 to 4 mm); skin is quite thin on the eyelids and quite thick on the palms and soles
4. The two fused layers of the skin — epidermis and dermis — are separated by the BASEMENT MEMBRANE

B. Functions

1. The skin has six major functions — it protects the body, excretes waste products, helps regulate body temperature, provides sensation, promotes vitamin D synthesis, and acts as a reservoir for blood
2. The skin protects the body chemically, physically, and biologically
   a. Chemically, acidic skin secretions inhibit bacteria from multiplying on the body's surface
      (1) Bactericidal substances in the sebum (a sebaceous gland secretion) kill some bacteria
      (2) Melanin, a chemical pigment, shields the skin from the sun's ultraviolet rays
   b. Physically, the KERATINIZED cells of the epidermis, hair, and nails provide a barrier to invading organisms
   c. Biologically, the epidermis contains macrophage-like Langerhans' cells that take part in immunity; dermal macrophages serve as a second line of defense against bacteria and viruses
3. The skin excretes waste products
   a. Although most nitrogenous wastes are eliminated in urine, small amounts are excreted in sweat
   b. Profuse sweating also causes excretion of large amounts of sodium chloride
4. The skin helps regulate body temperature (for details, see "Thermoregulation," page 50)
5. The skin provides CUTANEOUS sensation
   a. The skin contains sensory receptors — Meissner's corpuscles, PACINIAN CORPUSCLES, and free nerve endings

   b. These receptors receive stimuli that the brain interprets as temperature, pressure, or the presence of tissue-damaging elements (for details, see Chapter 9, Sensory System)
6. The skin plays a role in vitamin D synthesis
   a. When exposed to ultraviolet rays, the skin converts cholesterol molecules to vitamin D
   b. Vitamin D, in turn, participates in calcium METABOLISM
7. The skin also acts as a reservoir for blood; when needed, blood can be shunted from the skin to the general circulation (such as to supply vigorously working muscles)

C. Developmental considerations
1. In the embryo, the epidermis and dermis develop from the ectodermal and mesodermal germ layers, respectively
2. A newborn's skin is covered with *vernix caseosa,* a white cheesy substance that protects the skin from amniotic fluid in utero
3. During adolescence, sebaceous glands become more active from excessive hormonal secretions

ALERT

4. With advanced age, the skin and its derivatives change
   a. The skin loses elasticity, develops wrinkles, undergoes pigmentation changes, and heals more slowly; because of this, elderly people are more prone to develop skin cancer, pressure ulcers, and shingles than younger people
   b. The hair loses pigmentation and grows more slowly; the nails also grow more slowly
   c. Sweat and oil production diminishes

♦ II. Epidermis

A. General information
1. The *epidermis* is the skin's surface layer and outermost protective covering of the body
2. Composed of keratinized, stratified squamous epithelium, it consists of four types of cells — keratinocytes, melanocytes, Merkel's cells, and Langerhans' cells
   a. *Keratinocytes* are the most abundant type of epidermal cell; their chief role is to produce keratin, a water-insoluble protein that hardens structures (such as hair follicles)
   b. *Melanocytes* are clear cells that synthesize tyrosinase and melanin
   c. *Merkel's cells* are cup-shaped tactile nerve endings that serve as touch receptors
   d. *Langerhans' cells* are branched, star-shaped cells that resemble melanocytes but do not synthesize tyrosinase; arising in bone marrow, they migrate to the epidermis in a macrophage-like fashion

Microscopic structures of the skin

The epidermis has five strata: stratum basale, stratum spinosum, stratum granulosum, stratum lucidum, and stratum corneum. The dermis has a papillary region and a reticular region. Subcutaneous tissue, found beneath the dermis, is loose connective tissue that attaches the skin to underlying structures.

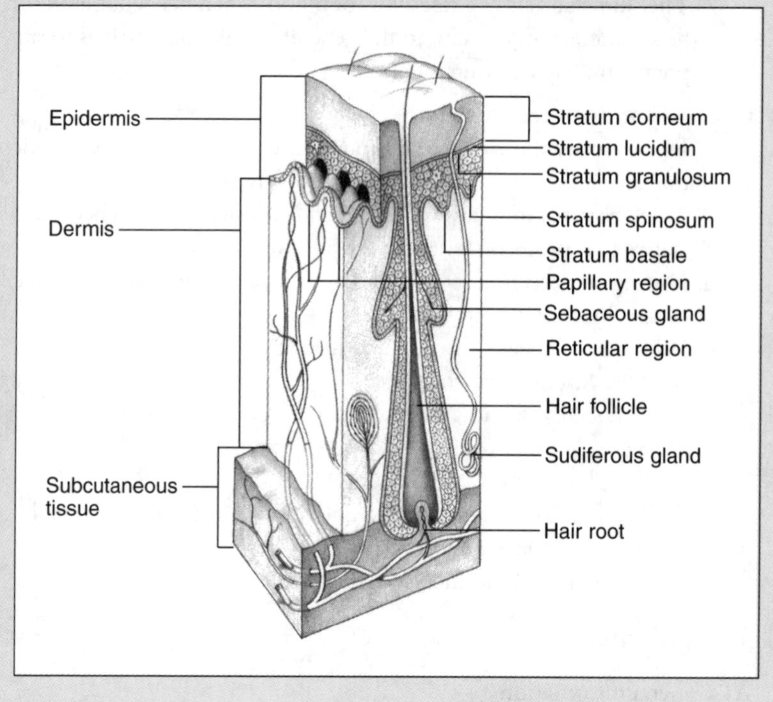

3. The epidermis has five layers, or strata (see *Microscopic structures of the skin*)

B. Epidermal layers
1. The *stratum basale* (basal layer) is the deepest layer of the epidermis
   a. Most cells in this layer are keratinocytes, which are arranged perpendicularly
   b. Merkel's cells occasionally appear among the keratinocytes
   c. Approximately 25% of the cells in the stratum basale are melanocytes
2. The *stratum spinosum* (spiny layer) is thicker than the stratum basale and lies just above it
   a. Besides keratinocytes, this layer contains Langerhans' cells
   b. Collectively, the stratum basale and stratum spinosum are called the STRATUM GERMINATIVUM (growth layer) because epidermal growth occurs in these layers

3. The *stratum granulosum* (granular layer) is a thin layer above the stratum spinosum
   a. It is composed of flattened cells and some Langerhans' cells
   b. Its name comes from the granular substance (keratohyalin) within the flattened cells
   c. Keratinization (the process by which cells produce keratin) begins in this layer
4. The *stratum lucidum* (clear layer) is a translucent band just above the stratum granulosum; it consists of several rows of flattened keratinocytes with indistinct or absent nuclei
5. The *stratum corneum* (horny layer) is the outermost epidermal layer
   a. It contains 20 to 30 layers of flattened, cornified nonnucleated cells
   b. The stratum corneum accounts for 75% of the epidermal thickness

♦ III. Dermis

A. General information
   1. The *dermis* (also called corium) is the layer of skin just below the epidermis
      a. It comprises the bulk of the skin
      b. It is composed of a strong, flexible connective tissue whose *matrix* is heavily embedded with collagen, elastin, and reticular fibers
      c. It contains many blood vessels, nerve fibers, and lymphatic vessels
      d. The dermis also contains most of the body's hair follicles, sweat glands, and oil glands
   2. The dermis sometimes is called the true skin because it nourishes the epidermis (which lacks blood vessels, lymphatic vessels, and connective tissue)
   3. Cells in the dermis include fibroblasts, macrophages, and occasionally mast cells and white blood cells
      a. *Fibroblasts* are differentiated cells of adult connective tissue
      b. *Macrophages* are large, highly phagocytic cells
      c. *Mast cells* are connective tissue cells capable of elaborating basophilic cytoplasmic granules containing histamine and heparin
      d. *White blood cells* (leukocytes) are formed elements of the blood involved in the inflammatory and immune responses
   4. The dermis may tear with excessive skin stretching; such damage results in silvery white scars called striae (commonly called stretch marks), especially during pregnancy
   5. Beneath the dermis is subcutaneous tissue
      a. Also called the hypodermis or superficial fascia, subcutaneous tissue is not skin; it is loose connective tissue that attaches the skin to underlying structures

b. Fat in subcutaneous tissue insulates the body

B. Dermal regions
1. The dermis has two regions
2. The *papillary region* is the upper region
a. It accounts for approximately 20% of the dermal thickness
b. Its surface contains small fingerlike projections called dermal papillae
(1) Many dermal papillae contain capillary loops; others contain free nerve endings (pain or touch receptors)
(2) Dermal papillae make blood vessels and nerves more readily available to the skin surface
3. The *reticular region* is the lower region of the dermis
a. It is composed of dense irregular collagenous connective tissue
b. The irregular arrangement of this tissue makes the dermis flexible and strong

♦ IV. Skin derivatives

A. General information
1. Skin derivatives derive from the epidermis
2. They help maintain homeostasis, or equilibrium of the body's internal environment
3. Skin derivatives include the hair, nails, sudoriferous glands, sebaceous glands, and ceruminous glands

B. Hair
1. Hair covers most parts of the body; only the lips, nipples, palms, soles, and parts of the external genitalia totally lack hair
a. Hair protects the body from heat loss and ultraviolet rays
b. It also shields the eyes and helps keep dust out of the upper respiratory tract
2. Hair follicles extend down into the dermis
a. A nerve ending surrounds the bulb of each hair follicle
b. Sebaceous glands secrete oily sebum directly onto the hair follicle, lubricating the hair shaft
c. Smooth-muscle fibers called *arrectores pilorum* cause cutis anserina (gooseflesh); each tiny arrector pili muscle moves the individual hair when it contracts
3. Nutrition and hormones affect hair growth and distribution
ALERT
a. Poor nutrition leads to a less nourishing blood supply to the hair
b. The male hormone testosterone encourages hair growth; growth may occur abnormally, as from a hormone-producing tumor

C. Nails
1. Nails are modified, heavily keratinized epidermal protective coverings on the dorsal surface at the end of each finger and toe

2. The skinfold over the proximal portion of the nail is called the *cuticle*
3. The *lunula* is a white, crescent-shaped region at the base of the nail plate

D. Sudoriferous glands
1. *Sudoriferous glands* (sweat glands) are long, coiled tubes located in the dermis or subcutaneous tissue that secrete sweat through a duct on the body's surface
2. They are crucial to maintaining normal body temperature; the sympathetic division of the autonomic nervous system regulates their function
3. The body contains approximately 2.5 million sudoriferous glands; only the lips, nipples, and parts of the external genitalia lack these glands
4. Sudoriferous glands are classified as eccrine or apocrine
   a. Eccrine glands are distributed over nearly the entire body surface
      (1) Most abundant on the palms, soles, and forehead, eccrine glands are more numerous than apocrine glands
      (2) Their SECRETORY COIL originates in the dermis, with a duct extending up to a funnel-shaped pore on the skin surface
      (3) Eccrine glands promote cooling through evaporation of their secretions
   b. Apocrine glands appear mainly in the axillary, anal, and genital areas
      (1) These large, branched, specialized glands empty into ducts that terminate in the upper portion of hair follicles rather than on the skin surface
      (2) Mammary glands, a type of modified apocrine gland, secrete milk

E. Sebaceous glands
1. Sebaceous glands (oil glands) are simple alveolar glands that secrete sebum (oil)
2. Sebum softens and lubricates the hair and skin, preventing hair from become brittle and impeding water loss from the skin; it also acts as a bactericide
3. Sebum usually travels via a duct to a hair follicle
   a. A duct blocked by sebum forms a whitehead
   b. As duct contents oxidize and dry, they form a blackhead
4. Only the palms and soles lack sebaceous glands
5. Hormones influence sebaceous gland secretion; sex hormones cause sebaceous glands to hypertrophy during puberty and atrophy in old age

F. Ceruminous glands
   1. Ceruminous glands are modified apocrine glands
   2. They line the external ear canal
   3. The combination of ceruminous and sebaceous gland secretions is called *cerumen* (earwax)

♦ V. Thermoregulation

A. General information
   1. The skin normally keeps the body temperature around 98.6° F (37° C); this homeostatic process is called thermoregulation
   2. Thermoregulation occurs by negative feedback mechanisms

B. Mechanisms
   1. When skin receptors sense a temperature stimulus (environmental heat or cold), they send impulses (input) to the control center in the brain
   2. The brain transmits impulses (output) to effector organs (sweat glands and blood vessels)
   3. The effector organs respond to the brain's message
      a. When the body is hot, the sweat glands produce perspiration and the blood vessels dilate
         (1) Evaporation of sweat from the surface dissipates heat
         (2) Vasodilation brings more warm blood to the skin, where it is cooled
      b. When the body is cold, blood vessels constrict to prevent heat loss

POINTS TO REMEMBER

♦ The integumentary system includes the skin and its derivatives.

♦ The skin's functions include protection, excretion, thermoregulation, sensation, vitamin D synthesis, and action as a blood reservoir.

♦ The epidermis is the skin's surface layer and the body's outermost protective covering. The dermis lies just below the epidermis and constitutes the bulk of the skin.

♦ Skin derivatives (hair, nails, and sudoriferous, sebaceous, and ceruminous glands) help maintain homeostasis.

♦ Thermoregulation is a negative feedback mechanism that helps the body maintain a relatively constant temperature.

STUDY QUESTIONS

To evaluate your understanding of this chapter, answer the following questions in the space provided; then compare your responses with the correct answers in Appendix B, page 329.

1. What are the two layers of the skin?

2. How does the skin act as a reservoir for blood?

3. What types of cells are found in the epidermis?

4. What types of cells are found in the dermis?

5. How do sudoriferous glands function?

6. How does the skin help regulate body temperature?

CRITICAL THINKING AND APPLICATION EXERCISES

1. Develop a chart that summarizes the chemical, physical, and biological mechanisms by which the skin protects the body.
2. Take closeup photographs of an infant, adolescent, and elderly person. Compare their skin, hair, and nails.
3. On a large poster, draw and identify the five epidermal layers and the two dermal regions.

CHAPTER

6

Skeletal System

Learning objectives

After studying this chapter, you should be able to:

- Identify the major components of the skeletal system.
- List the major functions of bones.
- Compare long bones, short bones, flat bones, and irregular bones.
- Describe the two types of bone formation and the factors that affect them.
- Contrast bone formation and resorption.
- Compare the various types of cartilage.
- Name the three main regions where the bones of the axial skeleton are located.
- Discuss the segments of the appendicular skeleton.
- Compare the basic structure and function of the three types of joints.

Chapter overview

The skeletal system forms the framework that supports and protects the body. It is made of four types of bones and three types of cartilage. Together with the muscular and nervous systems, the skeletal system is responsible for body movement. The health care professional needs a full understanding of skeletal anatomy and physiology to provide comprehensive care for patients with musculoskeletal disorders or injuries and related health problems.

♦ I. Bone

A. General information
   1. The skeleton is composed of 206 bones
   2. Bone is a hard form of connective tissue; it is composed of one of two types of osseous (bony) tissue
      a. Compact bone tissue is dense and smooth
      b. Cancellous bone tissue has a spongy or latticelike structure
   3. Bones support and protect the body, allow movement and hematopoiesis, and act as a mineral reservoir; they constantly undergo formation and breakdown
   4. Bones are classified by shape as long, short, flat, or irregular

B. Classification by shape
   1. LONG BONES are bones whose length exceeds their width
      a. Long bones of the upper body include the clavicle, humerus, radius, and ulna; long bones of the lower body include the femur, tibia, and fibula; the metatarsals, metacarpals, and phalanges also are long bones
      b. Each long bone consists of a shaft (diaphysis) and two extremities (epiphyses), which usually are articulated, or jointed
      c. The *diaphysis* is a tube of compact bone
      d. The medullary cavity lies within the diaphysis
         (1) It is filled with yellow marrow
         (2) Depending on the growth stage, it also may contain varying amounts of red marrow
      e. The *metaphysis* is the portion of developing long bone between the diaphysis (shaft) and epiphysis
      f. The *epiphyses* are separated from the diaphysis by cartilage at the *epiphyseal line*
      g. The *endosteum* is a thin layer of cells that lines the inner surface of compact bone, defining the medullary cavity
      h. The PERIOSTEUM is a tough fibrous membrane sheath surrounding the diaphysis
   2. *Short bones* are bones that lack a long axis; typically, they are cuboidal
      a. Ankle and wrist bones are examples of short bones
      b. Short bones are composed of spongy bone and marrow enclosed by a thin layer of compact bone; periosteum surrounds the compact bone (except on articular surfaces)

c. Sesamoid bones are a special type of short bone embedded in tendons; the kneecap (patella) is an example
3. *Flat bones* are thin bones consisting of two layers of compact bone separated by spongy bone and marrow
   a. Usually, they are curved, not flat
   b. The sternum, ribs, and most skull bones are flat bones
4. *Irregular bones* are bones that do not fit any other classification
   a. They consist of spongy bone enclosed by thin layers of compact bone
   b. Examples include the vertebrae, hip bones, and some skull bones

C. Functions
1. Bones support and stabilize the body; they contribute to its shape
2. They protect internal organs from injury
3. Bones act as levers for skeletal muscles to move the body and its parts; they permit locomotion, grasping of objects, and breathing
4. Bones serve as a reservoir for such minerals as calcium, copper, magnesium, phosphorus, potassium, sodium, and sulfur; bone cavities act as storage sites for fat
5. Bones play a role in *hematopoiesis,* or blood cell formation; hematopoiesis occurs chiefly in the red marrow of certain bones (for more information, see Chapter 11, Hematologic System)

D. Bone formation
1. Two types of bone formation exist: *endochondral* and *intramembranous;* OSTEOBLASTS are the active bone-forming cells in both types of formation
   a. These cells produce an organic matrix for bones and also secrete the enzyme alkaline phosphatase, which liberates phosphate ions from compounds at the site of bone formation
   b. These phosphate ions combine with calcium ions to form calcium phosphate
   c. Calcium phosphate is deposited in the bone matrix, causing the bone to become rigid
   d. Osteoblasts become incorporated into the bone as it forms; then they are transformed into osteocytes
2. In ENDOCHONDRAL BONE FORMATION, a cartilage model forms first; then osteoblasts invade the cartilage and convert it into bone
   a. Areas of bone formation are called *centers of ossification*
   b. In a long bone, ossification begins first in the shaft, or diaphysis; then centers of ossification form in the ends of the bone, or epiphyses
   c. The actively growing zone of cartilage between the diaphysis and epiphyses is called the *epiphyseal plate*

3. INTRAMEMBRANOUS BONE FORMATION occurs in many of the flat bones of the skull and in the clavicle; osteoblasts form these bones directly without a preliminary cartilage mass
   a. Bone-forming cells differentiate from precursor cells in connective tissue and begin to produce bone directly within the connective tissue
   b. The initial centers of ossification extend peripherally and eventually convert all the connective tissue to bone
4. Bone increases in length and thickness as an individual grows
   a. In endochondral formation, bone grows in length by continuous production of cartilage at the distal end of the epiphyseal plate and conversion of cartilage into bone in the proximal part of the epiphyseal plate; this is followed by remodeling of the bone to maintain its configuration
      (1) Toward the end of adolescence, the epiphyseal lines are converted into bone, a process called *closure of the epiphyses*
      (2) Once closure occurs, no further increase in bone length is possible
   b. In endochondral formation, bone increases in thickness and is remodeled as it grows
      (1) Addition of newly formed bone from the periosteum increases long bone diameter
      (2) Simultaneous RESORPTION of bone near the marrow cavity also increases long bone diameter
   c. In intramembranous formation, bone grows by the addition of newly formed bone from the periosteum and simultaneous resorption of bone near the marrow cavity; this process is similar to long bone growth, except that epiphyseal plates do not form

E. Bone remodeling
1. Through *bone remodeling,* new bone tissue replaces old bone tissue
2. In this process, OSTEOCLASTS constantly break down old bone tissue, while osteoblasts build new bone
3. Bone remodeling requires hormones, such as growth and sex hormones; minerals, such as calcium and phosphorus; and vitamins, such as vitamin D
4. Bone strength and thickness are related to stresses on the bone; heavy physical activity and weight bearing promote heavier and stronger bones by stimulating osteoblast formation and bone matrix production and by inhibiting osteoclast activity

F. Bone resorption

1. Osteoclasts carry out bone resorption; they promote bone remodeling by removing unwanted bone while new bone is forming in other areas
    a. Osteoclasts secrete protein-digesting lysosomal enzymes, which digest the organic bone matrix; they also secrete lactic and citric acids, which dissolve calcium phosphate and other bone minerals
    b. Osteoclasts also actively employ phagocytosis and digest small bone fragments
    c. Calcium and phosphate ions are released into the bloodstream, where they become part of the body's ion pool
2. Adrenal cortical hormones promote bone resorption

G. Developmental considerations

1. Bone formation exceeds resorption during childhood and adolescence, allowing the bones to grow
2. In young and middle adulthood, bone formation and resorption are balanced closely; bone size and density do not change
3. In old age, bone breakdown exceeds formation, which causes a gradual decrease in bone density

ALERT

    a. When bone breakdown greatly outstrips bone formation, *osteoporosis* can occur
    b. Osteoporosis is marked by decreased bone mass and an increased tendency to develop fractures, especially pathologic ones

♦ II. Cartilage

A. General information

1. Cartilage is a tough, resilient type of connective tissue
2. It consists of a dense network of collagenous and elastic fibers embedded in a gel-like substance
    a. New cartilage forms from cells called *chondroblasts*
    b. Mature cartilage cells are called *chondrocytes*
3. Cartilage supports and shapes various body structures; it also cushions bone

B. Types

1. The three types of cartilage are hyaline cartilage, fibrocartilage, and elastic cartilage
2. Hyaline cartilage has a characteristic translucent appearance
    a. Hyaline cartilage is the most abundant type; it provides flexibility and support
    b. Hyaline cartilage forms the nose, larynx, trachea, bronchi, and bronchial tubes; it also forms the epiphyseal discs and most articular cartilages

c. It appears at joints over the ends of long bones and at the ventral ends of the ribs

3. Fibrocartilage consists of bundles of collagenous fibers
   a. It provides strength and rigidity
   b. Fibrocartilage occurs in such joints as the temporomandibular joint; it is a component of intervertebral disks, which act as cushions between vertebrae
4. Elastic cartilage is more opaque, flexible, and elastic than hyaline cartilage; it lends strength and helps maintain the shape of certain organs, such as the auricle (external ear), auditory tube, and larynx

♦ III. Axial skeleton

A. General information
1. The AXIAL SKELETON consists of the bones that form the longitudinal axis of the body — those of the head, neck, and trunk
2. Its 80 bones are located in three major regions — the skull, vertebral column, and bony thorax (see *Bones of the human skeleton,* page 58)

B. Skull
1. Also called the cranium, the skull has several functions
   a. It protects the brain
   b. It provides cavities for sensory organs, such as the eyes, ears, and nose
   c. It has openings that allow passage of air and food
   d. It contains teeth and jaws for mastication
2. The skull consists of cranial bones (cranial vault, or calvaria) and facial bones
3. The eight cranial bones include the paired parietal and temporal bones and the unpaired frontal, occipital, sphenoid, and ethmoid bones
   a. These irregular bones consist of a spongy layer between internal and external tables (flat layers) of compact bone
   b. Internally, bony ridges divide the cranial bones at the base of the skull into three fossae, or depressed regions
4. Facial bones can be studied by viewing the skull from different positions (see *Views of the skull,* page 59)
   a. In an anterior view, prominent skull features include the forehead, nasion, superciliary arch, orbits, zygomatic bones, piriform aperture, upper and lower jaws, and paranasal sinuses
      (1) The forehead is formed by the frontal bone
      (2) The *nasion* (depression at the root of the nose) is formed by the intersection of the frontal bone and the two nasal bones

Bones of the human skeleton

The skeleton accounts for roughly 20% of the body mass. Composed of 206 bones, it is divided into the axial and appendicular divisions. The axial skeleton includes the skull, vertebrae, and bony thorax. The appendicular skeleton includes the bones of the shoulder and pelvic girdles and the upper and lower limbs. This illustration shows the major bones of both divisions.

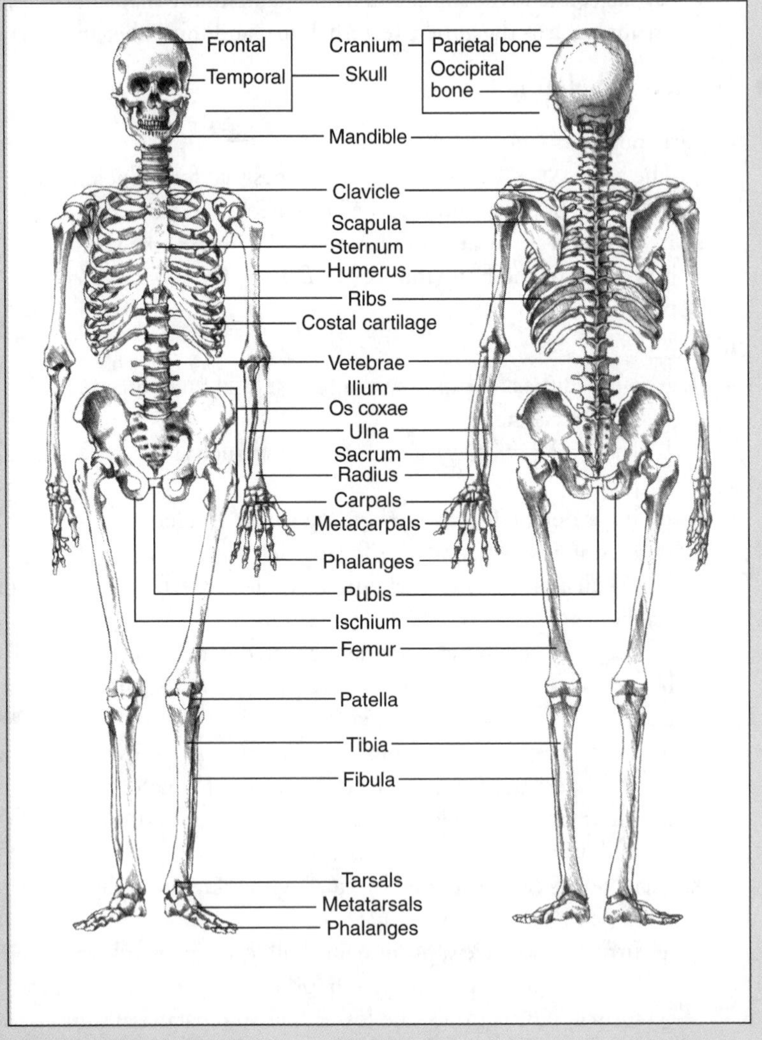

Illustration from Stevens, N., and Adler, J. *Introduction to Medical Terminology.* Springhouse, Pa.: Springhouse Corp., 1992.

Views of the skull

The cranium is composed of eight bones—the frontal bone, sphenoid bone, ethmoid bone, occipital bone, two parietal bones, and two temporal bones.

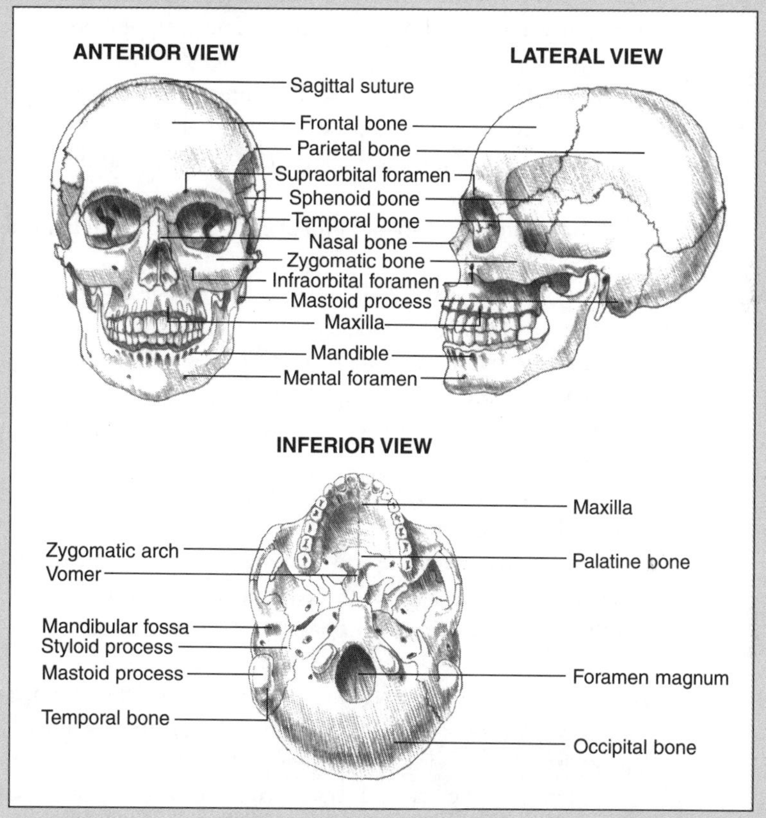

Top two illustrations from Stevens, N., and Adler, J. *Introduction to Medical Terminology.* Springhouse, Pa.: Springhouse Corp., 1992.

(3) The *superciliary arch* is the elevation that extends laterally from the GLABELLA (the region above the nasion and between the eyebrows)

(4) Orbits are the bony cavities that house the eyes

(5) The zygomatic (malar) bones form the prominences of the cheeks

(6) The piriform aperture is formed by the nasal bones and maxillae (upper jaw bones)

(7) The upper and lower jaws are formed by the maxillae and mandible, respectively
(8) The four pairs of paranasal sinuses are named for the bones in which they are found: frontal, ethmoid, sphenoid, and maxillary

b. In a lateral view, the frontal, parietal, and occipital bones are seen superiorly and the ethmoid, sphenoid, and temporal bones are seen inferiorly
(1) Laterally, the most prominent features are the zygomatic PROCESS, which articulates with the temporal process of the zygomatic bone, the coronoid process, and the mandibular CONDYLE
(2) The mastoid and styloid processes of the temporal bone also are visible
(3) The mental FORAMEN (an opening for passage of the mental nerve and vessels) can be seen in the mandible

c. In a posterior view, the paired parietal bones join the occipital and mastoid parts of the temporal bones
(1) When viewed inferiorly, the mastoid processes are prominent bilaterally
(2) When viewed superiorly, the sagittal SUTURE joins the lambdoid suture

5. Like sutures elsewhere in the body, *sutures* in the skull (the joints between skull bones) have closely united opposing surfaces
   a. Skull sutures include the coronal suture, sagittal suture, lambdoid suture, and squamous suture
   b. In adults, skull joints are immovable except for the mandible; connected with the skull by paired synovial joints, the mandible moves freely

6. The hyoid bone, which lacks direct articulation with any other bone, is located in the front of the neck between the mandible and larynx
   a. Although not part of the skull, the hyoid commonly is described in conjunction with it because of its relationship to the mandible and temporal bones
   b. The hyoid serves as a movable base for the tongue and an attachment for the neck muscles that help elevate the larynx during swallowing and speech

C. Vertebral column

1. The vertebral column (spine) extends from the skull to the pelvis
   a. It provides the primary axial support for the body
   b. It consists of 26 irregular bones called vertebrae; 24 of these are movable

c. The vertebral column has sagittal curves in the cervical, thoracic, lumbar, and sacral regions
   (1) The cervical and lumbar curves are convex anteriorly; the thoracic and sacral curves are convex posteriorly
   (2) These curves increase the strength, resilience, balance, and flexibility of the spine

2. A typical vertebra consists of an ovoid body, a vertebral arch (a portion of which is called the lamina), two transverse processes, two superior articular processes, two inferior articular processes, and one spinous process (see *Structures of the vertebra,* page 62)
   a. Muscle attaches at the spinous process and the two transverse processes
   b. The superior and inferior articular processes articulate with the vertebrae immediately above and below them

3. The vertebral column has 7 cervical vertebrae, 12 thoracic vertebrae, 5 lumbar vertebrae, the sacrum (formed by the fusion of 5 vertebrae), and the coccyx (formed by the fusion of 4 vertebrae)
   a. The *cervical vertebrae* (designated C1 to C7) constitute the skeleton of the neck; they are smaller than the other vertebrae
      (1) C1, called the atlas, is highly modified (different from other cervical vertebrae); a ring of bone, it lacks a body or spinous process
      (2) C2, called the axis, has a toothlike process called the *dens* that projects superiorly from the body; the dens forms a specialized type of articulation with the atlas above it
      (3) C3 through C7 consist of a body (the discoid, weight-bearing portion) anteriorly and a vertebral arch posteriorly
         (a) The body and arch form the *vertebral foramen;* collectively, these openings form the vertebral canal, which houses the spinal cord
         (b) Each of these vertebrae contains two *transverse processes,* lateral projections from the vertebral arch; and one *spinous process,* a posterior projection in the midline
         (c) The bony connections between the body and the transverse processes are called *pedicles;* the bony connections between the transverse and spinous processes are called *laminae*
   b. The *thoracic vertebrae* (designated T1 to T12) are located between the cervical and lumbar vertebrae
      (1) Each thoracic vertebra articulates bilaterally with the ribs
      (2) The first 10 have facets on the transverse processes that articulate with the TUBERCLES of the ribs

Structures of the vertebra

Most vertebrae share several important features. The body (centrum) is the disk-shaped, weight-bearing, ventral portion. Laminae are flat, broad structures that fuse to form the posterior portion of the vertebral arch. Pedicles project posteriorly from the vertebral body, forming the sides of the vertebral foramen, a large opening in the center of the vertebra formed by its body and arch; collectively, the vertebral foramens comprise the spinal canal (which houses the spinal cord). Processes project laterally at the points where a lamina and pedicle join; a spinous process projects posteriorly and inferiorly from the junction of the laminae. Two superior articular processes project upward from the laminae and articulate with the immediately superior vertebra; two inferior articular processes project downward from the laminae and articulate with the immediately inferior vertebra.

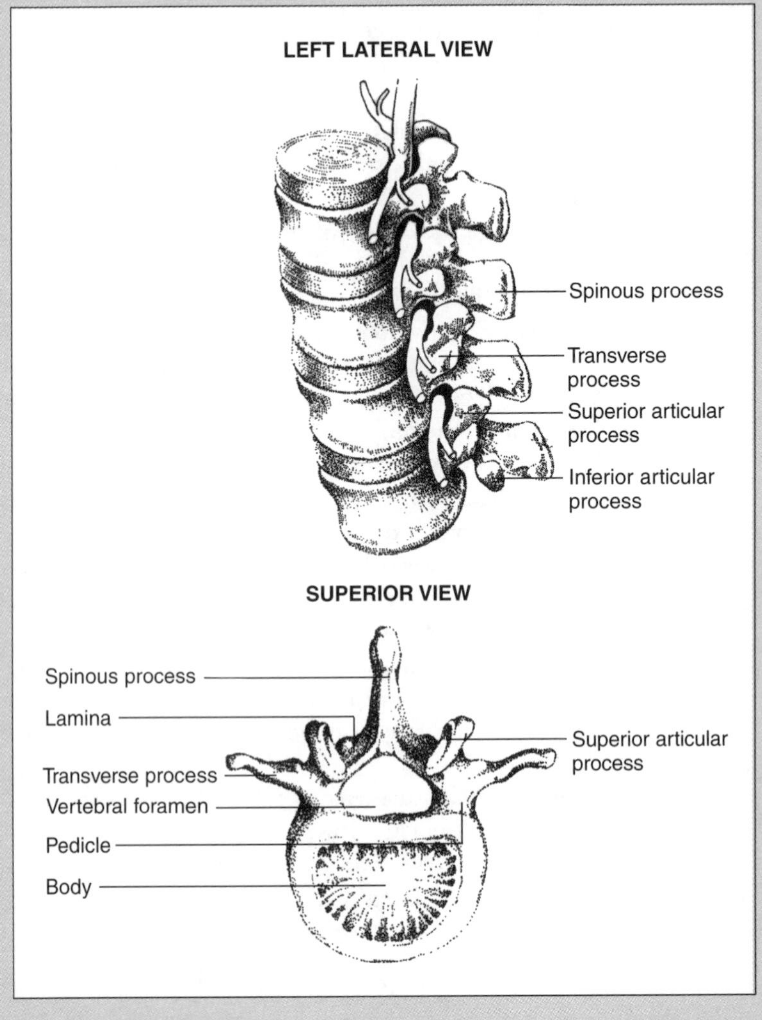

   c. The *lumbar vertebrae* (designated L1 to L5) are located between the thoracic vertebrae and the sacrum; they are the largest and strongest vertebrae
   d. The *sacrum,* a triangular bone formed by the fusion of five sacral vertebrae, lies in the posterior portion of the pelvic girdle between the hip bones
   e. The *coccyx,* a triangular bone formed by the fusion of the four coccygeal vertebrae, articulates superiorly with the sacrum
4. As vertebrae articulate, alignment of the vertebral foramina forms the vertebral canal
5. Several ligaments attach to the vertebrae
   a. The anterior longitudinal ligament is a broad sheath of connective tissue along the anterior surface of the vertebral bodies
   b. The posterior longitudinal ligament, narrower than the anterior one, lies along the posterior surface of the vertebral bodies inside the vertebral canal
   c. Other ligaments — the flaval ligaments, interspinous ligaments, and supraspinous ligaments — attach in various ways to the spinous processes

D. Bony thorax
1. The bony thorax, or rib cage, forms a protective enclosure for the heart, lungs, and great vessels of the thoracic cavity
2. It also supports the pectoral (shoulder) girdle and provides attachment points for various muscles
3. The bony thorax consists of the thoracic vertebrae (dorsally), the ribs (laterally), and the sternum and costal cartilages (anteriorly)
4. The bony thorax includes 12 pairs of ribs
   a. The first seven pairs (sometimes eight) connect to the sternum by costal cartilages; they are called true ribs
   b. The remaining five pairs are called false ribs
      (1) The first three pairs of false ribs connect to the costal cartilages immediately above them
      (2) The last two pairs of false ribs, which do not connect to the costal cartilages, are called floating ribs
5. The *sternum* is a flat bone that joins the ribs anteriorly to close the wall of the bony thorax
   a. It consists of the manubrium (triangular superior portion), body (middle and largest portion), and xiphoid process (inferior smaller portion)
   b. The manubrium has a superior depression called the suprasternal notch

♦ IV. Appendicular skeleton

A. General information

1. The APPENDICULAR SKELETON (so named because its bones are appended to the axial skeleton) consists of the pectoral (shoulder) and pelvic girdles and the bones of the upper and lower limbs
2. Its 126 bones include the clavicle, scapula, upper limb bones, hip bones, and lower limb bones (see *Bones of the human skeleton,* page 58)
3. The upper limb bones attach to the shoulder girdle; the lower limb bones attach to the pelvic girdle
   a. The shoulder girdle consists of the clavicle (anteriorly) and scapula (posteriorly)
   b. The pelvic girdle consists of the hip bones (*os coxae,* or innominate bones)

B. Shoulder girdle

1. The clavicle (collar bone) is a slender, curved flat bone that forms the anterior portion of the shoulder girdle
   a. At the medial end, the clavicle articulates with the manubrium portion of the sternum
   b. At the distal end, it articulates with the scapula
2. The scapula (shoulder blade) is a triangular flat bone
   a. Laterally, it contains a shallow cavity called the glenoid FOSSA, which articulates with the humerus of the arm to form the shoulder joint
   b. Superiorly, the scapula has two prominent bony projections — the coracoid process in front and the acromion process in back
   c. Posteriorly, the scapula attaches only to muscle, not to the thorax

C. Bones of the upper limbs

1. The upper limbs consist of 30 bones, including the humerus, ulna, radius, and hand bones
2. The *humerus* is the largest and longest bone of the upper arm
   a. It articulates with the scapula medially
   b. It also articulates with the radius and ulna distally (at the elbow)
3. The *ulna* is the longer of the two forearm bones
   a. It articulates with the humerus to form the elbow joint
   b. It also articulates with the radius at the proximal and distal ends
   c. The olecranon and coronoid processes are located at the proximal end of the ulna
   d. The styloid process is found on the medial side of the distal head of the ulna
4. The *radius* is the shorter of the two forearm bones
   a. Proximally, the upper concavity of the head of the radius articulates with the capitulum of the humerus

b. Medially, the head articulates with the radial fossa of the ulna
c. The radial TUBEROSITY (protuberance) is a projection immediately below the proximal head
d. Distally, the radius has a medial ulnar notch and a lateral styloid process

5. Hand bones include the carpus (wrist), metacarpus (palm), and phalanges (digits or fingers)
   a. The eight carpals (short bones) of the wrist are joined tightly by ligaments; they are limited to gliding movements
   b. The flexor retinaculum, which forms the carpal tunnel for passage of the flexor tendons, maintains wrist concavity
   c. The five metacarpals radiate from the carpus to form the framework of the palm; beginning with the thumb (pollex), they are numbered 1 through 5 (instead of named)
   d. Each hand has 14 *phalanges,* or tapering bones
      (1) The thumb has only proximal and distal phalanges
      (2) The other four fingers have proximal, middle, and distal phalanges

D. Pelvic girdle
1. Formed by the hip bones, the pelvic girdle attaches the lower limbs to the axial skeleton
2. In the front of the body, the hip bones articulate with each other; in the back of the body, they articulate with the sacrum
3. Together with the sacrum, the pelvic girdle forms the bony pelvis
4. At birth, each coxa contains three bones — ilium, ischium, and pubis
   a. Although these bones fuse in the adult, the names are used to describe the corresponding regions of the hip bones
   b. Paired coxal bones are referred to as the pelvic girdle
5. The *ilium* is a large, flaring bone located superiorly
   a. It forms the greater portion of the os coxa
   b. The bony projections commonly called the hips are the iliac crests
6. The arc-shaped *ischium* forms the posteroinferior part of the os coxa; its inferior surface thickens to form the ischial tuberosity
7. The pubis (pubic bone) forms the anterior part of the os coxa
   a. It joins the ischium posterolaterally to form the *obturator foramen,* a large opening
   b. The two pubic bones articulate anteriorly at the symphysis pubis
8. A deep, round socket (acetabulum) forms on the lateral surface of the os coxa; the acetabulum articulates with the head of the femur

E. Bones of the lower limbs
1. The lower limbs consist of 30 bones, including the femur, patella, tibia, fibula, and bones of the foot (talus, calcaneus, cuboid, and na-

vicular; medial, intermediate, and lateral cuneiforms; five metatarsals; and 14 phalanges)

2. Because these bones support the weight of the entire body and endure great force, they are thicker and stronger than those of the upper limbs
3. The femur (thigh bone) is the longest, thickest, and strongest bone in the body
   a. The ball-like proximal head of the femur articulates with the acetabulum of the pelvis
   b. The greater trochanter is a bony projection located superolateral to the neck of the femur; the lesser trochanter is located inferomedially
   c. Distally, the femur ends in the lateral and medial condyles, which articulate with the tibia
4. The patella (kneecap) articulates with the anterior surface between the condyles
5. The shape of the leg comes from the tibia and fibula
   a. The tibia is the leg's weight-bearing bone
      (1) Proximally, its medial and lateral condyles articulate with the femur
      (2) The large tibial tuberosity for attachment of the patellar ligament lies immediately below the condyles
      (3) Distally, the tibia articulates with the talus of the ankle
      (4) Medially, at the distal end, an inferior projection called the *medial malleolus* forms the medial bulge of the ankle
   b. The fibula bears no weight
      (1) It articulates proximally and distally with the tibia
      (2) An inferior projection called the lateral malleolus lies at the distal end of the fibula
6. The foot bones include the tarsals (ankle), metatarsals (instep), and phalanges (toes)
   a. The foot supports the body and acts as a lever during locomotion
   b. The seven tarsals are the talus, calcaneus, cuboid, and navicular bones and the medial, intermediate, and lateral cuneiforms; they correspond to the carpals in the wrist
   c. The five metatarsals are numbered 1 through 5, beginning with the great toe (hallux)
   d. The 14 phalanges in the toes correspond to those in the fingers
      (1) The great toe has only two phalanges, proximal and distal
      (2) The other toes have proximal, middle, and distal phalanges

♦ V. Articulations

A. General information

1. ARTICULATIONS, or joints, are the junction points between two or more bones
2. Usually composed of fibrous connective tissue and cartilage, joints permit movement
3. Joints are classified according to function and structure
   a. Functional classification is based on the degree of movement the joint allows; thus, a joint may be a synarthrosis (an immovable joint), an amphiarthrosis (a slightly movable joint), or a diarthrosis (a freely movable joint)
      (1) The axial skeleton has mainly synarthrotic and amphiarthrotic joints
      (2) The appendicular skeleton has mostly diarthrotic joints, with some amphiarthrotic joints; most limb joints are diarthrotic
   b. Structural classification is based on the type of material holding the bones of the joint together; thus, a joint may be fibrous, cartilaginous, or synovial

B. Synarthroses

1. *Synarthroses* are immovable joints that fall into three types — sutures, gomphoses, and synchondroses
   a. Sutures are fibrous joints with closely united opposing surfaces, such as the coronal suture
   b. *Gomphoses* have a conical process inserted into a socketlike portion (such as teeth in the dental alveoli); like sutures, they allow no movement
   c. *Synchondroses* usually are temporary joints in which the intervening hyaline cartilage converts to bone by adulthood; the epiphyseal plates of long bones are an example
2. Because the articular surfaces of the two bones are bound closely by fibrous connective tissue, little or no movement possible

C. Amphiarthroses

1. *Amphiarthroses* are joints in which cartilage connects one bone to another; they allow only slight movement
2. They fall into two categories — syndesmoses and symphyses
   a. *Syndesmoses* have intervening connective tissue that forms an interosseous membrane or ligament, such as the tibiofibular and radioulnar joints
   b. *Symphyses* have an intervening pad of fibrocartilage; examples are the intervertebral joints, the symphysis pubis, and the joint between the manubrium and sternum

D. Diarthroses

1. *Diarthroses* are joints in which the contiguous bony surfaces are covered by articular cartilage and joined by ligaments lined with synovial membrane; they are freely movable
2. Most joints of the upper and lower limbs are diarthroses
3. Diathrotic joints have five structural features
   a. *Articular cartilage* (hyaline cartilage) covers and cushions the articulating ends of bones
   b. The *joint cavity,* a potential space, separates the articulating surfaces of the two bones
   c. The articular capsule is a double-layered structure; the heavier outer layer is fibrous tissue lined with a vascular synovial membrane
   d. SYNOVIAL FLUID, a viscid fluid produced by the synovial membrane, lubricates the joint
   e. *Reinforcing ligaments,* consisting of fibrous connective tissue, connect bones within the joint and reinforce the joint capsule
4. Diarthrotic joints fall into various categories based on their structure and the type of movement they allow
   a. *Gliding joints* (also called plane or nonaxial joints) have flat or slightly curved articular surfaces
      (1) They allow gliding movements; however, movement may not be possible in all directions because these joints are bound by ligaments
      (2) Examples include the intercarpal and intertarsal joints of the hands and feet
   b. *Hinge joints* (also called uniaxial joints) are those in which a convex portion of one bone fits into a concave portion of another
      (1) Movement is limited to flexion and extension and resembles that of a metal hinge
      (2) Examples include the elbow and knee
   c. *Pivot joints* (also called uniaxial joints) are those in which a rounded portion of one bone fits into a groove in another bone
      (1) Movement is limited to uniaxial rotation of the first bone around the second
      (2) The head of the radius, which rotates within a groove of the ulna, is an example
   d. *Condyloid joints* (also called biaxial or ellipsoidal joints) are those in which the oval surface of one bone fits into a concavity in another
      (1) They permit flexion, extension, abduction, adduction, and circumduction
      (2) The radiocarpal and metacarpophalangeal joints of the hand are examples

e. *Saddle joints* (also called biaxial joints) resemble condyloid joints but allow greater freedom of movement; the carpometacarpal joints of the thumb are the only saddle joints in the body

f. *Ball-and-socket joints* (also called multiaxial joints) are those in which the spherical head of one bone fits into a concave "socket" of another

(1) They allow the greatest freedom of motion of all diarthrotic joints

(2) The shoulder and hip joints are the only ball-and-socket joints in the body

E. Joint contact and movement

1. Bursae, tendons, and ligaments hold the diarthroses' articular surfaces in contact with each other

a. Bursae and tendon sheaths prevent friction on adjacent structures during joint movement

(1) *Bursae* are flattened fibrous sacs that are lined with synovial membrane and filled with synovial fluid; they decrease stress on nearby tissues by acting as cushions

(a) They occur in areas where ligaments, muscles, skin, or tendons rub against bone

(b) An example is the subacromial bursa beneath the coracoacromial ligament in the shoulder

(2) *Tendon sheaths* are elongated bursae wrapped around a tendon subjected to friction; they occur at the wrist and ankle joints

b. *Tendons* are bands of fibrous connective tissue that attach muscles to bones; they enable bones to move when skeletal muscles contract

c. *Ligaments* are bands of strong, flexible, fibrous connective tissue that connect the articular ends of bones; they provide stability and may limit or facilitate movement

2. Diarthroses permit 13 basic types of movement

a. *Flexion* decreases the joint angle

b. *Extension* increases the joint angle

c. *Hyperextension* increases the joint angle beyond the anatomic position

d. *Circumduction* moves the limb in a circle

e. *Abduction* moves the limb away from midline

f. *Adduction* moves the limb toward midline

g. *Rotation* revolves the limb around a longitudinal axis, moving it toward midline (internal rotation) or away from midline (external rotation)

h. *Supination* turns the palm upward

i. *Pronation* turns the palm downward

j. *Inversion* turns the plantar surface inward
k. *Eversion* turns the plantar surface outward
l. *Retraction* moves the jaw backward
m. *Protraction* moves the jaw forward

ALERT

3. Injuries, such as sprains and strains, and disorders, such as arthritis and bursitis, can decrease joint movement

POINTS TO REMEMBER

- Bone is a hard form of connective tissue that is composed of compact and cancellous bone tissue.
- Bones support and protect the body, allow movement and hematopoiesis, and act as a mineral reservoir; they constantly undergo formation and breakdown.
- Hyaline cartilage, fibrocartilage, and elastic cartilage support and shape various body structures and cushion bones.
- The axial skeleton is made up of head, neck, and trunk bones, which form the longitudinal axis of the body. Its bones are divided among the skull, vertebral column, and bony thorax.
- The bones of the appendicular skeleton are appended to the axial skeleton. They include the bones of the shoulder and pelvic girdles and the upper and lower limbs.
- A synarthrosis is an immovable joint; an amphiarthrosis is a slightly movable joint; and a diarthrosis is a freely movable joint.

STUDY QUESTIONS

To evaluate your understanding of this chapter, answer the following questions in the space provided. Then compare your responses with the correct answers in Appendix B, pages 329 and 330.

1. Name the two types of bone tissues. ______________________________

____

____

2. What are the four classifications of bones based on shape? ____________

____

____

3. What functions does cartilage serve?______________________________

____

____

4. How is the axial skeleton different from the appendicular skeleton?______

____

____

5. How do the three types of joints differ?____________________________

____

____

CRITICAL THINKING AND APPLICATION EXERCISES

1. On a model of a skeleton, label six different types of surface markings.
2. Write a one-page paper describing the functions of osteoblasts and osteoclasts.
3. Create a chart that compares endochondral and intramembranous bone formations.
4. List at least 10 major bones of the upper limbs and 10 major bones of the lower limbs.
5. Demonstrate to a classmate each of the 13 types of movement permitted by diarthroses.

CHAPTER

7

Muscular System

LEARNING OBJECTIVES

After studying this chapter, you should be able to:

- Describe the main functions of muscle tissue.
- Name the four special properties of muscle tissue.
- Discuss nerve impulse transmission across the neuromuscular junction.
- Explain how the muscles obtain energy for contraction.
- Compare the three types of muscle tissue.
- Identify some locations of smooth muscle in the body.
- Differentiate between the origin point and the insertion point of a skeletal muscle.
- Explain the role of actin and myosin filaments in skeletal muscle contraction.

CHAPTER OVERVIEW

The muscular system animates the bones and joints of the skeletal system, which provide a framework for it. The skeletal muscles are responsible for every body movement. The cardiac and smooth muscles handle less visible motions, such as the pumping of the heart and the passage of urine or feces. Because the muscular system produces these vital actions, the health care professional must understand its normal structures and functions in order to comprehend the effects of muscular disturbances in patients.

♦ I. Muscle tissue

A. General information
   1. Muscle tissue accounts for roughly 50% of total body weight
   2. The three types of muscle tissue — smooth, cardiac, and skeletal — differ in cell structure, location, and function (see *Comparing muscle types,* page 74)
   3. Muscle tissue is composed of fibers that contain the proteins actin and myosin
      a. Myosin is the most abundant protein in muscle
      b. Myosin and actin are responsible for muscle contraction
   4. Each muscle is innervated by sensory and motor neurons

B. Functions
   1. Muscle permits movement, maintains posture, and generates heat
      a. The integrated function of muscles, bones, and joints produces body movements, such as walking and running
      b. Skeletal muscle contractions maintain posture by holding body parts in postural positions
      c. Muscles produce a large amount of heat during contraction
   2. Muscle tissue has four special properties that help maintain homeostasis
      a. *Excitability* allows a muscle to receive and respond to a stimulus so that the body can respond to internal and external environmental changes
      b. *Contractility* allows a muscle to shorten when it receives a stimulus of sufficient strength
      c. *Extensibility* allows a muscle to stretch
      d. *Elasticity* allows a muscle to return to its original shape after contraction

C. Muscle fiber stimulation
   1. Skeletal, cardiac, and smooth muscles are controlled by nerve impulses (for details, see Chapter 8, Nervous System); although they are stimulated and respond in somewhat different ways, skeletal muscle will be used as an example
   2. Nerve fibers called axons transmit impulses from the central nervous system (CNS) to muscle fibers
   3. The axon terminates near a small depression on the surface of the muscle fiber called the *motor end plate;* a small gap called the synapse separates the axon terminal and motor end plate
   4. The term NEUROMUSCULAR JUNCTION refers to the motor end plate and the axon terminal associated with it

Comparing muscle types

Skeletal, cardiac, and smooth muscles differ in their location, appearance, striations, type of control, contraction speed, and function as described in this table.

FEATURES	SKELETAL MUSCLE	CARDIAC MUSCLE	SMOOTH MUSCLE
Location	• Attached to skeleton	• Heart	• Walls of hollow organs, blood vessels, skin, and eyes
Appearance	• Cylindrical fibers that may extend the entire length of a muscle • Multiple peripherally located nuclei	• Cylindrical branched fibers • Single centrally located nucleus • Intercalated disks that join the cells to each other	• Spindle-shaped fibers • Single centrally located nucleus
Striations	• Present	• Present	• Absent
Control	• Voluntary	• Involuntary	• Involuntary
Contraction speed	• Fast	• Moderate	• Slow
Function	• Body movement	• Blood pumping	• Food movement through the GI tract, urinary bladder emptying, uterine and tubal muscle contraction, regulation of blood vessel diameter, pupil size regulation, hair movement, and nipple erection

D. Nerve impulse transmission to muscle fibers
  1. The axon terminal has vesicles that contain the neurotransmitter acetylcholine
     a. When a nerve impulse reaches the axon terminal, the vesicles release acetylcholine, which diffuses across the synapse and attaches to receptors on the motor end plate
     b. Acetylcholine generates a depolarization wave, or impulse, which stimulates muscle fiber contraction
  2. The enzyme cholinesterase is present in the muscle membrane of the motor end plate
     a. Cholinesterase rapidly breaks down the released acetylcholine into acetate and choline

   b. Acetylcholine breakdown prevents the nerve impulse from continuing to stimulate the skeletal muscle fiber and inducing a sustained contraction
3. The axon terminal takes up the choline, which then combines with acetate to form more acetylcholine
4. Acetylcholine is stored in axon terminal vesicles until another impulse stimulates its release

E. Muscle metabolism
1. All muscle contractions require energy, which they can obtain from the breakdown of adenosine triphosphate (ATP) in muscle fiber
2. As needed, skeletal muscle fibers can increase ATP production by the phosphagen system, glycogen–lactic acid system, and aerobic system
   a. The *phosphagen system* uses the breakdown of creatine phosphate for energy
   b. The *glycogen–lactic acid system* breaks down muscle glycogen into glucose, which it metabolizes to generate ATP (energy) and pyruvic acid
   c. The *aerobic system* oxidizes pyruvic acid into ATP, carbon dioxide, and water via cellular respiration
      (1) This process is called AEROBIC METABOLISM because it requires oxygen; it is slower than glycolysis, but provides more ATP (for details on metabolism, see Chapter 14, Gastrointestinal System)
      (2) The body uses this system when muscle contractions last longer than about 30 seconds
3. During vigorous exertion, the lungs and circulatory system may not be able to provide sufficient oxygen to muscles for aerobic metabolism
   a. In such a case, muscle cells must derive energy through ANAEROBIC METABOLISM, which breaks down muscle glycogen and blood glucose to lactic acid rather than pyruvic acid; anaerobic metabolism provides less ATP than aerobic metabolism, but it yields enough to sustain muscular activity (for details on metabolism, see Chapter 14, Gastrointestinal System)
      (1) Some lactic acid accumulates in the muscles, but most diffuses into the blood and is transported to the liver
      (2) In the liver, lactic acid is reconverted to glucose, which is transported as blood glucose back to the muscles to be reused for energy

b. With anaerobic metabolism, the muscles develop an oxygen debt that must be repaid through extra oxygen consumption after exertion has ceased
   (1) The person must breathe rapidly after exertion until the muscles have obtained sufficient oxygen to restore them to their resting state
   (2) Elevated oxygen use after exercise is called recovery oxygen consumption
c. When oxygen supplies increase after exertion, the muscle fibers are restored to their normal resting state
   (1) Depleted muscle glycogen is resynthesized from glucose
   (2) Creatine phosphate is reformed
   (3) Accumulated lactic acid in the muscle is reconverted to pyruvic acid and oxidized by the mitochondrial enzymes to carbon dioxide and water and ATP

♦ II. Smooth muscle

A. General information
   1. Smooth-muscle tissue consists of elongated, spindle-shaped, nucleated fibers (cells)
   2. It lacks the striations (striped appearance) of cardiac and skeletal muscle
   3. Smooth muscle lines the visceral organs and urinary bladder and surrounds the blood vessels, bronchi, and various ducts
   4. Smooth-muscle contractions are involuntary, slow, and sustained; they occur sequentially as the nerve impulse spreads from one muscle fiber to the next

B. Types
   1. *Single-unit smooth muscle* has numerous gap junctions between adjacent fibers
      a. *Gap junctions* occur in the heart and certain other smooth-muscle tissue containing electrically excitable tissue; the plasma membranes are situated close to each other, with hollow cylinders of protein linking the cells
      b. Fibers in single-unit smooth muscle form a continuous network that contracts spontaneously in response to an appropriate stimulus
      c. Contraction occurs in a wave over many adjacent fibers
      d. Single-unit smooth muscle appears in the walls of the stomach, intestines, uterus, and bladder

2. *Multi-unit smooth muscle* consists of individual fibers, each with its own motor nerve ending; motor nerves carry impulses away from the CNS
   a. Fibers in multi-unit smooth muscle lack gap junctions
   b. Stimulation of a multi-unit smooth-muscle fiber causes contraction of that fiber only
   c. Multi-unit smooth-muscle tissue occurs in such structures as the walls of blood vessels and the muscles of the hair follicles and eyes (such as those of the iris)

♦ III. Cardiac muscle

A. General information
   1. Cardiac muscle makes up most of the mass of the heart wall
   2. It consists of striated fibers; these short, branched cells have one or two nuclei
      a. The fibers are somewhat quadrangular in shape
      b. Their nuclei are located centrally
   3. Strong, thin bands called *intercalated disks* traverse the muscle fibers, separating them from each other
      a. These disks provide a low resistance for the flow of electric current through the heart
      b. They also strengthen the muscle and promote impulse conduction
   4. Cardiac muscle moves blood through the heart and into blood vessels
   5. Involuntary, cardiac muscle contracts at a steady rate, regulated by an internal pacemaker
   6. Cardiac muscle is innervated by nerve fibers from the autonomic (involuntary) nervous system

B. Specialized fibers
   1. Specialized cardiac muscle fibers called *nodal tissues* constitute the conduction system of the heart
   2. They permit rapid, rhythmic spread of a stimulus through cardiac muscle (for details on these muscle fibers, see Chapter 10, Cardiovascular System)

♦ IV. Skeletal muscle

A. General information
   1. Skeletal muscle is muscle that attaches to the skeleton; it permits voluntary movements
   2. The human body contains approximately 600 skeletal muscles, which account for roughly 36% of body weight in women and 42% in men (see *Major skeletal muscles,* page 78)
   3. Skeletal muscles contract rapidly and vigorously for short periods

Major skeletal muscles

The human body contains roughly 600 skeletal muscles. A muscle's name may reflect its size, shape, location, action, attachment points, number of divisions, or direction of its fibers. Skeletal muscles produce voluntary and reflex movements, generate body heat, and maintain posture. This illustration shows major muscles.

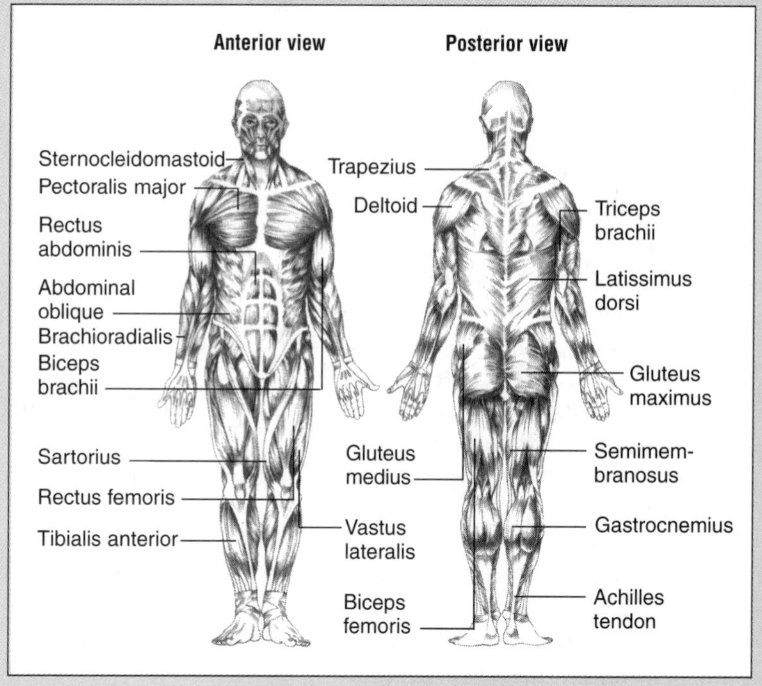

Illustration from Stevens, N., and Adler, J. *Introduction to Medical Terminology.* Springhouse, Pa.: Springhouse Corp., 1992.

4. They are innervated by nerve fibers from the somatic (voluntary) nervous system
5. The name of a skeletal muscle may come from its location, action, size, shape, points of attachment, number of divisions, or direction of fibers

B. Structure
1. Of all types of muscle tissue, skeletal muscle tissue has the longest fibers
2. Elongated and cylindrical, these fibers lie parallel to one another in bundles called FASCICULI
   a. Skeletal muscle fibers are multinucleated and have distinct transverse striations

   b. The *sarcolemma,* a plasma membrane, surrounds each fiber
3. Skeletal muscle fibers consist of threadlike structures called *myofibrils*
   a. Myofibrils run longitudinally through the fiber
   b. They are composed of thin and thick filaments
      (1) These filaments are stacked in compartments called SARCOMERES — the functional units of skeletal muscle
      (2) Thin filaments are composed of actin; thick filaments are composed of myosin
      (3) During muscle contraction, thin and thick filaments slide over each other, reducing sarcomere length

C. Functions
1. Skeletal muscles move body parts or the body as a whole
   a. Skeletal muscles produce movements by contracting; all movements of the body and its parts result from muscle contraction
   b. They shorten when they contract, pulling on the bones to which they are attached
      (1) Muscle contraction that moves a body part away from the midline of the body is called *abduction*
      (2) Muscle contraction that moves a body part toward the midline of the body is called *adduction*
   c. Skeletal muscles are responsible for voluntary and reflex movements
2. Skeletal muscle contractions generate most body heat because much of the body is composed of skeletal muscles
   a. ATP is released from cells to supply energy for muscle contraction; about 75% of this energy escapes as heat

ALERT

   b. Muscle fatigue occurs when a muscle cannot regenerate ATP
      (1) This fatigue results from muscle overstimulation
      (2) It causes muscle contractions to become gradually weaker and eventually nonexistent
3. Skeletal muscles also maintain posture; for instance, the combined contraction of skeletal muscles maintains an erect or seated posture

D. Attachment
1. Most skeletal muscles are attached to bones
   a. During contraction, one of the bones to which the muscle attaches stays relatively stationary while the other is pulled in the opposite direction
   b. The point where the muscle attaches to the stationary or less movable bone is called the *origin;* the point where it attaches to the more movable bone is called the *insertion* (see *Points of origin and insertion,* pages 80 to 83)

Text continues on page 83.

Points of origin and insertion

This table lists the points of origin and insertion for the major skeletal muscles.

MUSCLE	ORIGIN	INSERTION
Biceps brachii	• Long head: scapula (supraglenoid tubercle) • Short head: scapula (coracoid process)	• Radius (tubercle)
Biceps femoris	• Long head: ischial tubercle • Short head: linea aspera	• Fibula (lateral surface of head) • Tibia (lateral condyle)
Brachialis	• Humerus (anterior surface of distal half)	• Ulna (coronoid process)
Brachioradialis	• Humerus (lateral supracondylar ridge)	• Radius (styloid process)
Buccinator	• Mandible (alveolar process) • Maxillary bone	• Orbicularis oris • Skin at mouth angle
Deltoid	• Clavicle (lateral third) • Acromion process • Scapula (spine)	• Humerus (deltoid tubercle)
Diaphragm	• Rib cage (inferior border) • Xiphoid process • Costal cartilages • Vertebrae (lumbar)	• Central tendon of diaphragm
External abdominal oblique	• Ribs (external surface of lower eight)	• Iliac crest (anterior half) • Linea alba
External intercostal muscles	• Ribs (inferior border) • Costal cartilages	• Next inferior rib (superior border)
Gastrocnemius	• Femur (medial and lateral condyles)	• Calcaneus (via Achilles tendon)
Gluteus maximus	• Ilium (posterior gluteal line) • Sacrum and coccyx (posterior surfaces)	• Femur (gluteal tubercle) • Iliotibial band
Infraspinatus	• Scapula (infraspinatus fossa)	• Humerus (greater tubercle)
Internal abdominal oblique	• Inguinal ligament • Iliac crest • Lumbodorsal fascia	• Linea alba • Pubic crest • Ribs (lower four)

Points of origin and insertion (continued)

MUSCLE	ORIGIN	INSERTION
Internal intercostal muscles	• Ribs (inner surface) • Costal cartilages	• Next inferior rib (superior border)
Latissimus dorsi	• Vertebrae (spinous processes of lower six thoracic and all lumbar) • Sacrum • Ilium (posterior crest)	• Humerus (medial margin of intertubercular groove)
Levator scapulae	• Vertebrae (transverse processes of upper four cervical)	• Scapula (vertebral border, above spine)
Masseter	• Zygomatic arch	• Mandible (angle and ramus)
Medial pterygoid	• Sphenoid bone (lateral pterygoid plate) • Maxillary bone (tubercle)	• Mandible (inner surface)
Pectoralis major	• Clavicle (medial half) • Sternum • Ribs (costal cartilages of upper six) • External oblique (aponeurosis)	• Humerus (greater tubercle)
Plantaris	• Femur (lower surface, above lateral condyle)	• Calcaneus (via Achilles tendon)
Quadriceps femoris	• Rectus femoris: ilium (anterior inferior spine) • Vastus lateralis: femur (linea aspera, greater trochanter) • Vastus medialis: femur (linea aspera) • Vastus intermedias: femur (anterior surface of shaft)	• Tibia (via patella and patellar ligament)
Rectus abdominis	• Pubic crest	• Xiphoid process • Ribs (costal cartilages of fifth through seventh)
Rhomboideus major	• Vertebrae (spinous processes of second through fifth thoracic)	• Scapula (vertebral border, below spine)

(continued)

Points of origin and insertion (continued)

MUSCLE	ORIGIN	INSERTION
Rhomboideus minor	• Vertebrae (spinous processes of seventh cervical and first thoracic)	• Scapula (vertebral border, at base of spine)
Sartorius	• Anterior superior iliac spine	• Tibia (proximal medial surface, below tubercle)
Scalene muscles	• Cervical vertebrae (transverse processes)	• Ribs (first and second)
Soleus	• Fibula (posterior surface of proximal third) • Tibia (middle third)	• Calcaneus (via Achilles tendon)
Sternocleidomastoid	• Sternum (manubrium) • Clavicle (medial portion)	• Temporal bone (mastoid process)
Supinator	• Humerus (lateral epicondyle)	• Radius (proximal end, lateral surface of shaft)
Supraspinatus	• Scapula (supraspinatus fossa)	• Humerus (greater tubercle)
Temporalis	• Temporal fossa	• Mandible (coronoid process and ramus)
Tibialis anterior	• Tibia (lateral condyle, proximal two-thirds of shaft) • Interosseous membrane	• Tarsal (first cuneiform) • Metatarsal (first)
Tibialis posterior	• Tibia (posterior surface) • Fibula (posterior surface) • Interosseous membrane (posterior surface)	• Navicular bone • All three cuneiforms • Cuboid bone • Second through fourth metatarsals
Transversus abdominis	• Inguinal ligament • Iliac crest • Lumbodorsal fascia • Ribs (costal cartilages of last six)	• Linea alba • Pubic crest
Trapezius	• Occipital bone • Ligamentum nuchae • Vertebrae (spinous processes of seventh cervical and all thoracic)	• Clavicle (lateral third) • Acromion process • Scapula (spine)

Points of origin and insertion *(continued)*

MUSCLE	ORIGIN	INSERTION
Triceps brachii	• Long head: scapula (infraglenoid tubercle) • Lateral head: humerus (posterior surface, above radial groove) • Medial head: humerus (posterior surface, below radial groove)	• Ulna (olecranon process)

2. Muscles may attach to bones directly or indirectly
   a. In a direct attachment, the *epimysium,* or fibrous sheath, of the muscle fuses to the periosteum of the bone
   b. In an indirect attachment, the fascia extends past the muscle as a tendon or aponeurosis, which in turn attaches to bone; indirect attachments outnumber direct attachments

♦ V. Muscles of the axial skeleton

A. General information
   1. Muscles of the axial skeleton include those of the head and neck, those that move the vertebral column, and the thoracic muscles responsible for respiration
   2. Some references include the abdominopelvic muscles as muscles of the axial skeleton (for information on these muscles, see section VI, C on page 86)

B. Muscles of the head and neck
   1. These muscles include those of the face, tongue, and neck and those that permit mastication, or chewing
   2. Fourteen muscles are responsible for facial expression
      a. The *buccinator* compresses the cheek and pulls the corner of the mouth
      b. The *corrugator supercilii* draws the eyebrows together
      c. The *depressor anguli oris* pulls the mouth downward
      d. The *depressor labii inferioris* pulls the lower lip downward
      e. The *epicranius frontalis* raises the eyebrows and wrinkles the forehead skin
      f. The *epicranius occipitalis* draws the scalp backward
      g. The *levator labii superioris* raises the upper lip and opens the nostrils
      h. The *mentalis* raises the lower lip
      i. The *orbicularis oculi* closes the eyelids and tightens the forehead skin

j. The *orbicularis oris* closes the lips
k. The *platysma* depresses the jaw and tightens the skin of the neck
l. The *procerus* wrinkles the skin between the eyebrows
m. The *risorius* pulls the mouth backward
n. The *zygomaticus major* raises the angle of the mouth

3. Four muscles take part in mastication
   a. The *temporalis* and the *masseter* close the jaws
   b. The *pterygoideus medialis* closes the jaws and helps move them sideways
   c. The *pterygoideus lateralis* opens the jaws and helps move them sideways
4. The tongue has three skeletal muscles
   a. The *genioglossus* protracts, retracts, and depresses the tongue
   b. The *hyoglossus* depresses the tongue and draws its sides downward
   c. The *styloglossus* retracts and elevates the tongue
5. Neck muscles include the sternocleidomastoideus, suprahyoidei, and infrahyoidei
   a. The *sternocleidomastoideus* flexes the vertebral column and rotates the head to the opposite side
   b. Four suprahyoid muscles exist
      (1) The *digastricus* raises the hyoid (a single bone in the neck) and helps open the jaws
      (2) The *stylohyoideus* raises the hyoid and pulls it backward
      (3) The *mylohyoideus* raises the hyoid and floor of the mouth
      (4) The *geniohyoideus* pulls the hyoid forward
   c. Four infrahyoid muscles exist
      (1) The *sternohyoideus* pulls the hyoid downward
      (2) The *sternothyroideus* pulls the larynx downward
      (3) The *thyrohyoideus* pulls the hyoid downward and raises the larynx
      (4) The *omohyoideus* pulls the hyoid downward

C. Muscles that move the vertebral column
   1. These muscles are located along the spine
   2. They move the vertebral column
      a. The *semispinalis thoracis, semispinalis cervicis,* and *semispinalis capitis* are deep muscles that extend and rotate the vertebral column and head
      b. The *multifidi* extend and rotate the vertebral column
      c. The *rotatores* extend and rotate the vertebral column
      d. The *interspinales* extend the vertebral column
      e. The *scalenus* muscles flex and rotate the neck and aid inhalation
      f. The *intertransversarii* abduct the vertebral column

g. The *splenius capitis* and *splenius cervicis* act together to extend the head and neck and act singly to abduct and rotate the head toward the same side

h. The *erector spinae* muscles — the most prominent muscles that move the vertebral column — include a series of overlapping muscles

(1) The *iliocostalis lumborum, iliocostalis thoracis,* and *iliocostalis cervicis* extend the vertebral column and bend it to one side

(2) The *longissimus thoracis, longissimus cervicis,* and *longissimus capitis* extend the vertebral column and head and rotate the head toward the same side

(3) The *spinalis thoracis* and *spinalis cervicis* extend the vertebral column

D. Muscles of respiration

1. These muscles permit breathing
2. This group includes five muscles

a. The *diaphragm* allows inspiration (inhalation) by pulling the central tendon of the diaphragm down and enlarging the thoracic cavity

b. The *intercostales externi* muscles elevate the ribs, aiding inspiration

c. The *intercostales interni* muscles draw the ribs together, aiding expiration (exhalation)

d. The *subcostales* draws the ribs together, aiding expiration

e. The *transversus thoracis* draws the rib cage downward, aiding expiration

♦ VI. Muscles of the appendicular skeleton

A. General information

1. Muscles of the appendicular skeleton include those of the shoulder (pectoral) girdle, abdominopelvic cavity, and upper and lower limbs
2. Although abdominal muscles typically are not considered part of the appendicular skeleton, they are described here because they are part of the abdominopelvic cavity

B. Muscles of the shoulder girdle

1. These muscles move the scapulae (shoulder blades)
2. They include seven muscles

a. The *trapezius* elevates, depresses, rotates, adducts, and stabilizes the scapula

b. The *rhomboideus major* and *rhomboideus minor* adduct, stabilize, and rotate the scapula

c. The *levator scapulae* elevates and adducts the scapula and bends the neck laterally

d. The *pectoralis minor* draws the scapula forward and downward

e. The *serratus anterior* stabilizes, abducts, and rotates the scapula upward and helps to abduct and raise the arm
f. The *subclavius* stabilizes and depresses the shoulder

C. Muscles of the abdominopelvic cavity
1. These muscles include those of the abdominal wall and those that form the floor of the abdominopelvic cavity
2. The abdominal wall has five muscles
a. The *external abdominal oblique* muscle and *internal abdominal oblique* muscle compress the abdominopelvic cavity and help flex and rotate the vertebral column
b. The *transversus abdominis* compresses the abdominopelvic cavity
c. The *rectus abdominis* compresses the abdominopelvic cavity and flexes the vertebral column
d. The *quadratus lumborum* pulls the thoracic cage toward the pelvis
3. Muscles that form the floor of the abdominopelvic cavity and support the pelvic viscera include the *levator ani* and *coccygeus*

D. Muscles of the upper limbs
1. These muscles are classified according to the bones they move, such as those of the arm, forearm, wrist, hands, and fingers
2. Muscles that move the arm (humerus) are further subdivided into those with an origin on the axial skeleton and those with an origin on the scapula
a. Two muscles have an origin on the axial skeleton
(1) The *pectoralis major* flexes, adducts, and medially rotates the arm
(2) The *latissimus dorsi* extends, adducts, and medially rotates the arm; it also pulls the shoulder downward
b. Seven muscles have an origin on the scapula
(1) The *deltoideus* abducts, rotates, and extends the arm
(2) The *supraspinatus* abducts and causes slight lateral rotation of the arm
(3) The *infraspinatus* rotates and causes slight lateral adduction of the arm
(4) The *subscapularis* medially rotates the arm
(5) The *teres major* adducts, extends, and medially rotates the arm
(6) The *teres minor* laterally rotates the arm
(7) The *coracobrachialis* flexes and adducts the arm
3. Five muscles move the forearm
a. The *biceps brachii, brachialis,* and *brachioradialis* flex the forearm
b. The *triceps brachii* and *anconeus* extend the forearm
4. Muscles that move the wrist, hand, and fingers include anterior superficial muscles, anterior deep muscles, posterior superficial mus-

cles, and posterior deep muscles; the hand also has several intrinsic muscles

a. Five muscles are classified as anterior superficial muscles
   (1) The *pronator teres* pronates the forearm (rotates it forward)
   (2) The *flexor carpi radialis* flexes the wrist and abducts the hand
   (3) The *palmaris longus* flexes the wrist
   (4) The *flexor carpi ulnaris* flexes the wrist and adducts the hand
   (5) The *flexor digitorum superficialis* flexes the wrist and fingers
b. Three muscles are classified as anterior deep muscles
   (1) The *flexor digitorum profundus* flexes the wrist and fingers
   (2) The *flexor pollicis longus* flexes the thumb and helps flex the wrist
   (3) The *pronator quadratus* pronates the hand
c. Five muscles are classified as posterior superficial muscles
   (1) The *extensor carpi radialis longus* extends the wrist and abducts the hand
   (2) The *extensor carpi radialis brevis* extends the wrist and abducts the hand
   (3) The *extensor digitorum communis* extends the fingers and wrist
   (4) The *extensor digiti minimi* extends the little finger
   (5) The *extensor carpi ulnaris* extends the wrist and adducts the hand
d. Five muscles are classified as posterior deep muscles
   (1) The *supinator* supinates the forearm (rotates it backward)
   (2) The *abductor pollicis longus* abducts the thumb and hand
   (3) The *extensor pollicis brevis* extends the thumb
   (4) The *extensor pollicis longus* extends and abducts the thumb
   (5) The *extensor indicis* extends the index finger
e. Intrinsic muscles of the hand include the thenar, hypothenar, and midpalmar muscle groups
   (1) Thenar muscles include the *abductor pollicis brevis,* which abducts the thumb; *opponens pollicis,* which pulls the thumb in front of the palm; *flexor pollicis brevis,* which flexes and adducts the thumb; and *adductor pollicis,* which adducts the thumb
   (2) Hypothenar muscles include the *palmaris brevis,* which pulls the skin toward the middle of the palm; *abductor digiti minimi manus,* which abducts the little finger; *flexor digiti minimi brevis manus,* which flexes the little finger; and *opponens digiti minimi,* which moves the little finger in front of the palm
   (3) Midpalmar muscles include the *lumbricales manus,* which extend the interphalangeal joints and flex the metacarpopha-

langeal joints; *interossei dorsales manus,* which abduct the fingers; and *interossei palmares,* which adduct the fingers

E. Muscles of the lower limbs
   1. These muscles include the muscles that move the femur (thigh bone), the muscles that move the foot and toes, and the intrinsic muscles of the foot
   2. Numerous muscles move the femur
      a. The *iliopsoas* muscles (a compound muscle) flexes the thigh
      b. The *gluteus maximus* extends and laterally rotates the thigh
      c. The *gluteus medius* and *minimus* abduct and medially rotate the thigh
      d. The *tensor fasciae latae* helps to flex, abduct, and medially rotate the thigh
      e. The *piriformis* laterally rotates and helps to extend and abduct the thigh
      f. The *obturator internus, obturator externus, gemellus superior, gemellus inferior,* and *quadratus femoris* laterally rotate the thigh
      g. The *adductor magnus, adductor longus,* and *adductor brevis* adduct and laterally rotate the thigh
      h. The *pectineus* adducts, flexes, and laterally rotates the thigh
      i. The *gracilis* adducts the thigh and flexes the leg
      j. The *sartorius* flexes the thigh and leg
      k. The *quadriceps femoris* (a compound muscle) extends the leg and flexes the thigh
      l. The hamstrings group — *biceps femoris, semitendinosus,* and *semimembranosus* — flexes the leg and extends the thigh
   3. Muscles that move the foot and toes include those of the anterior compartment, lateral compartment, and posterior compartment; the last category includes superficial and deep muscles
      a. The anterior compartment includes four muscles
         (1) The *tibialis anterior* flexes the foot backward and inverts it (turns it inward)
         (2) The *extensor hallucis longus* flexes the foot backward, inverts the foot, and extends the great toe
         (3) The *extensor digitorum longus* flexes the foot backward and everts it (turns it outward); it also extends the toes
         (4) The *peroneus tertius* flexes the foot backward and everts it
      b. The lateral compartment includes the *peroneus longus* and *peroneus brevis,* which flex and evert the foot
      c. Superficial muscles of the posterior compartment are the *gastrocnemius, soleus,* and *plantaris;* these muscles flex the leg and foot
      d. Deep muscles of the posterior compartment include four muscles
         (1) The *popliteus* flexes and medially rotates the leg
         (2) The *flexor hallucis longus* flexes the foot and great toe

(3) The *flexor digitorum longus* flexes the foot and toes
(4) The *tibialis posterior* flexes and inverts the foot

4. Intrinsic muscles of the foot include one dorsal muscle and numerous plantar muscles; plantar muscles are subdivided into those of the superficial layer, second layer, third layer, and fourth layer
   a. The dorsal muscle, the *extensor digitorum brevis,* extends the second through fifth toes
   b. The plantaris group of the superficial layer includes three muscles
      (1) The *abductor hallucis* abducts the great toe
      (2) The *flexor digitorum brevis* flexes the second through fifth toes
      (3) The *abductor digiti minimi pedis* abducts the small toe
   c. The plantaris group of the second layer includes two muscles
      (1) The *quadratus plantae* helps flex the second through fifth toes
      (2) The *lumbricales pedis* flex the second through fifth toes
   d. The plantaris group of the third layer includes three muscles
      (1) The *flexor hallucis brevis* flexes the great toe
      (2) The *adductor hallucis* adducts the great toe
      (3) The *flexor digiti minimi brevis pedis* flexes the small toe
   e. The plantaris group of the fourth layer includes two muscles
      (1) The *interossei plantaris* adduct the toes toward the second toe
      (2) The *interossei dorsales pedis* abduct the toes from the second toe and medially and laterally moves the second toe

♦ VII. Skeletal muscle contraction

A. General information

1. Muscle contraction occurs in three periods
   a. During the latent period, nothing appears to happen
   b. During the contraction period, the muscle fibers shorten
   c. During the relaxation period, the muscle fibers lengthen
2. Skeletal muscle contraction involves calcium ion transport and nerve impulse transmission; relaxation normally follows contraction

B. Innervation

1. Skeletal muscle is under voluntary control; it contracts in response to impulses transmitted from the CNS by motor nerves
2. Each skeletal muscle is innervated by sensory neurons and at least one motor nerve, which contains hundreds of fibers from motor neurons
   a. Sensory (afferent) neurons receive impulses about the degree of muscle contraction and transmit them to the CNS; this allows proper coordination of muscle activity
   b. Motor (efferent) neurons convey impulses from the CNS to the muscle, triggering muscle contraction

c. As axons from a motor nerve enter a muscle, each branch innervates a muscle fiber; collectively, the neuron and the innervated fibers are termed the *motor unit*

3. Muscle fiber contraction of a motor unit is governed by the ALL-OR-NONE RESPONSE
   a. If the nerve impulse is intense enough to stimulate contraction, all the muscle fibers in the motor unit contract
   b. If the impulse is not intense enough to stimulate contraction of all the muscle fibers in the motor unit, none contract
4. Contraction strength depends on the number of motor units activated
   a. Weak contractions activate only a few motor units
   b. Stronger contractions activate more motor units

C. Contraction and relaxation
1. When a nerve impulse stimulates the muscle fiber at the neuromuscular junction, the impulse is propagated along the sarcolemma and transmitted through the transverse tubules (tubelike extensions of the sarcolemma) into the interior of the muscle fiber
2. The impulse causes the sarcoplasmic reticulum to release calcium ions
3. Calcium ions diffuse into the sarcoplasm and bind to troponin on the threadlike structures around the actin filaments, changing the position of these structures; as a result, tropomyosin no longer can prevent actin and myosin from binding
4. Myosin heads bind to the actin filaments, forming structures called CROSS BRIDGES that pull the actin filaments toward the center of the sarcomeres; this results in muscle fiber shortening, or contraction
5. When the motor unit no longer is stimulated, calcium ions separate from troponin and are transported back into the sarcoplasmic reticulum
6. The threadlike structures return to their original positions
7. Tropomyosin unbinds the cross bridges, and actin and myosin filaments separate, causing the sarcomeres (and muscle fibers) to lengthen

D. Muscle tone
1. Normal muscle is not relaxed completely; it maintains a slight, sustained contractility called *muscle tone,* which is a reflex contraction in response to stretching
   a. When a muscle is stretched, receptors in muscles, joints, and tendons respond by sending impulses to the nervous system
      (1) These afferent impulses are transmitted to the spinal cord and cause discharge of motor impulses that make the muscle fibers contract
      (2) The amount of stretching of the muscle fibers regulates the amount of reflex contraction

TEACHING TIPS

Patient with a strain or sprain

Be sure to include the following topics when teaching a patient with a strain or sprain.

- Explanation of the injury and its potential complications
- Preparation for diagnostic tests, such as X-rays
- RICE treatments: rest, ice, compression, and elevation
- Anti-inflammatory and analgesic drugs to relieve swelling and pain
- Physical therapy for rehabilitation
- Immobilization devices, such as elastic bandages, casts, and crutches
- Surgery for severe sprains
- Sources of information and support

(3) Overstretching of a muscle can cause a strain or other muscle injury (for teaching tips, see *Patient with a strain or sprain*)

b. Motor neurons then transmit impulses to the muscle fibers, causing them to contract and resist the stretching force; muscle tone is maintained by the contraction of muscles with opposing actions

(1) Flexor muscles respond to the pull of extensor muscles by contracting slightly

(2) Extensor muscles, in turn, respond to the pull of flexors, resulting in a slight state of tension in all muscle groups

2. Muscle tone maintains posture by maintaining continuous contraction of the head, neck, and back muscles
3. Muscle tone around joints maintains joint stability

♦ VIII. Cardiac muscle contraction

A. General information

1. In the heart, cardiac muscle contracts rhythmically to pump blood
2. The sarcoplasmic reticulum of the cardiac muscle fiber is less prominent than in skeletal muscle, and the T tubules are associated less closely with the sarcoplasmic reticulum
3. Cardiac muscle cells interconnect to form branching networks

B. Contraction and relaxation

1. Cardiac muscle cells have the same arrangement of actin and myosin and employ the same general mechanism of contraction and relaxation as skeletal muscle cells; however, some variations exist, especially in the manner of stimulation
2. Cardiac muscle contractions occur at a slower rate and last longer than skeletal muscle contractions because the T tubules and sarco-

plasmic reticulum are farther apart in cardiac muscles, making nerve impulse transmission less efficient

3. The blood supply to — and mitochondria in — cardiac muscle fibers are more abundant than those in skeletal muscle fibers
   a. Cardiac muscle fibers obtain sufficient ATP for energy from aerobic metabolism of nutrients in the mitochondria
   b. These fibers do not rely on anaerobic metabolism during increased activity and do not develop an oxygen debt as skeletal muscle fibers do
4. Cardiac muscle fibers are not organized into motor units like skeletal muscle fibers
   a. Interconnections called *intercalated disks* between the branching cardiac muscle fibers permit action potentials to pass from cell to cell
   b. These muscle fibers function as an integrated unit
5. The autonomic nervous system regulates cardiac rate and rhythm, but cardiac muscle fibers can generate impulses and contract rhythmically even when deprived of nervous stimulation
6. During cardiac muscle contraction, electrocardiography can measure the electrical activity associated with depolarization and depolarization of cardiac muscle (for details about cardiac contraction and electrical conduction, see Chapter 10, Cardiovascular System)

♦ IX. Smooth-muscle contraction

A. General information
1. In smooth-muscle fibers, the sarcoplasm contains fewer actin and myosin filaments than do skeletal muscle fibers; because smooth-muscle filaments are not organized into sarcomeres, the fibers do not appear striated
2. The sarcoplasmic reticulum is not well developed in smooth-muscle fibers; these fibers do not have a network of T tubules, but cytoplasmic vacuoles that connect with the surface of the fibers may serve the same function
3. The sarcoplasm contains a network of *intermediate filaments* attached to cytoplasmic structures called *dense bodies;* actin filaments attach to dense bodies during contraction

B. Contraction and relaxation
1. Contraction and relaxation of smooth muscle is basically the same as in skeletal muscle; however, some variations exist
2. Actin and myosin filaments slide together during contraction, pulling on the network of intermediate filaments and dense bodies; this causes the smooth-muscle fibers to shorten

3. Smooth muscle contracts and relaxes more slowly than skeletal muscle does
4. Smooth-muscle contraction requires less energy than skeletal muscle contraction
5. Smooth-muscle fibers receive motor impulses from the autonomic nervous system; they are not under voluntary control

POINTS TO REMEMBER

- The three types of muscle tissue — smooth, cardiac, and skeletal — differ in cell structure, location, and function. All three types are controlled by nerve impulses.
- Muscle permits movement, maintains posture, and generates heat.
- All muscle contractions require energy, which is obtained from the breakdown of ATP in muscle fiber. When needed, skeletal muscle fibers can increase ATP production by the phosphagen and glycogen–lactic acid systems, and by aerobic and anaerobic metabolism.
- Smooth muscle lines the visceral organs and urinary bladder and surrounds the blood vessels, bronchi, and various ducts. It produces involuntary, slow, and sustained contractions.
- Cardiac muscle makes up the heart wall. Under involuntary control, it moves blood through the heart and into blood vessels
- Skeletal muscle is attached to the skeleton and causes voluntary movements in the axial and appendicular skeletons.
- Each skeletal muscle is innervated by sensory neurons and motor neurons. Its contraction is governed by the all-or-none response.
- Cardiac muscle contractions occur at a slower rate and last longer than skeletal muscle contractions. They use aerobic — not anaerobic — metabolism.
- In smooth-muscle contraction, actin and myosin filaments slide together, pulling on the network of intermediate filaments and dense bodies. Contraction occurs more slowly and uses less energy than it does in skeletal muscle.

Study Questions

To evaluate your understanding of this chapter, answer the following questions in the space provided. Then compare your responses with the correct answers in Appendix B, page 330.

1. What is muscle excitability? ______________________
2. Which types of muscle tissue are striated? ______________________
3. Which types of muscle tissue are involuntary? ______________________
4. What proteins are involved in muscle contraction? ______________________
5. What are the two types of smooth muscle? ______________________
6. How are skeletal muscles named? ______________________
7. What is the all-or-none response? ______________________
8. How do cross bridges work? ______________________

CRITICAL THINKING AND APPLICATION EXERCISES

1. Create a poster that illustrates one system by which a muscle obtains energy.
2. Under a microscope, view samples of smooth-, cardiac, and skeletal muscle cells. Note their differences and similarities.
3. Ask a partner to perform various movements as you identify the skeletal muscles involved. Then, you and your partner switch roles.
4. Using an anatomical model, demonstrate how opposing muscles contract and relax during movement.
5. Prepare a chart that compares the differences in contraction and relaxation for each type of muscle.

CHAPTER

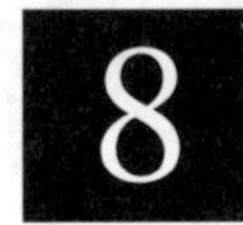

Nervous System

Learning objectives

After studying this chapter, you should be able to:

- Name the two major anatomic divisions of the nervous system.
- Identify the major functions of the nervous system.
- Describe the structure of a neuron.
- Compare the functions of each type of supporting cell.
- Contrast chemical and electrical synapses.
- Identify the four major regions of the brain.
- Explain the functions of the 12 pairs of cranial nerves.
- Discuss the autonomic and somatic nervous systems, neurotransmission, and reflexes.

Chapter overview

By serving as the body's control and communication center, the nervous system directs every body system and governs all movement, sensation, thought, and emotion. It senses internal and external changes, analyzes and stores this sensory information, makes decisions about it, and responds to it — all within a very brief time. To promote a properly functioning nervous system, which is vital to homeostasis, the health care professional must be familiar with its anatomy and physiology.

♦ I. Basic principles

A. General information
   1. The nervous system allows communication among different parts of the body and between the body and the external environment
   2. Anatomically, the nervous system is divided into the *central nervous system* (CNS), which includes the brain and spinal cord, and the *peripheral nervous system* (PNS), which includes all nervous tissue outside the CNS
   3. Functionally, the nervous system is divided into the *sensory (afferent) division,* which conveys impulses from the periphery to the CNS, and the *motor (efferent) division,* which conveys impulses from the CNS to the periphery

B. Functions
   1. The chief functions of the nervous system are to monitor, integrate, and respond to environmental stimuli
   2. The nervous system carries out these functions in three general steps
      a. Sensory receptors monitor changes inside and outside the body
      b. The nervous system processes (integrates) the information gathered by sensory receptors
      c. The nervous system activates the appropriate muscle or gland to respond to the sensory information
   3. With the endocrine system, the nervous system also helps maintain homeostasis
      a. The nervous and endocrine systems regulate certain aspects of the body's internal environment; for instance, the nervous system regulates the heart rate, and the endocrine system produces epinephrine
      b. Although certain functions are controlled chiefly by the nervous system and others by the endocrine system, the two systems generally work together; signals from either system affect functions in the other system

♦ II. Nervous tissue and cells

A. General information
   1. Nervous tissue is composed of nervous system cells that are packed densely and intertwined
   2. Nervous system cells fall into two categories — neurons and neuroglia (supporting cells)

B. Neurons
   1. Neurons are highly specialized cells that conduct nerve impulses

2. Each neuron has a *cell body* (perikaryon, or soma) and a large spherical nucleus with a prominent nucleolus and abundant granular cytoplasm (see *Structure of a neuron*)
   a. Most neuronal cell bodies are located within the CNS
   b. A few are found in the PNS, clustered in structures called ganglia
3. Cytoplasmic processes called AXONS and DENDRITES extend outward from the cell body
   a. Typically, a neuron has only one axon; the axon carries impulses away from the cell body
   b. A neuron typically has many short, thick, diffusely branched extensions called dendrites; dendrites receive impulses from other cells and carry them toward the cell body
   c. In the CNS, bundles of neuron processes (axons and dendrites) are called tracts; in the PNS, they are called nerves
4. The MYELIN SHEATH is a white, fatty (phospholipid) segmented covering that wraps around nerve fibers
   a. Most axons in the PNS are myelinated (covered by a myelin sheath)
   b. The CNS contains myelinated and unmyelinated axons
      (1) Portions of the CNS containing myelinated axons are called WHITE MATTER
      (2) Portions containing unmyelinated axons are called GRAY MATTER
   c. In the PNS, the myelin sheath is enveloped by a sheath of Schwann cells called the NEURILEMMA; in the CNS, nerve fibers lack a neurilemma
5. Neurons can be classified by structure or function
   a. Neurons are multipolar, bipolar, or unipolar in structure
      (1) *Multipolar neurons* have one axon and numerous dendrites; they are the most common type of neuron
      (2) *Bipolar neurons* have one axon and one dendrite; they serve as receptor cells in special sense organs
      (3) *Unipolar neurons* (pseudounipolar neurons) have a single process that divides into a proximal fiber (axon) and a distal fiber (dendrite)
   b. Based on function, neurons are classified as sensory, motor, or association neurons
      (1) *Sensory (afferent) neurons* transmit impulses from sensory receptors in the skin or internal organs toward the CNS; unipolar, their cell bodies lie within sensory ganglia (however, special sense organs have bipolar neurons)
      (2) *Motor (efferent) neurons* carry impulses away from the CNS; except for some neurons in the autonomic system, motor neurons are multipolar, with cell bodies located in the CNS

Structure of a neuron

The main parts of a neuron are the cell body and its cytoplasmic processes — axons and dendrites. The cytoplasm of the cell body contains a large nucleus with a prominent nucleolus and delicate threads called neurofibrils. In a typical neuron, one axon and many dendrites extend from the cell body. The axon conducts nerve impulses away from the cell body; dendrites conduct impulses toward the cell body. The axon may vary from quite short to quite long (up to 1 m [3.3′]). A typical axon has terminal branches and is covered by a myelin sheath. Segments of this sheath are separated by gaps called nodes of Ranvier.

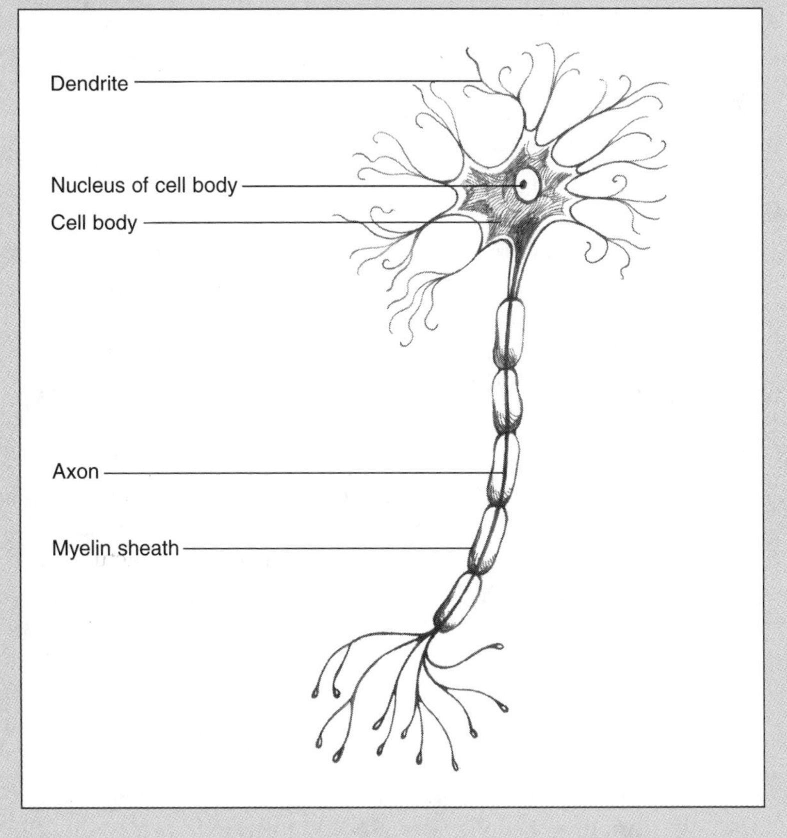

(3) *Association (connecting) neurons* (or interneurons) convey impulses between motor and sensory neurons; the most numerous type, these neurons are typically multipolar and confined to the CNS

6. *Sensory receptors* (also called dendritic end organs) are modified dendritic endings of sensory neurons
   a. They are specialized to respond to environmental stimuli

b. They are described mainly by location, type of stimulus detected, or structure
   (1) *Exteroceptors,* located at or near the body surface, are sensitive to outside stimuli, such as touch, pressure, and sound
   (2) *Interoceptors,* or *visceroceptors,* respond to stimuli arising from the viscera (internal organs) and blood vessels
   (3) *Proprioceptors* respond to internal stimuli and alert the brain to body movements; they exist in skeletal muscles, tendons, joints, and possibly the inner ear (equilibrium receptors)
   (4) *Mechanoreceptors* respond to pressure, touch, sound, vibration, and tissue stretching in the lungs, blood vessels, and bladder
   (5) *Thermoreceptors,* typically found in the skin, respond to temperature changes
   (6) *Photoreceptors,* found in the retina, respond to light
   (7) *Chemoreceptors* respond to chemical stimuli, such as changes in blood gas levels
   (8) *Nociceptors* (or pain receptors) are sensitive to excessive heat and pressure, extreme cold, and chemicals released at inflammation sites; most sensory receptors also function as nociceptors
   (9) *Cutaneous receptors* are commonly found in epithelial and connective tissue; most sensory receptors are cutaneous receptors

C. Supporting cells
   1. Supporting cells have less specialized functions than neurons; unlike neurons, they do not conduct impulses, but they can reproduce
   2. Supporting cells include astrocytes, microglia, oligodendrocytes, ependymal cells, Schwann cells, and satellite cells
      a. *Astrocytes* attach to neurons and capillaries; these abundant cells help supply nutrients to neurons and control ions present around the neuron
      b. *Microglia* are a special type of macrophage; they protect the CNS against microorganisms and engulf dead neural tissue
      c. *Oligodendrocytes* are small, branching cells; their cytoplasmic extensions wrap tightly around nerve fibers to form a myelin sheath
      d. *Ependymal cells* are ciliated cells that line the cavities of the brain and spinal cord; they continually form the CEREBROSPINAL FLUID (CSF), a plasma-like fluid that bathes, cushions, and protects the brain and spinal cord
      e. *Schwann cells* are phagocytic cells that form myelin sheaths around nerve fibers; they are separated by gaps called nodes of Ranvier

f. *Satellite cells,* found in the PNS, may help maintain the chemical balance of neurons

♦ III. Synapse

A. General information
   1. The SYNAPSE is a junction across which electrical or chemical impulses are transferred from one neuron to another
      a. Most synapses occur between the axon of one neuron and the dendrites or cell body of another neuron
      b. Some synapses occur between nerve endings and EFFECTOR CELLS (gland cells or muscle cells)
   2. Synapses are one-way junctions, ensuring that the nerve impulse travels in only one direction

B. Electrical synapse
   1. An electrical synapse provides rapid transmission of impulses from one neuron to the next
   2. Contact between adjacent cell membranes occurs
   3. Abundant in such tissues as cardiac and smooth muscle, electrical synapses allow rhythmic, sequential responses

C. Chemical synapse
   1. A chemical synapse is specialized to release and receive *neurotransmitters,* chemicals that modify or cause impulse transmission across the synapse
   2. When an impulse arrives, vesicles at the end of the axon empty the neurotransmitter into the synaptic gap
   3. The neurotransmitter crosses the gap and combines with receptors on the other neuron, which receive the impulse

♦ IV. Central nervous system

A. General information
   1. The CNS consists of the brain and spinal cord
   2. It is protected by bony enclosures (the skull and vertebrae), the membranous MENINGES, and the watery CSF

B. Brain
   1. The brain has four main regions — CEREBRUM, *diencephalon,* CEREBELLUM, and *brain stem* (see *Structures of the brain,* page 103)
   2. The cerebrum and cerebellum have an outer CORTEX of gray matter (unmyelinated nerve fibers) surrounding a central core of white matter (myelinated nerve fibers)
      a. This pattern changes with descent through the brain stem and spinal cord

b. In the caudal (tail) end of the brain stem and spinal cord, white matter surrounds gray matter

3. The *cerebrum* occupies the superior portion of the cranial cavity
   a. The largest region of the brain, the cerebrum is divided into right and left hemispheres, connected by nerve fibers
   b. The cerebrum performs motor, sensory, and integrative functions
   c. The wrinkles and folds of the cerebral surface—ridges of tissue (gyri), shallow grooves (sulci), and deeper grooves (fissures)—greatly increase its surface area
      (1) The *median longitudinal fissure* separates the hemispheres
      (2) The *transverse fissure* separates the hemispheres from the cerebellum
4. The *diencephalon* is surrounded by the cerebrum
   a. It forms the central core of the forebrain and connects the cerebrum with the brain stem
   b. The diencephalon consists of the thalamus, hypothalamus, and epithalamus
      (1) The *thalamus* forms the superolateral walls of the third ventricle; it serves as a relay station for sensory information
      (2) The *hypothalamus* extends from the optic chiasm to the posterior margin of the mamillary bodies; it regulates the autonomic nervous system (ANS)
      (3) The *epithalamus,* located dorsally, forms the floor of the third ventricle
         (a) It contains an external projection called the pineal gland
         (b) Internally, a mass of capillaries called the CHOROID PLEXUS produces CSF
5. The *cerebellum,* the second largest region of the brain, is posterior and inferior to the cerebrum; it is attached to the pons
   a. It consists of two lateral hemispheres, divided into three lobes each
   b. The cerebellum has an outer cortex of gray matter and an inner core of white matter
   c. The main function of the cerebellum is to regulate and coordinate all complex motor activities
6. The *brain stem* is immediately inferior to the cerebrum, just anterior to the cerebellum
   a. It lies between the cerebrum and spinal cord
   b. It consists of the midbrain, pons, and medulla oblongata
      (1) The *midbrain* is situated between the diencephalon superiorly and the pons inferiorly; it consists of the *cerebral peduncles,* two bundles made up of nerve tracts
      (2) The *pons* lies between the midbrain and medulla oblongata, forming part of the anterior wall of the fourth ventricle

Structures of the brain

The main divisions of the brain are the cerebrum, diencephalon, cerebellum, and brain stem. The cerebrum, the largest division, controls motor activities, interprets sensation, and serves as the center of intellect, language, memory, and consciousness. The cerebellum, the second largest division, is located behind the brain stem; it coordinates movements. The diencephalon, located between the cerebrum and midbrain (part of the brain stem), consists of the thalamus, hypothalamus, and epithalamus. These structures control various body functions essential to homeostasis (such as temperature regulation). The brain stem is composed of the pons, medulla, and midbrain. The pons helps regulate respiration. The medulla is comprised of vital centers for cardiac, vasomotor, and respiratory control. The midbrain serves as a reflex center. This illustration shows a midsagittal cross section of the main features of the brain.

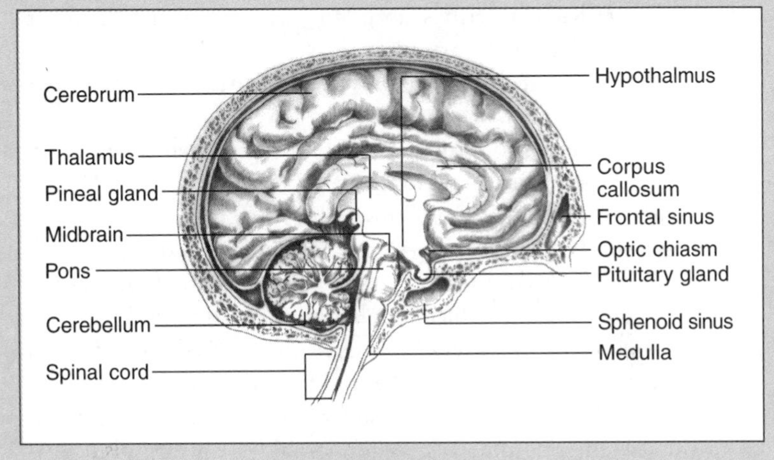

(3) The *medulla oblongata* is the most inferior portion of the brain stem; it joins the spinal cord at the level of the *foramen magnum,* an opening in the occipital portion of the skull

c. The brain stem has three general functions
   (1) It produces the rigid autonomic behaviors necessary for survival; for example, it increases the heart rate
   (2) It provides pathways for nerve fibers between higher and lower neural centers
   (3) It serves as the origin for 10 of the 12 pairs of cranial nerves

7. The brain also contains four *ventricles,* or small cavities
   a. The right and left lateral ventricles are embedded in the right and left cerebral hemispheres, respectively; they communicate with the narrow third ventricle in the diencephalon by a small opening called the interventricular foramen (foramen of Monro)

b. The third ventricle is continuous with the fourth ventricle via the cerebral aqueduct that traverses the midbrain
c. The fourth ventricle is continuous with the central canal of the spinal cord
(1) It is located dorsal to the pons and medulla and ventral to the cerebellum
(2) Three openings (or apertures) allow continuity between the fourth ventricle and subarachnoid space (the fluid-filled area around the brain)
d. The ventricles serve as a site of CSF formation

C. Spinal cord
1. The *spinal cord* is an oval-shaped cylinder that lies within the spinal cavity; it extends from the medulla to the first or second lumbar vertebra (see *Spinal cord and spinal nerves*)
2. The cord has a butterfly-shaped inner core of gray matter and an outer layer of white matter
a. Bilateral posterior projections of gray matter, called *posterior (dorsal) horns,* contain sensory neurons
b. Bilateral anterior projections of gray matter, called *anterior (ventral) horns,* contain motor nerves
3. The spinal cord provides pathways for nerve impulses to and from the brain and performs sensory, motor, and reflex functions
a. Bundles of sensory (afferent) nerve fibers in the cord, called *ascending tracts,* conduct impulses up the cord to the brain
b. Bundles of motor (efferent) nerve fibers, called *descending tracts,* conduct impulses down the cord from the brain
c. The gray matter of the spinal cord contains reflex centers for spinal reflexes (for details, see Section VII, E on page 121)
4. Thirty-one pairs of spinal nerves arise from the cord and exit the vertebral column through openings called *foramina*
5. The *cauda equina,* a collection of nerve roots at the inferior end of the cord, travels through the vertebral canal; typically, it exits the cord between the twelfth thoracic and third lumbar vertebrae

D. Meninges
1. The brain and spinal cord are covered by three connective tissue membranes called the *meninges*
2. The meninges protect the brain and spinal cord, enclose the venous sinuses, contain CSF, and form partitions within the skull
3. The outer meningeal membrane is called the *dura mater* ("tough mother"), or pachymeninx
a. The portion of the dura mater that covers the brain has two layers; the portion that covers the spinal cord has only one layer

Spinal cord and spinal nerves

The spinal cord is a cylindrical structure in the vertebral canal that extends from the foramen magnum at the base of the skull to the upper lumbar region of the vertebral column. Along with the brain, it constitutes the central nervous system. The spinal cord conducts nerve impulses to and from the brain and controls reflexes. Its inner core consists of gray matter (unmyelinated nerve fibers); its outer core consists of white matter (myelinated nerve fibers). Thirty-one pairs of spinal nerves arise from the cord. As this illustration shows, these nerves are designated (from top to bottom) as C1 through S5, plus the coccygeal nerve. At the inferior end of the cord, nerve roots cluster in the cauda equina.

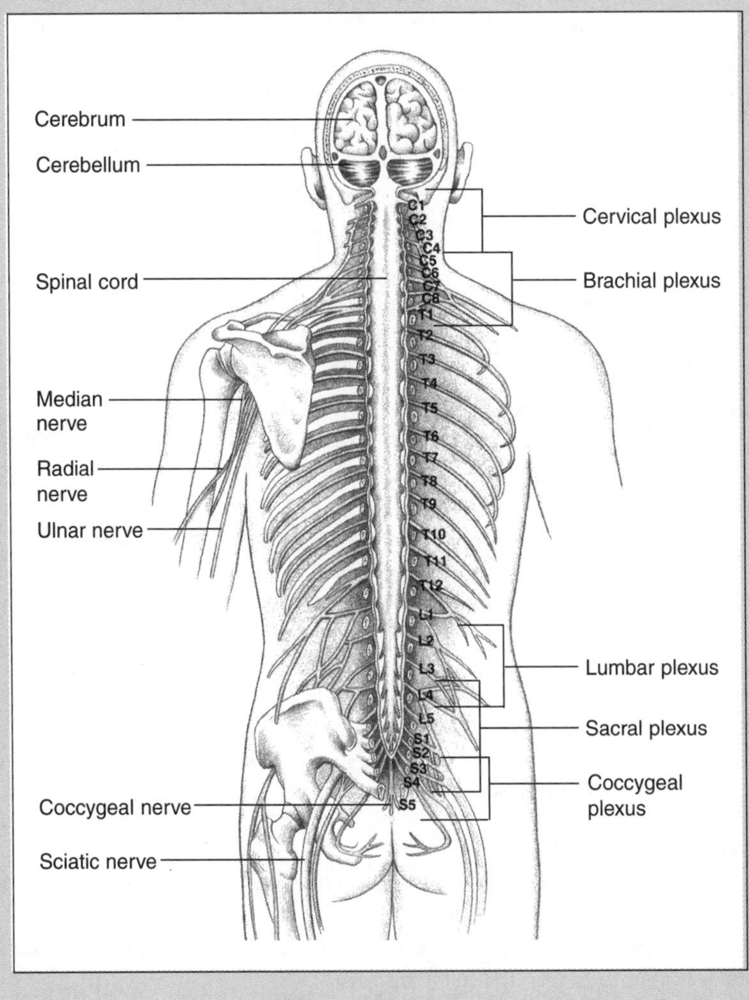

b. The two layers that cover the brain are fused except where they enclose the dural sinuses (which collect venous blood from the brain and convey it to the internal jugular veins of the neck)
c. The dura mater forms septa (partitions) that anchor the brain to the skull in four locations

4. The middle meningeal membrane, called the *arachnoid* ("resembling a spider's web"), is a loose covering
   a. The narrow subdural space separates the arachnoid from the dura mater
   b. The subarachnoid space separates the arachnoid from the innermost meningeal layer; it contains CSF and all major arteries and veins of the brain
   c. The arachnoid villi protrude through the dura mater into the dural sinuses
5. The *pia mater* ("gentle mother") is the innermost meningeal layer
   a. Transparent, it contains blood vessels and reticular and elastic fibers
   b. It adheres to the outer surface of the brain and cord
   c. Collectively, the arachnoid and pia mater are called the *leptomeninges*

E. CSF
1. CSF cushions the CNS, protecting it from damage; its composition is similar to that of blood plasma
2. CSF forms continuously in clusters of capillaries called *choroid plexuses,* found in the roof of each ventricle
3. CSF flows through the ventricles, exits through openings in the roof of the fourth ventricle, and circulates around the brain and spinal cord
   a. CSF is absorbed into the venous sinuses through the *arachnoid villi*
   b. CSF also is absorbed directly into the veins on the surface of the brain
   c. Normally, the rates of CSF production and absorption are balanced so the CSF volume remains constant and the CSF pressure remains normal

♦ V. Peripheral nervous system

A. General information
1. The PNS consists of all nervous tissue outside the CNS; it includes the nerves and ganglia
2. It provides the link between the CNS and body functions via continuous nerves and nerve tracts

3. The PNS includes 12 pairs of cranial nerves and 31 pairs of spinal nerves
4. Its two major divisions, the autonomic and somatic nervous systems, control different functions

B. Cranial nerves
1. These paired nerves arise from the undersurface of the brain and exit the skull through the foramina
2. The first two pairs of nerves originate in the forebrain; the remaining 10 pairs, in the brain stem
3. Cranial nerves are described by type (sensory or motor) and function; starting with the most anterior nerve, they are designated by Roman numerals and by name (see *Cranial nerve functions,* pages 108 and 109)

C. Spinal nerves
1. The 31 pairs of spinal nerves originate in the spinal cord and exit through the vertebrae (see *Spinal cord and spinal nerves,* page 105)
   a. They include 8 cervical, 12 thoracic, 5 lumbar, and 5 sacral pairs and 1 pair of coccygeal nerves
   b. They are designated according to the level of the vertebral column at which they emerge; for instance, T1 refers to the first spinal nerve exiting from the thoracic segment of the vertebral column
2. Each spinal nerve contains a dorsal (sensory, or afferent) root and a ventral (motor, or efferent) root
   a. Cell bodies of afferent fibers lie outside the spinal cord in the dorsal root GANGLION
   b. Cell bodies of efferent fibers lie within the ventral gray column of the cord
3. Spinal nerves divide into branches called *rami;* those exiting the anterior portion are called ventral rami and those exiting the posterior portion are called dorsal rami
   a. The ventral rami of the first four cervical nerves form the *cervical plexus;* this plexus connects with the skin and muscles of the head, neck, and upper part of the shoulders, cranial nerves XI and XII, and phrenic nerves
   b. The ventral rami of spinal nerves C5 to C8 and T1 (with contributions from C4 and T2) form the *brachial plexus;* this plexus provides the entire nerve supply to the arms and several neck and shoulder muscles
   c. The ventral rami of spinal nerves L1 to L4 form the *lumbar plexus,* which supplies the anterolateral abdominal wall, external genitals, and part of the legs

Cranial nerve functions

The 12 cranial nerves perform a wide range of sensory and motor functions, as described here.

NERVE NUMBER AND NAME	TYPE	FUNCTION
I (olfactory)	Sensory	• Provides a sense of smell
II (optic)	Sensory	• Provides vision
III (oculomotor)	Motor	• Moves the eyes and raises the eyelids • Adjusts the amount of light entering the eyes and focuses the lenses • Provides a sense of eye muscle movement
IV (trochlear)	Motor	• Moves the eyes • Provides eye muscle movement
V (trigeminal)	Motor and sensory	• Moves the muscles of mastication and those in the floor of the mouth • Provides sensory input from the eye surface, tear glands, upper eyelids, forehead, and scalp • Provides sensory input from the upper teeth, gingivae, and lip; palate lining; and facial skin • Provides sensory input from the lower teeth, gingivae, and lip; scalp; and skin over the jaw
VI (abducen)	Motor	• Moves the eyes • Provides eye muscle movement
VII (facial)	Motor and sensory	• Allows facial expression • Innervates tear and salivary glands • Provides a sense of taste to anterior tongue
VIII (vestibulo-cochlear)	Sensory	• Provides a sense of hearing • Provides a sense of equilibrium
IX (glosso-pharyngeal)	Motor and sensory	• Allows swallowing by controlling pharynx muscles • Innervates salivary glands • Provides a sense of taste to the posterior tongue • Provides sensory input from the pharynx, tonsils, and carotid arteries

Cranial nerve functions *(continued)*

NERVE NUMBER AND NAME	TYPE	FUNCTION
X (vagus)	Motor and sensory	• Allows speech and swallowing by controlling pharynx muscles • Innervates muscles of the heart and smooth muscles of thoracic and abdominal organs • Provides sensory input from the pharynx, larynx, esophagus, and thoracic and abdominal organs
XI (spinal accessory)	Motor	• Allows movement of the soft palate, pharynx, and larynx • Allows movement of the neck and back
XII (hypoglossal)	Motor	• Allows tongue movement

d. The ventral rami of spinal nerves L4 to L5 and S1 to S4 form the *sacral plexus,* which supplies the buttocks, perineum, and legs

ALERT

4. Damage to a spinal nerve can lead to muscular paralysis or loss of sensation in the area supplied by the nerve
   a. Most spinal nerves innervate specific areas of the skin called dermatomes
   b. By testing each dermatome, the health care professional can determine which spinal nerve has been affected

D. Autonomic nervous system
1. The ANS controls involuntary (or automatic) body functions, such as the activity of cardiac muscle, smooth muscle, and glandular epithelial tissue; although it consists entirely of motor nerves, sensory neurons participate in its function
2. It has two subdivisions — the sympathetic and parasympathetic systems
   a. Anatomically and functionally, the two systems are distinct
   b. Although the systems generally serve the same organs, they have a counterbalancing effect; each system can inhibit the organs excited by the other (for details, see *Responses to autonomic nervous system stimulation,* page 111)
3. The *sympathetic system* originates from the lateral horns of the first thoracic through first lumbar segments of the spinal cord
   a. It helps the body cope with events in the external environment

   b. It functions mainly during stress, triggering the FIGHT-OR-FLIGHT RESPONSE (increased heart and respiratory rate; cold, sweaty palms; and pupil dilation)
4. The *parasympathetic system* consists of the vagus nerve, which originates in the medulla of the brain stem, and spinal nerves originating in the sacral region of the spinal cord
   a. It activates the gastrointestinal system
   b. It also supports restorative, resting body functions through such actions as replenishing fluid and electrolytes
5. The arrangement of neurons in the ANS differs from that in the somatic nervous system (see *Physiologic process: Neuron pathways in the peripheral nervous system,* page 112)

E. Somatic nervous system
1. The somatic nervous system consists of motor and sensory nerves
2. It controls skeletal muscles (those under voluntary or conscious control)
3. The somatic nervous system produces a motor response through efferent fibers from the CNS, which transmit impulses to the skin and skeletal muscles

♦ VI. Neurotransmission

A. General information
1. *Neurotransmission* is the conduction of impulses throughout the nervous system; it occurs through the actions of neurons, which detect and transmit stimuli in the form of electrochemical impulses
2. Electrical transmission occurs within the nerve fiber
   a. Each neuron has an electrical potential (RESTING MEMBRANE POTENTIAL) caused by different concentrations of sodium and potassium ions on each side of the membrane; normally the neuron is *polarized* (positive outside and negative inside)
   b. Stimulation of a nerve alters membrane permeability, allowing sodium to enter and suddenly causing the membrane to become *depolarized* (positive inside and negative outside)
   c. The spread of increased permeability and electrical current along the membrane is a nerve impulse
3. Chemical transmission occurs between two neurons or between a neuron and a muscle
   a. When the impulse reaches the end of a neuron, a *neurotransmitter* is released, which causes the impulse to cross the synapse
   b. When the impulse is received by the next neuron, another chemical breaks down the neurotransmitter to prevent sustained impulse transmission

Responses to autonomic nervous system stimulation

Most effector organs are innervated by the parasympathetic and sympathetic divisions of the autonomic nervous system. These divisions usually produce opposite responses, as shown in the examples below.

EFFECTOR ORGANS	PARASYMPATHETIC RESPONSES	SYMPATHETIC RESPONSES
Eye		
Radial muscle of iris	None	Contraction (mydriasis)
Sphincter muscle of iris	Contraction for near vision	None
Heart	Decreased rate and contractility	Increased rate and contractility
Lung (bronchial muscle)	Contraction	Relaxation
Stomach		
Motility and tone	Increased	Decreased (usually)
Sphincters	Relaxation	Contraction (usually)
Intestine		
Motility and tone	Increased	Decreased
Sphincters	Relaxation	Contraction
Urinary bladder		
Bladder muscle	Contraction	Relaxation
Trigone and sphincter	Relaxation	Contraction
Skin		
Erector pilli	None	Contraction
Sweat glands	Generalized secretion	Slight localized secretion
Adrenal medulla	None	Secretion of epinephrine and norepinephrine
Liver	None	Glycogenolysis
Pancreas (acini)	Increased secretion	Decreased secretion
Adipose tissue	None	Lipolysis
Juxtaglomerular cells	None	Increased renin secretion

4. Neurotransmitters are chemicals that are essential for neurotransmission; neuropeptides regulate or modulate their actions
5. Sensory impulses ultimately reach the brain for interpretation; motor impulses are transmitted from the brain to the muscles or other effect or organs

Text continues on page 114.

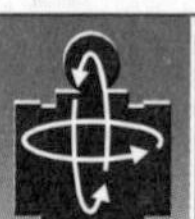

PHYSIOLOGIC PROCESS

Neuron pathways in the peripheral nervous system

The peripheral nervous system consists of the autonomic nervous system (ANS), which has parasympathetic and sympathetic divisions, and the somatic nervous system. Each of these systems has different neuron pathways, as described below.

ANS pathways consist of two neurons: one neuron extends from the central nervous system (CNS) to a ganglion (preganglionic neuron); the other extends from the ganglion to the effector organ or gland (postganglionic neuron). Somatic nervous system pathways consist of only one neuron.

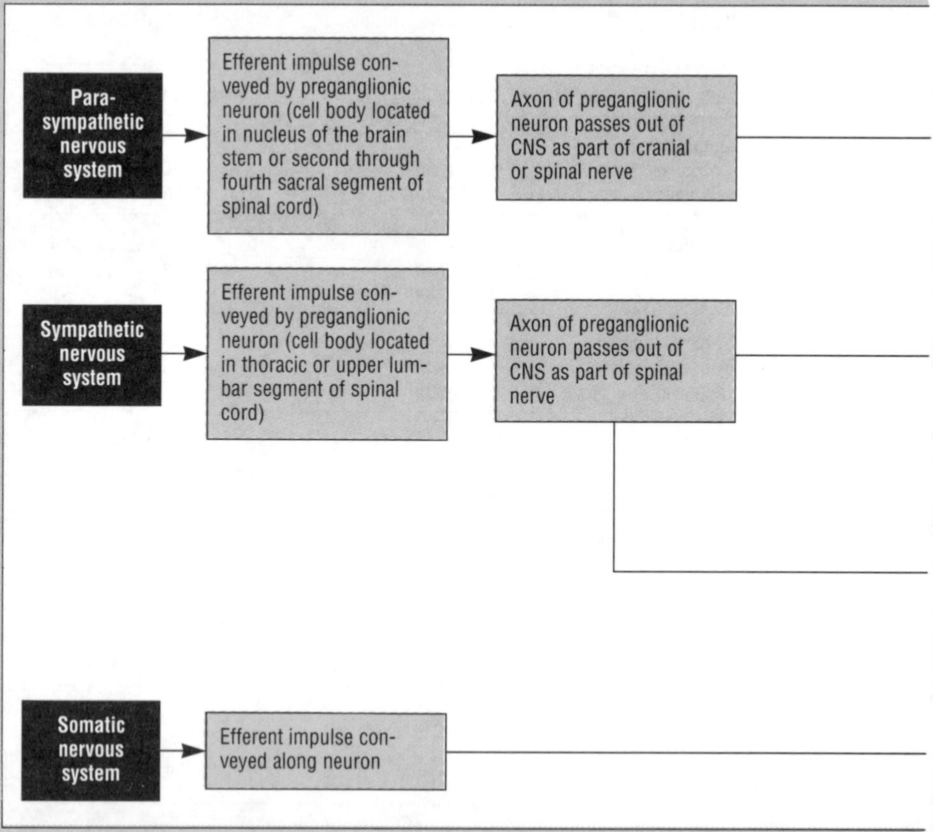

Parasympathetic nervous system → Efferent impulse conveyed by preganglionic neuron (cell body located in nucleus of the brain stem or second through fourth sacral segment of spinal cord) → Axon of preganglionic neuron passes out of CNS as part of cranial or spinal nerve

Sympathetic nervous system → Efferent impulse conveyed by preganglionic neuron (cell body located in thoracic or upper lumbar segment of spinal cord) → Axon of preganglionic neuron passes out of CNS as part of spinal nerve

Somatic nervous system → Efferent impulse conveyed along neuron

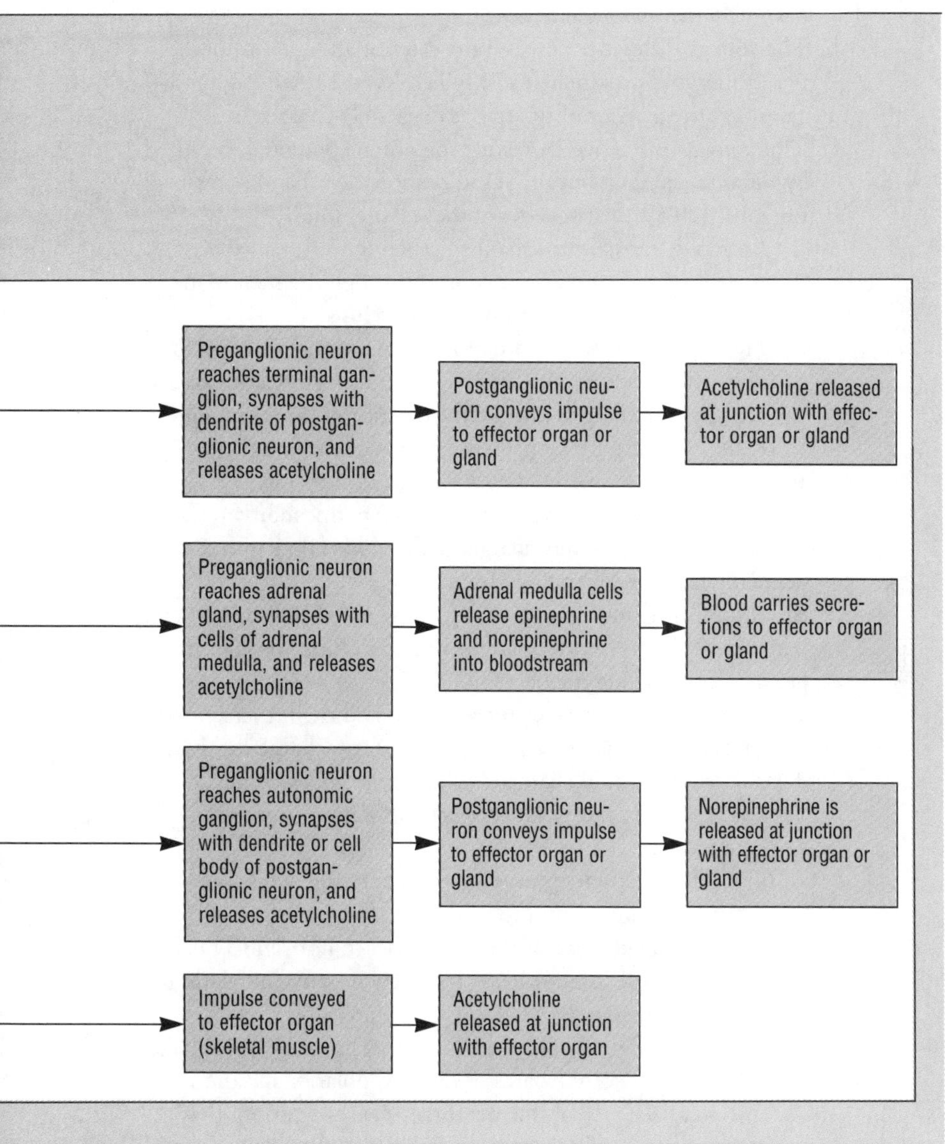
Preganglionic neuron reaches terminal ganglion, synapses with dendrite of postganglionic neuron, and releases acetylcholine
Postganglionic neuron conveys impulse to effector organ or gland
Acetylcholine released at junction with effector organ or gland
Preganglionic neuron reaches adrenal gland, synapses with cells of adrenal medulla, and releases acetylcholine
Adrenal medulla cells release epinephrine and norepinephrine into bloodstream
Blood carries secretions to effector organ or gland
Preganglionic neuron reaches autonomic ganglion, synapses with dendrite or cell body of postganglionic neuron, and releases acetylcholine
Postganglionic neuron conveys impulse to effector organ or gland
Norepinephrine is released at junction with effector organ or gland
Impulse conveyed to effector organ (skeletal muscle)
Acetylcholine released at junction with effector organ

B. Transmission within nerve fibers

1. POLARIZATION is the electrical state during which a nerve fiber is not transmitting an impulse
   a. The exterior of the nerve fiber has a positive charge; the interior has a negative charge
   b. The voltage difference between the exterior and interior of the nerve fiber is approximately -70 millivolts (the minus sign indicates that the interior of the cells is negatively charged)
   c. This voltage difference, or resting membrane potential, is caused by the unequal distribution of sodium ions (Na^+) and potassium ions (K^+) on the two sides of the cell membrane
      (1) An active transport mechanism called the SODIUM-POTASSIUM PUMP transports potassium ions in through the membrane and simultaneously transports sodium ions out
      (2) The pump carries in approximately two potassium ions for every three sodium ions carried out, causing a relative excess of positively charged ions on the exterior of the membrane
2. DEPOLARIZATION is the electrical state during which a nerve fiber's resting membrane potential moves toward zero
   a. Stimulation causes a change in membrane permeability in the stimulated area; positively charged sodium ions flow into the nerve fiber, enhancing depolarization
   b. Any stimulus strong enough to depolarize the membrane and initiate a nerve impulse will cause the depolarization wave, or impulse, to travel along the nerve fiber
   c. The membrane potential changes to zero and then reverses, with the interior of the nerve fiber having a positive charge relative to the exterior; this rapid change is called an *action potential*
      (1) The reversed polarity causes the membrane permeability to change again
         (a) Sodium ions are prevented from entering, while potassium ions are allowed to exit
         (b) This quickly returns the nerve fiber to its original polarity, with the interior being relatively negative in relation to the outside
      (2) Before the original polarization returns, however, the voltage difference between the area of reversed polarity and the adjacent polarized area of the membrane causes a current flow
         (a) This current flow depolarizes the adjacent area of the membrane; the action potential occurs there, causing a current flow to the next polarized area
         (b) The process continues along the entire length of the membrane, causing a depolarization wave that travels along the nerve fiber

(c) As the nerve impulse travels in a depolarization wave, the previously depolarized area becomes repolarized and its resting membrane potential is restored

d. In an unmyelinated nerve fiber, the impulse progresses without interruption along the entire length of the nerve fiber

e. In a myelinated nerve fiber, impulse conduction is similar, but is influenced by the myelin sheath

(1) The wave of depolarization "jumps" between the gaps in the myelin sheaths, bypassing the myelin-covered segments of the nerve fiber between the nodes of Ranvier

(2) This transmission process, called SALTATORY CONDUCTION ("jumping"), is much more rapid than the progressive depolarization wave that moves along an unmyelinated nerve fiber

f. Nerve impulse transmission is followed by a brief interval, called the REFRACTORY PERIOD, when the nerve fiber is unresponsive and cannot transmit another impulse until its membrane is repolarized

C. Transmission across synapses

1. Nerve impulses are transmitted across synapses from neuron to neuron by chemicals that stimulate neurons
2. Neurons are organized in chains but are not in direct contact with each other
   a. Small gaps called synapses separate the neurons
   b. At the synapse, the axon terminal of the presynaptic neuron (the one transmitting the impulse) is close to the cell body or dendrite of the postsynaptic neuron (the next neuron in the chain) or to the muscle or organ it innervates
3. When the nerve impulse reaches the presynaptic axon terminal, it stimulates vesicles there to release a neurotransmitter
   a. The neurotransmitter diffuses across the synapse and binds to receptors on the membrane of the postsynaptic neuron; this changes the permeability of the postsynaptic neuron, which initiates membrane depolarization and impulse transmission
   b. The neurotransmitter released from the axon terminals is inactivated rapidly by various mechanisms to prevent a sustained response
4. Each type of neuron releases its own specific type of neurotransmitter
5. Because neurotransmitters are released only from axon terminals, transmission across a synapse is only possible from an axon to a dendrite, to the cell body of the next neuron, or to a muscle or other effect or organ
6. Some neurons release *inhibitory neurotransmitters,* which inhibit — rather than stimulate — impulse transmission

a. An inhibitory neurotransmitter causes the membrane of the postsynaptic neuron to become more permeable to potassium and chloride (Cl^-) ions, without affecting the permeability to sodium
b. Potassium ions diffuse out and chloride ions diffuse in, increasing the negative charge of the postsynaptic neuron membrane
c. Then the membrane depolarizes less readily, which inhibits impulse transmission

D. CNS neurotransmitters

1. Neurotransmitters are essential for neurotransmission in the CNS; other substances also may be involved
   a. *Neuropeptides* are molecules composed of short chains of amino acids that usually appear in the axon terminals at synapses; they modify or regulate neurotransmitter activity
   b. Other substances, such as the amino acids glycine and glutamic and aspartic acids, may play a role in neurotransmission
2. All neurotransmitters, neuropeptides, and related substances must be inactivated after they are released to limit their duration of activity
3. The chief neurotransmitters in the CNS are acetylcholine, norepinephrine, dopamine, serotonin, and gamma-aminobutyric acid (GABA)
   a. *Acetylcholine* is stored in the synaptic vesicles of certain neurons, called *cholinergic neurons;* cholinergic neurons include all preganglionic neurons of the sympathetic and parasympathetic nervous systems, all postganglionic parasympathetic neurons, and postganglionic neurons that innervate sweat glands and some blood vessels
      (1) Acetylcholine is released in response to nerve stimulation and activates postganglionic neurons
      (2) It is inactivated rapidly by the enzyme cholinesterase, which breaks it down into acetate and choline
         (a) Some acetate diffuses away and is used by cells for energy
         (b) Axon terminals take up the choline, which then combines with acetate to form more acetylcholine
         (c) This acetylcholine is stored in synaptic vesicles for later release in response to further nerve stimulation
   b. *Norepinephrine* is stored in the synaptic vesicles of *adrenergic neurons,* which include most postganglionic neurons of the sympathetic nervous system
      (1) Norepinephrine is one of a group of neurotransmitters collectively called *catecholamines*
      (2) It is released from the axon terminals of most postganglionic neurons
      (3) Norepinephrine is inactivated in two ways

(a) Some is taken back into the synaptic vesicles in the axon terminals (REUPTAKE)

(b) Some is inactivated by the enzymes catechol O-methyltransferase (COMT) and monoamine oxidase (MAO)

c. Dopamine is a precursor of norepinephrine and also is a catecholamine

(1) This neurotransmitter stimulates postsynaptic neurons after being released from axon terminals

(2) It is inactivated in the same two ways as norepinephrine

d. *Serotonin* is a derivative of the amino acid tryptophane

(1) It is stored in the synaptic vesicles of axon terminals

(2) Serotonin is released in response to nerve stimulation and stimulates postsynaptic neurons

(3) It is inactivated by reuptake and by enzymatic (MAO) breakdown

e. *GABA* is an inhibitory neurotransmitter produced from glutamic acid, an amino acid; it is inactivated by enzymatic breakdown

4. Neuropeptides are closely related to neurotransmitters; they are chains of amino acids (peptides) that regulate or modulate the actions of neurotransmitters

a. A neuropeptide called *substance P*, found in sensory nerves and in the spinal cord, facilitates the transmission of pain sensations to the brain

b. Other neuropeptides, such as enkephalins, endorphins, and dynorphins, inhibit the perception of pain impulses transmitted to the brain

E. ANS neurotransmitters

1. *Acetylcholine* is a key neurotransmitter in the ANS

a. It is released from the axons of preganglionic neurons connected with the ANS, including all preganglionic neurons, postganglionic parasympathetic neurons, and postganglionic sympathetic neurons that innervate sweat glands and cause vasodilation in certain blood vessels in skeletal muscle (sympathetic vasodilator nerves)

b. Acetylcholine stimulates postganglionic neurons, which in turn release acetylcholine or the neurotransmitter norepinephrine from their axons

c. As a postganglionic neurotransmitter, it also activates effector organs

d. Acetylcholine is broken down rapidly by cholinesterase to prevent a sustained response (for details, see Section VI, D in this chapter)

2. *Norepinephrine* also is a key neurotransmitter in the ANS; it is related to epinephrine, which is produced by the adrenal medulla

a. Most postganglionic sympathetic neurons release norepinephrine

b. After norepinephrine is released from nerve endings, some is inactivated by reuptake into axons and some by the action of COMT and MAO

c. Because norepinephrine inactivation does not occur as rapidly as acetylcholine inactivation, the effects of sympathetic stimulation persist longer than those produced by parasympathetic stimulation

d. Sympathetic stimulation also triggers release of epinephrine and norepinephrine from the adrenal medulla, which augments the effects of the norepinephrine produced by postganglionic sympathetic neurons

3. Neurotransmitter receptors exist in effector organs

a. Acetylcholine released from postganglionic autonomic nerve endings produces its effect by combining with specific receptors on effector organs called *cholinergic receptors*

b. When released from the postganglionic sympathetic neurons, norepinephrine produces its effects by combining with specific receptors on effector organs called adrenergic receptors

(1) Adrenergic receptors are divided into *alpha* and *beta receptors*

(a) Alpha receptors contain two subgroups, $alpha_1$ and $alpha_2$

(b) Beta receptors contain two subgroups, $beta_1$ and $beta_2$

(2) Most effector organs contain alpha or beta receptors; some contain both

(a) Organs that contain beta receptors commonly contain $beta_1$ and $beta_2$ receptors, but usually one type predominates

(b) Blood vessel walls contain $alpha_1$ receptors, which cause vasoconstriction and tend to dominate over the counterbalancing effects of $alpha_2$ receptors, which are located primarily in terminals of postganglionic sympathetic neurons

(3) Usually, norepinephrine stimulates alpha adrenergic receptors

(4) Epinephrine stimulates $alpha_1$, $alpha_2$, $beta_1$, and $beta_2$ receptors

(5) Alpha and beta receptors respond differently to adrenergic stimulation

(a) Stimulation of $alpha_1$ receptors produces contraction (vasoconstriction) of smooth-muscle walls of blood vessels

(b) Stimulation of $alpha_2$ receptors produces the opposite effect by inhibiting norepinephrine release from sympathetic nerve endings

(c) Stimulation of $beta_1$ receptors, which predominate in cardiac muscle, causes the heart to beat faster and more forcefully

(d) Stimulation of $beta_2$ receptors, which predominate in the smooth muscle of bronchial walls and blood vessels, dilates bronchi and relaxes blood vessels

♦ VII. Control centers

A. General information

1. The control centers for most nervous system functions are located in the brain
2. In the brain, the cerebrum, cerebellum, diencephalon, and brain stem control specialized groups of functions
3. The spinal cord is primarily a reflex response center; it is modulated by the brain
4. Most simple REFLEXES result from neurotransmission through the REFLEX ARC a three-neuron chain composed of sensory, connecting, and motor neurons

B. Cerebrum

1. The cerebrum, which controls all advanced mental activities, is divided into two hemispheres
   a. The two cerebral hemispheres are divided into the frontal, varietal, temporal, and occipital lobes by large fissures
   b. The hemispheres are joined by a connecting bridge of nerve fibers, the corpus callosum
2. The *cerebral cortex,* which covers the surface of each hemisphere, is composed of gray matter that contains the cell bodies of neurons and white matter that contains their myelinated nerve fibers
3. Masses of gray matter called *basal ganglia* are located deep within each cerebral hemisphere; basal ganglia form part of the *extrapyramidal system,* which controls the coordination of muscle groups that function together to perform voluntary motion
4. The *internal capsule* is white matter, consisting of bundles of nerve fibers, that passes through the basal ganglia carrying sensory and motor impulses to and from the cerebral cortex
5. Certain parts of the cortex, called FUNCTIONAL AREAS, are related to specialized functions; however, their functions are not sharply separated because of the extensive interconnections between the areas
6. The motor area controls voluntary motor activity
   a. The area contains neurons that control specific body parts
      (1) Neurons in the upper part of the motor area control muscles in the lower part of the body
      (2) Neurons in the lower part of the area control muscles in the head, neck, and upper part of the body
   b. The number of neurons supplying a muscle depends on the type of movement it performs

(1) Muscles capable of fine movements, such as finger muscles, have large areas of cortical representation
(2) Muscles capable only of relatively gross movements, such as large limb and back muscles, are represented with smaller areas

7. The sensory area receives sensory impulses
   a. The upper part of the sensory cortex receives impulses from the lower part of the body
   b. The lower part of the sensory cortex receives impulses from the upper part of the body
8. Each cerebral hemisphere receives sensory impulses from, or supplies motor impulses to, the opposite side of the body because almost all the *fiber tracts* (bundles of nerve fibers carrying impulses) cross to the opposite side of the brain, brain stem, or spinal cord as they ascend (or descend) the CNS
9. Cortical areas associated with vision are located in the occipital lobe; those associated with hearing are located in the temporal lobes
10. Motor areas related to speech are located in the frontal lobes; cortical areas related to olfactory sensations are on the undersurface of the temporal lobes
11. Other cortical areas surrounding the primary areas are called *association areas;* although they are concerned with the same types of functions as the primary areas, they are more involved with interpretation, learning, and memory
12. The frontal areas primarily involve personality and judgment

C. Cerebellum
1. The cerebellum receives sensory impulses from muscles, joints, and tendons that convey a sense of position; it also receives impulses from the inner ear that involve balance and equilibrium
2. Cerebellar motor impulses regulate muscle groups that coordinate position and balance
3. The cerebellum is connected to the brain stem by bundles of fibers called the *cerebellar peduncles*
   a. Cerebellar peduncles transmit nerve impulses to the spinal cord, medulla, and brain
   b. The peduncles transmit impulses from the cerebellum to the thalamus for eventual transmission to the cortex

D. Diencephalon and brain stem
1. The diencephalon connects to the top of the brain stem and contains the slitlike third ventricle
   a. The thalamus, which forms the lateral walls of the third ventricle, contains relay stations that receive sensory impulses and transmit them to the cortex

b. The hypothalamus contains neurons that control hormone output from the endocrine glands and regulate the activity of the ANS; these neurons are responsible for such basic body functions as temperature regulation, food and water intake, and sexual behavior

2. The brain stem is divided into the midbrain, pons, and medulla
   a. The midbrain contains cell bodies of cranial nerves and large nerve fiber bundles that convey impulses to and from the cerebral hemispheres
   b. The pons is a transverse bridge of fibers connecting the brain stem with the cerebellum; the pons also contains fiber tracts extending to and from the cerebral hemispheres, neurons of several of the cranial nerves, and neurons involved with spontaneous respiratory movements
   c. The medulla is the lowest part of the brain stem; it forms the floor of the fourth ventricle, which is partially covered by the cerebellum
      (1) The medulla contains nerve cell bodies of cranial nerves and nerve fiber bundles, which relay impulses to higher and lower levels in the nervous system
      (2) The medulla also serves as an autonomic reflex center to maintain homeostasis; it contains the cardiac center (which adjusts the force and rate of myocardial contractions), respiratory center (which regulates breathing depth and rate), and vasomotor center (which regulates blood pressure)

E. Spinal cord
1. The major reflex center in the CNS, the spinal cord mediates most reflexes
2. *Reflexes* are automatic actions, such as a knee jerk elicited by tapping the patellar tendon

ALERT

   a. Hyperactive reflexes may result from a disease or injury of certain descending motor tracts
   b. Hypoactive reflexes may indicate degeneration or damage of the sensory or motor nerves
3. Three common types of somatic (skeletal muscle) reflexes are the *stretch reflex* (involving two neurons and one synapse), the *flexor reflex* (involving sensory, motor, and connecting neurons and more than one synapse), and the *crossed-extensor reflex* (involving the flexor reflex and a contralateral reflex arc)
4. Most simple reflexes result from nerve impulse transmission through a three-neuron chain between sensory, connecting, and motor neurons; these neurons form the reflex arc (see *The reflex arc,* page 122)
   a. The sensory (afferent) neuron carries the impulse into the spinal cord through the dorsal root to the connecting neuron in the posterior horn of the spinal cord gray matter

The reflex arc

A simple reflex arc requires a sensory (afferent) neuron and a motor (efferent) neuron as well as a connecting neuron in the spinal cord.

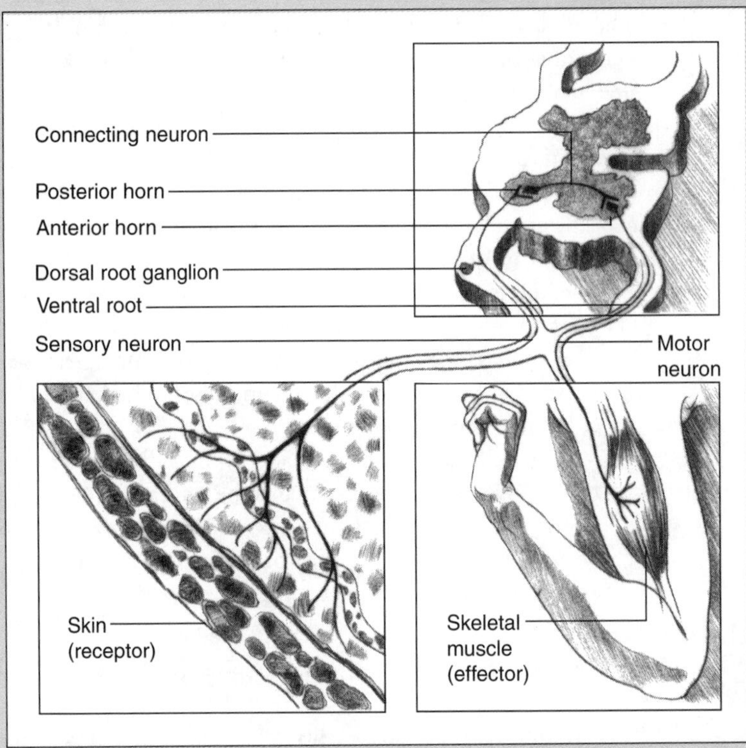

b. The connecting neuron relays the impulse to a motor neuron in the anterior horn of the gray matter
c. The motor neuron sends out a motor (efferent) impulse via an axon in the ventral root of the spinal cord; this impulse causes muscle contraction
d. Although a reflex arc is described in terms of a three-neuron chain, large numbers of sensory, connecting, and motor neurons are involved
e. In many reflexes, impulses initiated by sensory neurons also are relayed up and down the spinal cord by connecting neurons, causing a coordinated response from many different groups of motor neurons

5. Different types of reflexes may occur
   a. The person may be aware of the reflex response because the stimulus that initiated the reflex and the perception of the response are conveyed to the cortex; for example, the patellar reflex is automatic but also is perceptible
   b. Some reflexes, such as those that regulate heart rate and blood pressure, function automatically; the person is not aware of the reflex control of these physiologic functions
   c. Some reflexes can be inhibited or modified by conscious effort, such as control of urination and defecation reflexes
   d. Some reflexes, called CONDITIONED REFLEXES or *conditioned responses,* can be learned as a result of past associations, such as salivation induced by the sight or smell of specific foods

POINTS TO REMEMBER

- The nervous system allows communication among different parts of the body and between the body and the external environment
- The nervous system is divided into the CNS and PNS. It has a sensory (afferent) division, which conveys impulses from the periphery to the CNS, and a motor (efferent) division, which conveys impulses from the CNS to the periphery.
- Of the nervous system cells, neurons conduct impulses; neuroglia (supporting cells) do not.
- Synapses are one-way junctions across which electrical or chemical impulses are transferred from one neuron to another.
- The CNS consists of the brain and spinal cord. The PNS includes 12 pairs of cranial nerves, 31 pairs of spinal nerves, and two major divisions (the autonomic and somatic nervous systems).
- Through neurotransmission, impulses are conducted throughout the nervous system by neurons.
- CNS neurotransmitters include acetylcholine, norepinephrine, dopamine, serotonin, and GABA. ANS neurotransmitters include acetylcholine and norepinephrine.
- The brain is the control center for most nervous system functions. The spinal cord primarily controls reflex responses.

STUDY QUESTIONS

To evaluate your understanding of this chapter, answer the following questions in the space provided. Then compare your responses with the correct answers in Appendix B, page 330.

1. Which body system works with the nervous system to maintain homeostasis?

2. What are the two major components of the CNS?

3. How are neurons different from neuroglia?

4. What are the major regions of the brain?

5. What do the autonomic and somatic nervous systems have in common?

6. What are the main components of a simple reflex arc?

CRITICAL THINKING AND APPLICATION EXERCISES

1. On a model of the CNS, identify areas that contain gray matter and areas that contain white matter.
2. Make a diagram of CSF movement through the CNS.
3. Using a dermatome chart, test various areas for sensation and note which nerves supply these areas.

CHAPTER

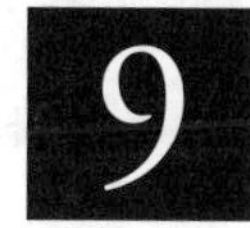

Sensory System

Learning objectives

After studying this chapter, you should be able to:

- Describe the major structures and functions of the eye.
- Trace the path of a retinal image from the retina through the visual pathways to the brain.
- Explain how the eyes adapt for near vision.
- Define binocular vision and explain how it contributes to depth perception.
- Describe the major structures of the external ear, middle ear, and inner ear.
- Discuss how sound wave transmission to the inner ear produces sound.
- Explain how vestibular structures maintain equilibrium.
- Compare the perceptions of taste and smell.
- Locate general sense receptors and explain how they produce sensations of touch, pressure, temperature, and pain.
- Contrast the three types of pain.

CHAPTER OVERVIEW

Through the sensory system, the body perceives — and reacts to — its environment. This system provides the senses of sight, sound, balance, smell, taste, touch, pressure, temperature, and pain. Without these protective senses, the body would be constantly in danger. Therefore, to maximize patients' health, the health care professional must understand the structures and functions of the sensory system.

♦ I. Sensory system divisions

A. General information
   1. The sensory system may be divided into the special senses — vision, hearing, equilibrium, smell, and taste — and the general senses — touch, pressure, temperature, and pain
   2. The special senses are so called because their receptors are found in complex organs in a relatively small area of the body
   3. The general senses are so called because their receptors are found throughout the body
   4. When stimulated, receptors generate nerve impulses, which are carried to the central nervous system (CNS) by sensory neurons; the brain then processes this information and makes a suitable response

B. Special senses
   1. The senses of vision, hearing, smell, and taste are considered special senses because their receptors are located in complex organs in a relatively small area of the body
      a. Vision receptors exist in the retina of the eye
      b. Hearing receptors exist in the inner ear
      c. Smell receptors exist in the upper nose
      d. Taste receptors exist in the tongue
      e. Receptors for equilibrium exist in the ear
   2. Equilibrium is considered a special sense because it is maintained by the sensory organ of hearing

C. General senses
   1. The general senses include touch, pressure, temperature, and pain
   2. Receptors for these senses are distributed widely in the skin and other body tissues
      a. Because the number of receptors for each sense varies greatly, not all parts of the body are equally sensitive

b. The fingertips and tip of the tongue, for example, are much more sensitive than the back of the neck

♦ II. Eyes and vision

A. General information
1. The eye is a complex structure composed of three layers of tissue — the cornea and sclera, a middle choroid coat, and an inner retina — and a lens
2. The space between the cornea and lens is divided by the iris into the anterior and posterior chambers
3. The eyes, the sensory organs for vision, collect light waves and transmit them as nerve impulses along the visual pathways to the brain, which translates them into images
4. The eyes normally form a clear retinal image of an object 20′ (6.1 m) away; they must make several changes to adapt for near vision
5. BINOCULAR VISION contributes to depth perception (ability to judge relative distances of objects)

B. Structures
1. The organ of vision, the eye is a spherical structure that measures about 1" (2.5 cm) in diameter; it contains 70% of the body's sensory receptors
2. Accessory structures of the eye include the eyebrows, eyelids, conjunctiva, lacrimal glands, and eye muscles (superior, inferior, lateral, and medial rectus muscles and superior and inferior oblique muscles)
   a. The conjunctiva is the thin vascular membrane that lines the inner surface of the eyelids and sclera; it is attached to the sclerocorneal junction but does not extend over the cornea
   b. Lacrimal glands discharge fluid secretions to moisten the conjunctiva; the fluid collects in the lacrimal ducts, which have openings on the ridges of the eyelids near the nose, and is discharged into the nose
   c. The eye muscles are paired and work together to perform eye movement
3. The eye has three layers of tissue and a lens
4. The outermost layer (fibrous tunic) contains the sclera and cornea
   a. The *sclera* represents the bulk of the fibrous tunic
      (1) It is composed of opaque, white, dense connective tissue
      (2) Posteriorly, it is continuous with the dura mater of the brain; anteriorly, it is continuous with the cornea
   b. The *cornea* is a convex, transparent structure that bulges where it joins the sclera

(1) The cornea is covered with an internal layer (endothelium) and an external layer (epithelium) of epithelial tissue
(2) It refracts light (bends light waves)

5. The middle layer (uvea or vascular tunic) has three regions — choroid, ciliary body, and iris
   a. The *choroid* is a highly vascular coat that surrounds most of the eye
      (1) Posteriorly, it stops at the point where the optic nerve exits the eye
      (2) Anteriorly, it is continuous with the ciliary body
   b. The *ciliary body* is a thick ring of smooth muscle that encircles the lens and helps maintain its shape
   c. The *iris* is the most anterior portion of the uvea
      (1) It is the colored portion of the eye
      (2) Shaped like a flat doughnut, it is continuous with the ciliary body
6. The innermost layer (sensory tunic) of the eye is the *retina*
   a. Its outer pigmented layer lies adjacent to the choroid
   b. Its inner neural layer is transparent and contains photoreceptors (rods and cones) that process external images
   c. Nerve fibers from the retina converge to form the optic nerve, which penetrates the posterior surface of the sclera
7. The *lens* is a transparent, encapsulated, biconvex structure
   a. It attaches to the ciliary muscle by suspensory ligaments
   b. Its thickness can be adjusted to focus for near and far vision by contraction or relaxation of the ciliary muscle, which varies the tension on the suspensory ligament
8. The eye also is divided into anterior and posterior cavities
   a. The anterior cavity contains an anterior and a posterior chamber
      (1) The *anterior chamber* is bounded anteriorly by the cornea and posteriorly by the iris and lens
      (2) The *posterior chamber* is bounded by the iris, ciliary body, and lens
      (3) The anterior and posterior chambers contain aqueous humor
         (a) *Aqueous humor* is a clear, watery fluid similar in composition to blood plasma
         (b) It is secreted by the epithelium of the ciliary bodies, diffuses around anterior eye structures, and is absorbed into a drainage system at the periphery of the anterior chamber
   b. The posterior cavity is located dorsal to the lens; it contains a clear gel called the *vitreous humor,* a thick, gelatinous fluid

C. Aqueous humor formation and circulation
1. Aqueous humor is a lymphlike fluid secreted by the ciliary body
2. After the fluid flows into the posterior chamber of the eye, it flows into the anterior chamber by passing through the pupil; it is ab-

sorbed into *Schlemm's canal,* a ring-shaped canal that encircles the eyeball at the sclerocorneal junction

3. The portion of the eyeball between the anterior chamber and Schlemm's canal is porous and contains a network of channels, called the *trabecular meshwork,* that leads to the canal
   a. Aqueous humor flows through the trabecular meshwork into Schlemm's canal
   b. Then the fluid enters the veins that drain blood from the eyeball

ALERT

4. Normally, aqueous humor secretion balances its absorption, and the pressure in the anterior chamber remains relatively constant at about 20 to 25 mm Hg (about one-fifth of systemic arterial pressure); elevated intraocular pressure may lead to vision loss when the pressure is transmitted to the vitreous humor, where it damages retinal neurons

D. Light refraction
1. Light rays that enter a transparent medium at an oblique angle to the surface are refracted as they pass into another medium of different density, such as from air to glass or from air to the eye
2. The degree of REFRACTION depends on the angle of the light rays and the difference in the refractive indices (measures of the density of the media) of the two media through which light rays pass
   a. The more oblique the angle of the light rays, the greater the refraction
   b. The greater the difference in the refractive indices, the greater the refraction; for example, light rays passing from air (with a REFRACTIVE INDEX of 1) to glass (with a refractive index of 1.4) are bent more than rays passing from water (refractive index of 1.33) to glass because the difference between the refractive indices of air and glass is greater
3. The cornea is an efficient refracting medium because its refractive index (1.33) is significantly higher than that of air (1), which the light rays travel through before striking the cornea
4. Light rays also can be refracted by lens curvature; the greater the curvature, the more the rays are refracted
   a. Concave lenses (those curved inward), such as the type used to correct nearsightedness, cause light rays to diverge
   b. Convex lenses (those curved outward), such as the cornea and lens of the eye, cause light rays to converge
5. Parallel rays from an object more than 20′ (6.1 m) away that strike a convex lens come into focus at the FOCAL POINT *(principal focus);* the distance from the lens to its focal point is the FOCAL LENGTH of the lens
6. The converging power of a convex lens is expressed in *diopters,* the reciprocal of the focal length of the lens expressed in meters
   a. A lens with a focal length of 1 m (3.3′) has a strength of 1 diopter

b. A lens with a focal length of 50 cm (½ m) has a strength of 2 diopters because the reciprocal of ½ is 2/1, or 2

7. The refractive power of a concave lens cannot be expressed in focal length because this lens causes light rays to diverge instead of converge at a focal point
   a. Refraction power of a concave lens is determined by its ability to counteract the converging power of a convex lens; its power is expressed by a minus sign
   b. A concave lens that counteracts the converging power of a 0.5-diopter lens has a refractive power of -0.5 diopters

E. Image formation
1. The eye has a refractive power of about 60 diopters
   a. The cornea performs most of the refraction because it is a convex lens and has a high refractive index (1.33)
   b. The lens has much less refractive power than the cornea because it is surrounded by media (aqueous and vitreous humors) that have almost the same refractive index as the cornea
   c. However, the lens can change its focal length and can bring images into sharp focus on the retina through ACCOMMODATION
2. After passing through the cornea, aqueous humor, lens, and in vitreous humor, light waves hit the retina
3. Receptor cells of the retina (rods and cones) contain a photosensitive visual pigment (rhodopsin) that decomposes on light exposure, stimulating an impulse that is conveyed to the brain
   a. Rods are the most numerous photoreceptors
      (1) They are concentrated at the periphery of the retina
      (2) Rods are sensitive to low levels of illumination but cannot discriminate color
   b. Rods do not function in bright light because it decomposes most of their rhodopsin
      (1) This explains why a person cannot see well for a short time after going from bright light into darkness
      (2) After a brief period of darkness, rhodopsin reforms and the rods start functioning again
   c. Cones are less sensitive to light
      (1) They are concentrated in the center of the retina
      (2) Cones provide daylight color vision
   d. Cones come in three types, responding to red, green, or blue light
      (1) Stimulation of various receptor combinations transmits impulses that the brain interprets as color

ALERT

      (2) Color blindness occurs when one or more types of cones are absent or defective

4. Images form in the eye similar to the way they form in an autofocus camera (see *Physiologic process: Image perception and formation,* page 132)
   a. The image on the retina is inverted
   b. The brain reverses the image and perceives the object right side up

F. Visual pathways

1. An image forms on the retina when light stimulates the rods and cones
2. Each half of the retina receives visual input from the opposite visual field
   a. The right half of each retina receives input from the left visual field
   b. The left half of each retina receives input from the right visual field
3. Two optic nerves converge at the base of the brain to form the optic chiasma
   a. The nerve fibers continue behind the chiasma, forming the OPTIC TRACTS
   b. These tracts connect to neurons in the brain stem, which convey visual impulses to the occipital cortex by means of fiber tracts called the optic radiations
4. Nerve fibers from the medial halves of both optic nerves cross in the optic chiasma, and fibers from the lateral halves of the optic nerves continue into the optic tracts without crossing
5. Each half of the retina receives an image of objects from the visual field on the opposite side
   a. The right optic tract contains nerve fibers from the right half of each retina
   b. The left optic tract contains nerve fibers from the left half of each retina

G. Near vision

1. In an eye with normal refractive power, the retina forms a clear image of an object 20′ (6.1 m) away
2. Viewing of objects closer than 20′ from the eye (near vision) requires three automatic changes: accommodation, pupillary constriction, and eye convergence
3. Accommodation (adjustment of the refractory power of the lens) depends on the elasticity of the lens, which is surrounded by a strong capsule attached to suspensory ligaments
   a. When the eye is at rest, suspensory ligaments hold the lens under tension, compressing and flattening it

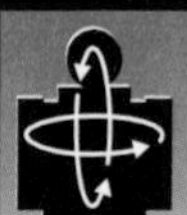

PHYSIOLOGIC PROCESS

Image perception and formation

The structures of the eye perform a series of steps that allow image perception and formation, as described and illustrated below.

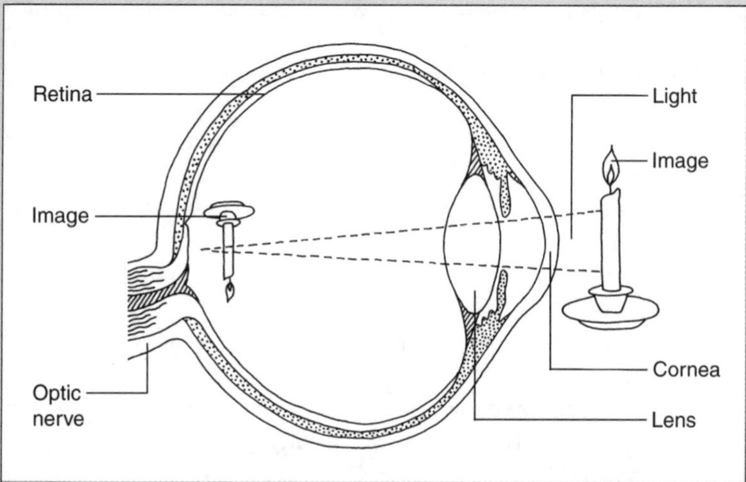

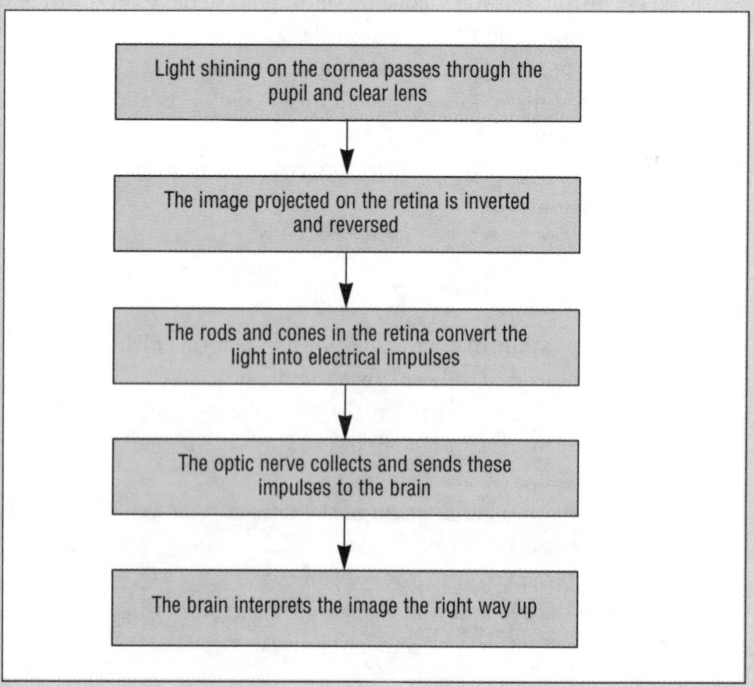

   b. During accommodation, the ciliary muscles contract, pulling the suspensory ligaments forward and relaxing their tension on the lens capsule; this makes the lens bulge and become more convex
   c. Accommodation increases the refractive power of the eye, which is necessary for near vision
4. *Pupillary constriction* blocks light rays that normally pass through the lens periphery; such rays are refracted more than those passing through the center because the refractive index at the periphery (1.36) is slightly different than that at the center (1.42)
   a. Blocking these rays increases the sharpness of the image because all the rays are focused more sharply on the retina
   b. The pupils also constrict in response to bright light to protect the eyes
5. CONVERGENCE allows the individual to see an object close up with both eyes without seeing double because the two images are focused on corresponding points on the two retinas

H. Binocular vision
1. *Binocular vision* (single vision with two eyes) permits depth or distance perception and creates a larger field of vision
2. During convergence, when the image falls at corresponding points on both retinas, each eye views the object from a slightly different angle
3. The two slightly different images are relayed to the brain, where they are synthesized (fused) into a single image, which conveys an impression of depth that the separate retinal images lack

♦ III. Ears and hearing

A. General information
1. The ears, the sensory organs for hearing, gather sound waves and transmit them as nerve impulses to the brain; the brain interprets these impulses as hearing
2. The auditory apparatus consists of the external ear, middle ear, and inner ear
   a. The external ear collects sound
   b. The middle ear conducts sound
   c. The inner ear contains structures that transmit sound waves and maintain equilibrium

B. Structures
1. The ear contains various structures involved in hearing and maintaining equilibrium
2. It includes the external (outer) ear, middle ear, and inner ear
3. The *external ear* consists of the auricle (pinna) and the external auditory canal

a. The *auricle* is composed of elastic cartilage covered by thin skin; its outer rim is called the *helix*
b. The *external auditory canal,* a narrow chamber about 1″ (2.5 cm) long, connects the auricle with the tympanic membrane
   (1) The outer portion of the canal is framed by elastic cartilage; the inner portion lies within the temporal bone
   (2) The skin that lines the external auditory canal contains ceruminous glands; these modified apocrine sweat glands secrete a brown earwax called cerumen

4. The *middle ear,* or tympanic cavity, is a mucosa-lined structure within the petrous (hard) portion of the temporal bone
   a. It is bounded distally by the ear drum (tympanic membrane) and medially by the oval and round windows
      (1) The *oval window* is a small opening in the wall between the middle and inner ears into which the footpiece of the stapes fits; it transmits vibrations to the inner ear
      (2) The *round window,* also an opening in the wall between the middle and inner ears, is enclosed by a membrane called the secondary tympanic membrane; like the oval window, it transmits vibrations to the inner ear
   b. The middle ear joins with the nasopharynx via the eustachian tube
   c. The middle ear contains three small ossicles (bones) called the *malleus* (hammer), *incus* (anvil), and *stapes* (stirrup)
      (1) The malleus attaches to the tympanic membrane
      (2) The stapes attaches to the oval window
      (3) The incus, located between the malleus and stapes, articulates with these structures during transmission of vibratory motion from the ear drum to the fluid of the inner ear; the vibration excites receptor nerve endings in the inner ear
      (4) Two small muscles attached to the ossicles contract automatically in response to loud noises
         (a) This contraction dampens ossicle vibrations, which normally are transmitted to the inner ear
         (b) It protects inner ear structures from damage

5. The inner ear, or osseous (bony) labyrinth, is located in the temporal bone; it consists of the vestibule, semicircular canals, and cochlea
   a. The *vestibule* is the central portion; it serves as the entrance to the inner ear and houses the saccule and utricle
      (1) It is posterior to the cochlea and anterior to the semicircular canals
      (2) Laterally, it contains the oval and round windows
      (3) The *saccule* and *utricle* are membranous sacs suspended in a fluid called perilymph (which is similar to cerebrospinal flu-

id); they sense gravity changes and linear and angular acceleration

b. The three *semicircular canals* project from the posterior aspect of the vestibule
   (1) Each canal is oriented in one of three planes — superior, posterior, or lateral (horizontal)
   (2) The semicircular duct, which traverses the canals, is continuous with the utricle anteriorly
   (3) The crista ampullaris, located at the end of each canal, contains hair cells and supporting cells; it is stimulated by sudden movements or changes in the rate or direction of movement

c. The *cochlea* is a spiraling, bony cone that extends from the anterior part of the vestibule
   (1) The cochlear duct, located inside the cochlea, is a triangular, membranous structure that houses the *organ of Corti;* this organ contains auditory receptor cells (hair cells), supporting cells, and nerve fibers
      (a) Receptor cells are embedded in the basilar membrane of the cochlear duct; their free surfaces project into the endolymph of the duct
      (b) A gelatinous membrane called the *tectorial membrane* overhangs and touches these hair cells
      (c) Stimulation of these cells causes sound wave transmission
   (2) The cochlear cavity has three chambers — the *scala vestibuli* and *scala tympani* (which are continuous with each other at the apex and contain perilymph) and the *scala media* (which contains endolymph, a substance similar to intracellular fluid)

C. Sound wave transmission

1. Hearing requires sound wave reception and conduction to the organ of Corti, where the waves are converted into nerve impulses; then the nerve impulses are transmitted to the auditory area in the cerebral cortex
2. Sound waves may arise from any vibration source, such as the vocal cords or a musical instrument
3. Sound waves differ in pitch, which reflects the number of cycles (vibrations) per second (CPS); the higher the pitch, the greater the number of CPS
   a. The human ear can detect tones as low as 30 CPS and as high as 20,000 CPS
   b. It is most sensitive to sounds that range from 500 to 4,000 CPS
4. Sound waves may be transmitted to the inner ear by vibrations of the tympanic membrane and ossicles (AIR CONDUCTION) or by vibra-

tions of the skull, which bypass the tympanic membrane and ossicles (BONE CONDUCTION)

5. In air conduction, the external ear funnels sound waves into the ear canal, where they strike the tympanic membrane, causing it to vibrate
   a. These vibrations are transmitted through the middle ear to the oval window, which is covered by the foot plate of the stapes
   b. Because the surface area of the tympanic membrane is 20 times greater than that of the oval window, sound waves are concentrated and amplified at the foot plate
   c. Foot plate vibrations are transmitted to the perilymph of the vestibular canal and then into the perilymph of the tympanic canal
   d. Each inward movement of the oval window causes a corresponding outward movement of the round window at the base of the tympanic canal, causing waves in the perilymph
   e. Perilymph vibrations in the vestibular and tympanic canals set up corresponding vibrations in the basilar membrane of the cochlea duct
      (1) Basilar membrane vibrations cause the processes of the hair cells in contact with the tectorial membrane to bend, which stimulates these cells; the cells stimulate neurons that synapse on the hair cells
      (2) Sounds of different frequencies cause vibrations in different parts of the basilar membrane, which stimulate hair cells in different parts of the organ of Corti
   f. The cochlear branch of the vestibulocochlear nerve (cranial nerve VIII) collects nerve impulses initiated by stimulated hair cells and transmits them to the brain
6. In bone conduction, the sound waves pass through the bones of the skull and cause perilymph and basilar membrane vibrations, which activate the hair cells in the same way that they are activated in air conduction

ALERT

7. Weber's test and the Rinne test evaluate sound conduction; both tests are performed with a tuning fork
   a. During Weber's test, a patient with conductive hearing loss (loss due to interference with external or middle ear structures) hears sound on the affected side by bone conduction; a patient with sensorineural hearing loss (loss due to damage to inner ear structures, cranial nerve VIII, or temporal lobe) hears sound on the unaffected side
   b. During the Rinne test, a patient with conductive hearing loss hears sound longer through bone conduction than air conduction; one with sensorineural hearing loss hears sound longer through air conduction than bone conduction, but in an abnormal ratio

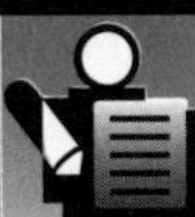

TEACHING TIPS

Patient with a hearing loss

Be sure to include the following topics when teaching a patient with a hearing loss.

- Sound and hearing loss measurement
- Type and possible cause of hearing loss (conductive, sensorineural, or mixed)
- Common ototoxic substances and their effect on hearing
- Weber's, Rinne, and other diagnostic tests
- Cerumen removal from ears
- Hearing aid use
- Surgical options, such as stapedectomy and cochlear implant
- Hearing loss prevention, including use of hearing protectors
- Tips to help family members communicate with hearing-impaired patient
- Sources of information and support

c. Patients with either type of hearing loss require education (for teaching tips, see *Patient with a hearing loss*)

D. Sound perception and localization
1. The auditory center in the cerebral cortex interprets the pitch of a sound based on the part of the organ of Corti that is stimulated by vibrations
2. Differences in loudness result from variations in hair cell stimulation; loud sounds stimulate more hair cells, which generate more impulses than soft sounds
3. The brain interprets the direction of sound based on slight differences in the arrival time and intensity of the sound in each ear

E. Maintenance of equilibrium
1. The sense of EQUILIBRIUM, or balance, is vital for maintaining stability during movement or at rest
2. The vestibular apparatus of the inner ear controls the sense of equilibrium and position
3. The vestibular apparatus consists of the membranous semicircular canals, which respond to motion, and the utricle and the saccule, which respond to position changes
4. The three tubes of the semicircular canals are connected to the utricle; each tube lies at right angles to the other two
   a. One end of each semicircular canal expands slightly where it joins the utricle and contains groups of specialized receptors called *hair cells* as well as supporting cells
      (1) These hair cells are similar to those in the organ of Corti
      (2) They are covered by gelatinous material called *cupula*

(3) They are stimulated by endolymph movement in the semicircular canals during body movement

b. These hair cells transmit nerve impulses over the vestibular branch of the vestibulocochlear nerve to the medulla, where they are interpreted as motion; impulses also are relayed to the cerebellum, where they initiate reflex movements of body muscles and eye muscles

3. The utricle and saccule convey a sense of head position to the brain by sending impulses to the cerebellum through the vestibulocochlear nerve
   a. The utricle and saccule are filled with endolymph and contain hair cells; the free ends of the hair cells are embedded in a mass of gelatinous material, which contains calcium carbonate crystals called otoliths
   b. Gravity presses on the otoliths and the cilia of the hair cells, stimulating nerve impulses that the brain interprets as the normal head position
   c. During head movement, the weight of the otoliths shifts and the cilia bend, transmitting nerve impulses that are perceived by the brain as a change in head position
   d. The impulses also initiate automatic reflex reactions that restore the head to its normal position

ALERT

4. Loss of equilibrium may result from a nervous system disorder, such as acoustic neuroma or multiple sclerosis, or an ear disorder, such as labyrinthitis or Ménière's disease

♦ IV. Nose and smell

A. General information
   1. Olfactory receptors are specialized neurons with dendrites that are modified to respond to odors
   2. These receptors are located in the roof of the nasal cavity; they relay impulses to the olfactory bulbs in the cranial cavity, which transmit impulses to cortical neurons where odor is perceived

B. Structures
   1. The nose contains olfactory (smell) receptors
      a. Olfactory receptors are located in the mucosal epithelium that lines the upper part of the nasal cavity
      b. Pain receptors also are located in the nasal cavity; because they respond to chemicals (such as ammonia), they sometimes are confused with olfactory receptors
   2. Olfactory receptors are bipolar neurons
      a. Each olfactory receptor has a dendrite that terminates in several long cilia called olfactory hairs

b. Olfactory hairs convey mucus, secreted by the mucosa, back to the nasopharynx
3. Olfactory receptors have a life span of 60 days

C. Sensation of smell

ALERT

1. Air must pass through the nose to stimulate the olfactory receptors
2. A person cannot smell if the nostrils are blocked by mucus, polyps, or other substances, because no air can enter the nose to stimulate the olfactory receptors
3. Olfactory receptors are sensitive to very low concentrations of odors, but they rapidly adapt to odors
   a. After smelling an odor for a short time, the individual no longer perceives it as intensely
   b. This loss of odor sensitivity results from reduced responsiveness of the olfactory receptors and diminished perception of the odor in the olfactory portion of the cerebral cortex
   c. However, the cerebral cortex stores memories of odors; after smelling an odor once, an individual can recognize it readily if smelled again

♦ V. Taste buds and taste

A. General information

1. Taste receptors are located in the taste buds in the mouth
2. Taste buds are oval bodies that contain three types of epithelial cells — supporting cells, taste receptor cells, and basal cells
3. Cranial nerves VII (facial), IX (glossopharyngeal), and X (vagus) conduct taste sensations to the brain, which perceives taste

B. Structures

1. Taste receptors are concentrated in the tongue, but also exist in the soft palate and throat
2. Four types of taste receptors exist; each type can sense one of four basic tastes: sweet, sour, bitter, and salt
   a. Sweet tastes are perceived on the tip of the tongue
   b. Sour tastes are perceived along the sides of the tongue
   c. Bitter tastes are perceived on the back of the tongue
   d. Salty tastes are perceived on the tip and sides of the tongue

C. Taste sensation

1. For taste to occur, substances must be in solution in saliva
2. Taste perception results from taste bud stimulation as well as olfactory receptor stimulation from air passage through the nose

ALERT

3. Smell, texture, and temperature contribute to the perception of taste
4. If the sense of smell is not functioning properly (for example, if the nose is congested from a cold), the taste perception may be diminished or unusual

♦ VI. General senses

A. General information
   1. The general senses include touch, pressure, temperature, and PAIN
   2. Receptors for these senses are distributed widely throughout the skin and other body tissues
   3. Because the number of receptors for each general sense varies widely, body parts are not equally sensitive to stimulation

B. Touch and pressure
   1. Receptors for these sensations lie in nerve endings around hair follicles and in the papillary layer of the skin
   2. When stimulated, these receptors transmit a nerve impulse that is carried by a cranial nerve to the brain or by a spinal nerve to the spinal cord and then to the brain
   3. In the brain, the general sensory area located behind the central fissure interprets these impulses as touch or pressure

C. Temperature
   1. Cold receptors lie near the surface of the skin
   2. Heat receptors lie deep in the skin
   3. When stimulated, these receptors transmit a nerve impulse via the same transmission route as that of touch and pressure receptors
   4. These impulses are perceived and interpreted in a similar manner to impulses stimulated by touch and pressure

D. Pain
   1. Pain receptors are located throughout the body in the skin, muscles, tendons, and joints

ALERT

   2. Pain serves a protective function by alerting the individual to withdraw from a harmful stimulus; loss of the ability to feel pain makes the individual vulnerable to injury
   3. Pain impulses are transmitted by myelinated and unmyelinated nerve fibers via the same transmission route as the other general senses
      a. Impulses conducted rapidly by myelinated fibers are perceived as sharp pain
      b. Impulses conducted more slowly by unmyelinated fibers are perceived as dull, aching pain

ALERT

   4. Different types of pain result from stimulation of different areas
      a. Pain in the skin, subcutaneous tissues, muscles, bones, and joints is called *somatic pain*
      b. Pain in the internal organs (from distention, smooth-muscle spasm, or inadequate blood supply) is called *visceral pain*
      c. Internal organ pain that seems to come from the body surface at a distant site is called REFERRED PAIN; for example, the pain of a myocardial infarction may be felt in the neck

(1) Referred pain results because pain impulses from receptors in an internal organ enter the same part of the spinal cord as impulses from somatic pain receptors on the body's surface
(2) The pain impulses are conveyed along pain pathways in the spinal cord to the brain
(3) The brain misinterprets these sensations as coming from the pain receptors on the body surface rather than from those in the internal organ

POINTS TO REMEMBER

- The sensory system includes the special senses (vision, hearing, equilibrium, smell, and taste) and the general senses (touch, pressure, temperature, and pain).
- The eyes are complex, sensory organs for vision. They collect light waves and transmit them as nerve impulses along the visual pathways to the brain, which translates them into images.
- The ears, which are the sensory organs for hearing, are composed of an external, middle, and inner ear. The ears gather sound waves and transmit them as nerve impulses to the brain; the brain interprets these impulses as hearing.
- The nose contains olfactory receptors, which convey impulses that the brain interprets as specific smells.
- The mouth contains taste receptors, which conduct taste sensations to the brain via cranial nerves VII, IX, and X.
- Receptors for touch, pressure, and temperature are located primarily in the skin. Pain receptors are found in the skin, subcutaneous tissues, muscles, bones, and joints (somatic pain) and in the internal organs (visceral pain).

STUDY QUESTIONS

To evaluate your understanding of this chapter, answer the following questions in the space provided. Then compare your responses with the correct answers in Appendix B, pages 330 and 331.

1. How are special senses different from general ones? ______________________

____

____

2. What are the major functions of the retina? ______________________

____

____

3. How is near vision different from binocular vision? ______________

____

____

4. What are the functions of the major structures of the ear? _________

____

____

5. What allows the brain to perceive differences in the loudness of sounds?

____

____

6. How are the senses of smell and taste related? _________________

____

____

7. How are pain impulses transmitted? ___________________________

____

____

CRITICAL THINKING AND APPLICATION EXERCISES

1. Diagram the visual pathways from the eye to the brain.
2. Conduct a hearing test on a partner, comparing air conduction and bone conduction.
3. Write a one-page paper describing how the body maintains a sense of equilibrium.
4. Put on a blindfold, pinch your nostrils shut, and see if you can taste a food your partner provides. Then open your nostrils and try again. Characterize the difference in taste perception.

CHAPTER

10

Cardiovascular System

Learning objectives

After studying this chapter, you should be able to:

- List the functions of the cardiovascular system.
- Briefly describe the structures of the heart.
- Characterize the major differences between the superior and inferior chambers of the heart.
- Explain the cause of normal heart sounds and the pulse.
- Identify the tissues that comprise the heart's conduction system.
- Describe the events in the cardiac cycle.
- Compare the three major types of blood vessels.
- Contrast the pulmonary and systemic circulatory systems.
- Define blood pressure and compare its systolic and diastolic components.
- Explain how changes in cardiac output and peripheral resistance can affect blood pressure.
- Explain how Starling's law, baroreceptors, chemoreceptors, and hormones help regulate cardiac output and blood pressure.
- Describe four factors that affect fluid flow between the capillaries and interstitial tissues.

CHAPTER OVERVIEW

In the cardiovascular system, the heart pumps constantly refreshed blood through thousands of miles of blood vessels, delivering nutrients to cells and removing their wastes. To receptorsunderstand this system, the health care professional must be familiar with the structures of the heart and vessels as well as the cardiac cycle, cardiac conduction system, various types of circulation, blood pressure, and cardiac output. This information forms the basis for knowledgeable cardiovascular care.

♦ I. Basic principles

A. Cardiovascular structures
1. This system consists of the heart and blood vessels
2. The heart pumps the blood through the blood vessels
3. Blood vessels include arteries, arterioles, capillaries, venules, and veins

B. Cardiovascular functions
1. The *cardiovascular system* moves blood throughout the body
2. It helps maintain proper body pH and electrolyte composition
3. It also helps regulate body temperature

♦ II. Heart

A. General information
1. The heart is a hollow, fist-sized, muscular organ located slightly to the left of the body's midline in the mediastinum, between the second rib and fifth intercostal space
2. A physiologic pump, the heart moves the body's entire volume of blood to and from the lungs (pulmonary circulation) and to and from the tissues (systemic circulation)
3. The heart actually acts as two separate pumps; the right side acts as a pulmonary pump, the left side as a systemic pump

B. Pericardium
1. The *pericardium* is a fibroserous sac that covers the heart
2. It has two portions
   a. The *fibrous pericardium* is the outer portion
      (1) Composed of tough, white, fibrous tissue, it fits loosely around the heart and is relatively inelastic
      (2) It protects the heart and serous membrane
   b. The *serous pericardium* is the thin, smooth inner portion; it has two layers

(1) The *parietal layer* lines the inside of the fibrous pericardium
(2) The *visceral layer* (epicardium) adheres to the outer surface of the heart

3. The *pericardial space* separates the parietal and visceral layers of the serous pericardium; it contains serous fluid, which lubricates the surfaces of the space and aids heart movements during contraction

ALERT

4. Pericarditis (inflammation of the pericardium) stems from infection
   a. Inflammation causes the pericardial space to lose fluid
   b. This lets the heart muscle rub against the pericardium as it beats, causing a friction rub

C. Heart wall
1. The heart wall has three distinct tissue layers
2. The *epicardium* is the outer layer
   a. It is composed of a sheet of squamous epithelial cells overlying connective tissue
   b. It is the visceral layer of the pericardium
3. The *myocardium* is the muscular middle layer
   a. It makes up the bulk of the heart wall
   b. Thick and contractile, the myocardium has unique striated muscle fibers that cause the heart to contract
4. The *endocardium* is the inner layer of the heart wall; it consists of endothelial tissue with small blood vessels and several bundles of smooth muscle

D. Heart chambers
1. The heart has two upper chambers and two lower chambers (see *Structures and vessels of the heart,* page 146)
2. The upper chambers are the *left atrium* and *right atrium*
   a. The atria are separated by the interatrial septum
   b. They receive blood returning to the heart
   c. They pump blood only to the lower chambers of the heart
3. The lower chambers are the *left ventricle* and *right ventricle*
   a. The ventricles are separated by the interventricular septum
   b. They are larger and thicker walled than the atria; the left ventricle has thicker walls than the right ventricle
   c. Composed of highly developed musculature, the ventricles receive blood from the atria
   d. The right ventricle pumps blood to and from the lungs
   e. The left ventricle pumps blood through all other vessels of the body
4. *Valves* separate the cardiac chambers from the bases of the aorta and pulmonary artery; they permit blood to flow in one direction only — away from the heart
5. Each side of the heart pumps blood through a different branch of the circulatory system

Structures and vessels of the heart

This illustration shows a cross-sectional view of the structures of the heart.

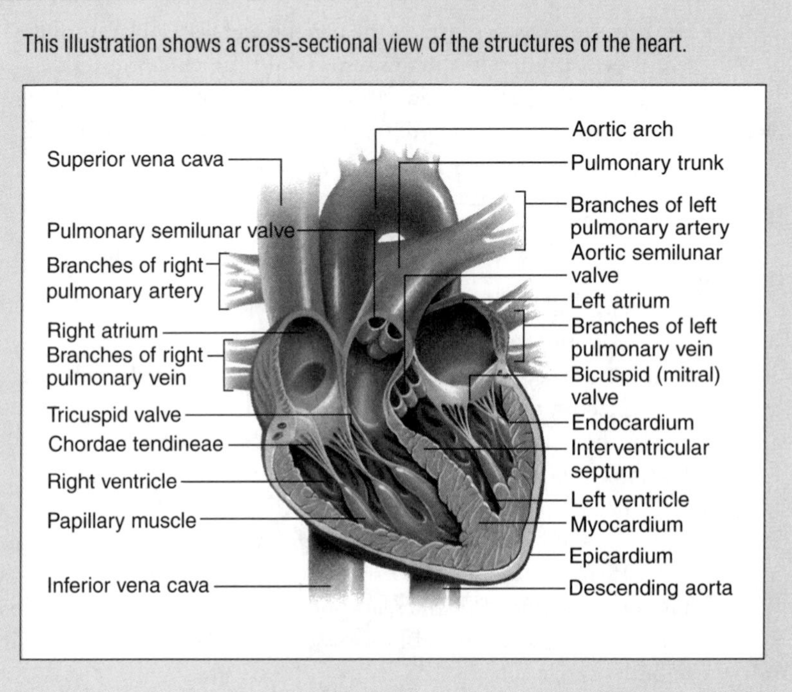

a. The right atrium and ventricle pump blood through the pulmonary circulation
b. The left atrium and ventricle pump blood through the systemic circulation
c. The muscular walls of the left ventricle are thicker than those of the right ventricle because it pumps blood through the systemic circulation at a much higher pressure than that of the pulmonary circulation

6. The right and left coronary arteries supply blood to the heart muscle; these arteries arise by separate orifices from the part of the aortic wall that is attached to the cusps of the aortic semilunar valves
7. The *cardiac conduction system* sends impulses through the heart muscle to cause synchronized contractions of the atria and ventricles, which pump blood throughout the body

♦ III. Cardiac cycle

A. General information

1. Impulses generated by the conduction system cause synchronized contractions of the atria and ventricles

2. Each cardiac contraction (SYSTOLE) is followed by a period of relaxation (DIASTOLE); the atria and ventricles dilate during their respective diastoles
   a. The atria and ventricles contract and relax in sequence
      (1) *Atrial systole* refers to atrial muscle contraction; atrial diastole refers to relaxation
      (2) *Ventricular systole* refers to ventricular muscle contraction; ventricular diastole refers to relaxation
   b. When used without reference to a specific cardiac chamber, the terms *systole* and *diastole* refer to the ventricular systole and diastole
   c. Events that occur during a single systole and diastole of the atria and ventricles make up the CARDIAC CYCLE
3. Actions during the cardiac cycle cause certain characteristic heart sounds and a palpable pulse

B. Systole and diastole

1. When the atria are contracting, the ventricles are relaxed
   a. The *atrioventricular (AV) valves* (valves between the atrial and ventricular chambers) are open during atrial systole
   b. The atria eject blood into the ventricles through the open AV valves
2. When the atria relax, the ventricles contract
   a. Ventricular contraction exerts pressure on the blood in the ventricles, increasing the intraventricular pressure
   b. This rising pressure forces the AV valves to close, preventing blood from flowing backward into the atria
   c. For a short time after the AV valves close, the intraventricular pressure is not high enough to force the *semilunar valves* (valves between the heart and the aorta and pulmonary artery) open; the ventricles are completely closed chambers
   d. Continued ventricular contraction increases the intraventricular pressure until it exceeds the pressure of blood in the aorta and pulmonary artery
   e. This increased intraventricular pressure forces open the semilunar valves and ejects the blood from the ventricles
3. While the ventricles are contracting, venous blood from the systemic and pulmonary circulations is flowing into the relaxed atria
   a. This blood is held in the atria because the AV valves are closed during ventricular systole
   b. As blood fills the atria, the intra-atrial pressure rises slightly
4. Pressure in the aorta and pulmonary artery peaks during ventricular systole as the ventricles eject blood, which distends these vessels
5. After expelling this blood, the ventricles begin to relax

a. The blood ejected from the ventricles into the aorta and pulmonary artery loses its forward momentum caused by the force of ventricular contraction
   (1) Loss of momentum causes the blood to flow back toward the ventricles
   (2) Blood fills the cup-shaped cusps of the semilunar valves, forcing the valves shut and preventing blood from refluxing into the ventricles; this maintains high pressure in the aorta and pulmonary artery
   (3) The stretched walls of the aorta and pulmonary artery return to their former dimensions by the end of ventricular diastole; this elastic recoil compresses the blood and maintains pressure on it, causing it to continue moving through the vessels in the intervals between ventricular contractions

b. Ventricular pressure falls during ventricular diastole; eventually, it falls below the intra-atrial pressure
   (1) Then the AV valves open, allowing the accumulated blood in the atria to flow into the ventricles
   (2) The same type of pressure changes occur in the right ventricle and pulmonary artery as those in the left ventricle and aorta; however, the pressures are much lower

6. The events of the cardiac cycle are repeated with each heartbeat

C. Heart sounds

1. Each cardiac cycle, or heartbeat, is associated with characteristic heart sounds (*lub-dub* followed by a pause)
2. These sounds can be heard by placing the ear or a stethoscope against the chest
   a. The *lub* results from vibrations caused by AV valve closure during ventricular systole
   b. The *dub* results from vibrations caused by semilunar valve closure during ventricular diastole
   c. The pause is the interval between successive cardiac contractions

D. Pulse

1. If the heart is contracting normally, pulse assessment is a convenient way to measure the heart rate; the *pulse rate* typically is assessed in a large artery
2. The pulse is produced by a shock wave from ventricular ejection of blood into the aorta; this shock wave is transmitted through the walls of the large arteries, somewhat like the vibrations transmitted along a metal pipe struck by a hammer
3. The pulse rate is assessed by palpating an artery that lies near the body surface over a bone or other firm tissue and counting the number of pulsations felt in 1 minute

♦ IV. Cardiac electrical conduction

A. General information
   1. The conduction system controls the heartbeat
   2. It consists of various structures composed of cardiac muscle cells specialized to conduct electrical impulses
   3. Cardiac muscle fibers are polarized; positive charges outside the fibers are balanced by negative charges inside
   4. The electrical impulse that causes heart contraction (systole) spreads as a wave through the cardiac muscle; it causes activated areas of the fibers to accumulate negative charges on the outside and positive charges on the inside (depolarization)
   5. During diastole, the cell membranes become depolarized as positive charges on the cell surfaces are restored and the cell interiors again accumulate negative charges

B. Conduction system
   1. The heart contains a specialized system of nodal tissue for generating and conducting impulses that cause rhythmic contractions
   2. The conduction system consists of nodal tissue that contains few myofibrils
   3. The cardiac conduction system has four main components: the sinoatrial node and internodal tracts, atrioventricular (AV) node, the bundle of His, and the PURKINJE FIBERS
      a. The SINOATRIAL (SA) NODE is located in the posterior wall of the right atrium near the opening of the superior vena cava
         (1) The SA node serves as the heart's PACEMAKER
         (2) It initiates depolarization waves that set the pace of cardiac contraction (called SINUS RHYTHM)
         (2) These rhythmic impulses are conducted to the AV node by small bundles of fibers called internodal tracts
      b. The *AV node* is located in the lower right interatrial septum, near the tricuspid valve (one of the AV valves)
         (1) It acts as an electrical bridge between the atria and ventricles, receiving and passing on impulses from the SA node
         (2) The impulses slow in the AV node
         (3) Impulse slowing allows the atria to contract and the ventricles to fill with blood
         (4) From the AV node, depolarization waves pass rapidly to the *AV bundle (bundle of His),* bundle branches, and Purkinje fibers, a network of muscle fibers spreading through the ventricular myocardium
      c. The *bundle of His* originates in the AV node and divides into the right and left bundle branches

Cardiac conduction route

In the cardiac conduction system, the impulse begins in the sinoatrial node, travels through the heart chambers, and reaches ventricular muscle. The illustration below traces the conduction route through these cardiac structures.

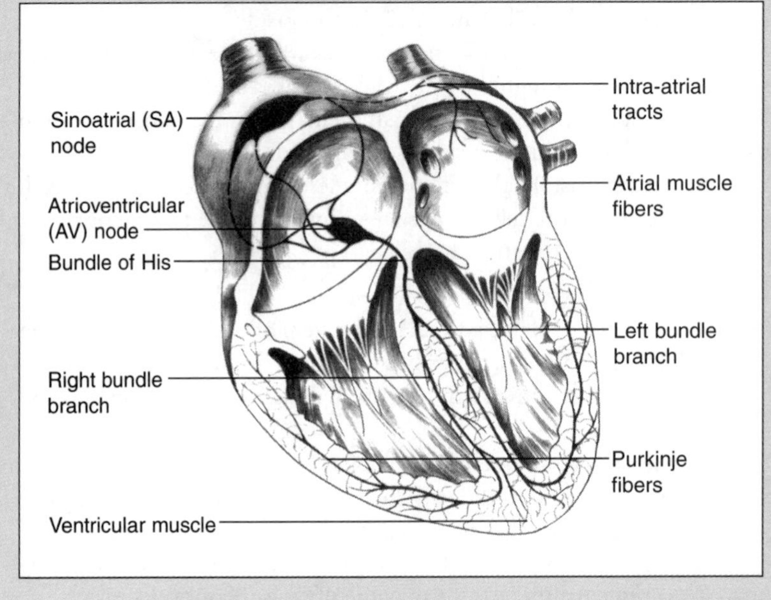

(1) These branches extend down the right and left sides of the interventricular septum

(2) The impulse from the AV node continues through the bundle of His to the right and left bundle branches, which ensure excitation of AV septal cells

d. The Purkinje fibers connect the right and left bundle branches to the papillary muscles and the lateral walls of the ventricles; the fibers are more elaborate in the left ventricle than in the right ventricle

(1) The impulse moves through the Purkinje fibers, eventually reaching the ventricular muscles

(2) Ventricular muscle stimulation begins in the intraventricular septum and moves downward, causing ventricular depolarization and contraction (see *Cardiac conduction route*)

C. Conduction tracing

1. The electrocardiogram (ECG) traces serial changes in electrical conduction associated with depolarization and repolarization of cardiac muscle fibers

TEACHING TIPS
Patient with an arrhythmia

Be sure to include the following topics when teaching a patient with an arrhythmia.
- Normal cardiac conduction
- Patient's specific arrhythmia
- Diagnostic tests, such as an electrocardiogram and electrolyte levels
- Activity instructions, such as obtaining moderate exercise regularly
- Dietary changes, such as increased potassium intake and moderate use of alcohol and caffeine
- Treatments, such as antiarrhythmic drugs, pacemaker implant, and electrocardioversion
- Guidelines for use and maintenance of pacemaker or automatic implantable cardioverter defibrillator, if needed
- How to take pulse rate
- Sources of information and support

2. These changes are recorded as a series of positive and negative deflections, commonly called waveforms, which produce characteristic patterns (see *Characteristic PQRST patterns,* page 152)
3. The ECG can detect arrhythmias (abnormal heart rate or rhythm), which result from any disruption of normal conduction (for teaching tips, see *Patient with an arrhythmia*)

♦ V. Blood vessels

A. General information
1. *Blood vessels* are tubules that convey blood between the heart and every functioning cell in the body
2. The three main types of blood vessels are arteries, veins, and capillaries
   a. Arteries give rise to smaller vessels called arterioles
   b. Veins give rise to smaller vessels called venules
   c. Arterioles and venules decrease in size to become capillaries

B. Arteries
1. *Arteries* are large vessels that carry blood from the heart to the lungs and tissues
2. Their walls have three layers and are thicker than those of veins and capillaries
   a. The *tunica adventitia* is the outer wall layer
   b. The *tunica media* is the thick middle layer
   c. The *tunica intima* is the inner layer

Characteristic PQRST patterns

Electrocardiogram wave patterns are identified by letters; each waveform corresponds to specific electrical events in the cardiac cycle.

- The P wave reflects the initial wave of depolarization associated with atrial systole.
- The Q, R, and S waves (collectively called the QRS complex) reflect impulse transmission through the right and left bundles into the terminal branches, leading to ventricular systole.
- The T wave reflects ventricular repolarization during diastole.
- The PR interval (time from the beginning of the P wave to the beginning of the QRS complex) represents the time needed for an impulse to pass from the atria to the ventricles through the bundle of His.
- The ST segment (time from the end of the S wave to the beginning of the T wave) represents the time between the end of the spread of the impulse through the ventricle and repolarization of the ventricle.

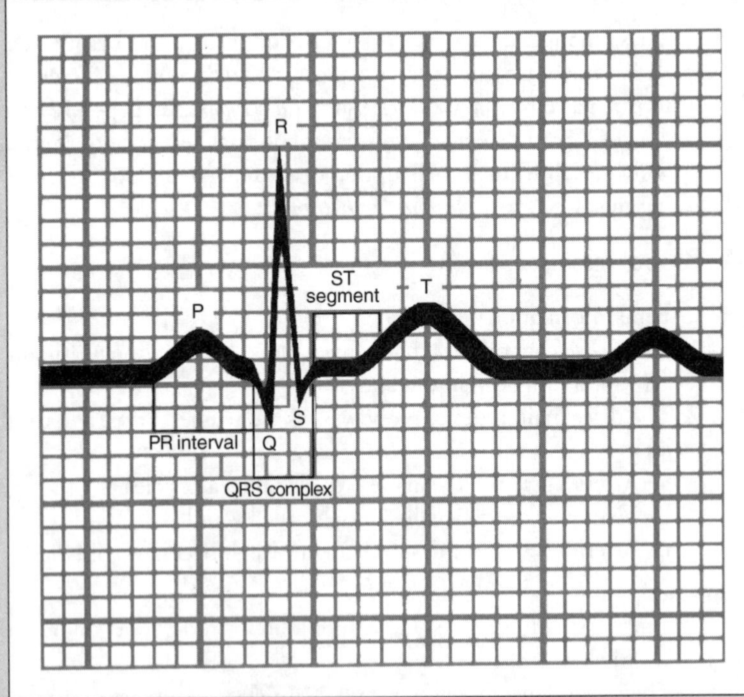

3. The large arteries close to the heart are called elastic arteries because their tunica media contains more elastic fibers than those of the other arteries
4. The medium and small arteries branching from the large arteries are called muscular arteries
   a. The tunica media of these arteries contains more smooth-muscle and fewer elastic fibers than those of the large arteries
   b. These arteries also are called distributing arteries because they distribute blood to the various organs
5. In arteries, vascular resistance to blood flow is low; mean arterial pressure (average of diastolic and systolic pressures) remains around 100 mm Hg
6. *Arterioles* are the smallest arteries; they lie between arteries and capillaries
   a. Their walls consist mainly of muscle; they consist of the same three coats as arteries, but are smaller in diameter
   b. Contraction of arteriolar muscle helps control the flow of blood into the capillaries
   c. Intravascular pressure is lower in arterioles than in arteries; mean pressure is about 85 mm Hg

C. Veins
1. *Veins* are vessels that transport blood from the lungs and tissues to the heart; they are the largest vessels
2. The walls of veins, like those of arteries, are composed of a tunica adventitia, tunica media, and tunica intima; however, the tunica media of a vein is much thinner than that of an artery
3. Veins have valves, composed of tunica intima, that prevent backflow of blood away from the heart
4. The superior and inferior venae cavae are the main tributaries that collect venous blood for return to the heart
5. Mean pressure in the veins is less than 15 mm Hg
6. Venules are the smallest veins; they carry blood from the capillaries to the veins
   a. The smallest venules have only a tunica intima and tunica adventitia
   b. In some larger venules, the tunica media contains spiraling smooth-muscle fibers
   c. Blood pressure is only about 15 mm Hg when blood begins to return to the heart

D. Capillaries
1. *Capillaries* are microscopic vessels that connect arterioles with venules to form a network throughout the body
2. Capillary walls are extremely thin, consisting only of tunica intima

a. In some cases, they consist only of a single endothelial cell
b. Capillary walls serve as the exchange site for various substances between blood and tissue cells

3. Vascular resistance to blood flow is very low in capillaries; mean pressure is about 35 mm Hg

♦ VI. Circulation

A. General information

1. The cardiovascular system includes the cardiac circulation, pulmonary circulation, systemic circulation, and hepatic circulation
2. In pregnant females, the cardiovascular system also includes the fetal circulation

B. Cardiac circulation

1. In the heart, blood enters the right atrium via the superior vena cava, inferior vena cava, and CORONARY SINUS (see *Coronary circulation*)
   a. As blood passes through the right AV (tricuspid) valve, it flows from the right atrium into the right ventricle
   b. It exits through the pulmonary (semilunar) valve and enters the pulmonary circuit
2. Blood returns from the pulmonary circuit to the left atrium
   a. As it passes through the left AV (bicuspid or mitral) valve, it flows from the left atrium into the left ventricle
   b. Blood exits the left ventricle via the aortic (semilunar) valve and enters the systemic circuit
3. The heart's functional blood supply comes from the right and left coronary arteries, which branch from the base of the aorta
   a. The left coronary artery branches into the anterior interventricular artery and circumflex artery
   b. The right coronary artery branches into the posterior interventricular artery and marginal artery
   c. Extensive capillary beds join coronary arteries with cardiac veins, which empty into the coronary sinus

C. Pulmonary circulation

1. Pulmonary circulation starts with the blood flowing from the right ventricle into the pulmonary trunk
2. The pulmonary trunk bifurcates into the right and left pulmonary arteries, which carry deoxygenated blood to the lungs
3. In the lungs, the pulmonary arteries divide into the lobar arteries
   a. Lobar arteries (three on the right and two on the left) branch profusely to form arterioles and pulmonary capillaries
   b. Pulmonary capillaries drain into venules that join with pulmonary veins (two on the right and two on the left)

Coronary circulation

These illustrations show the anterior and posterior views of the blood vessels of the heart.

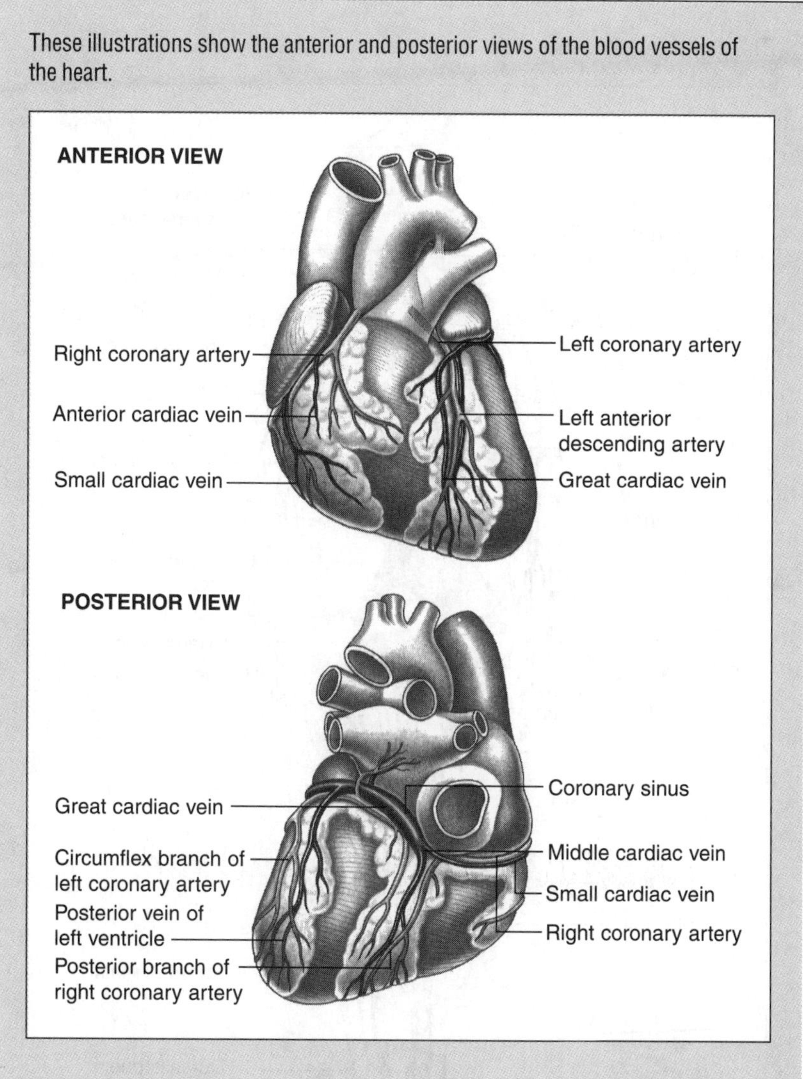

4. Pulmonary veins empty into the left atrium of the heart

D. Systemic circulation
   1. The systemic circulation supplies blood to all body tissues (see *Arteries and veins of the systemic circulation,* page 156)
   2. Starting at the heart, blood flow begins in the ascending aorta, which gives rise to the right and left coronary arteries
   3. The ascending aorta forms an arch, which has three branches

Arteries and veins of the systemic circulation

This illustration shows the major arteries and veins of the systemic circulation.

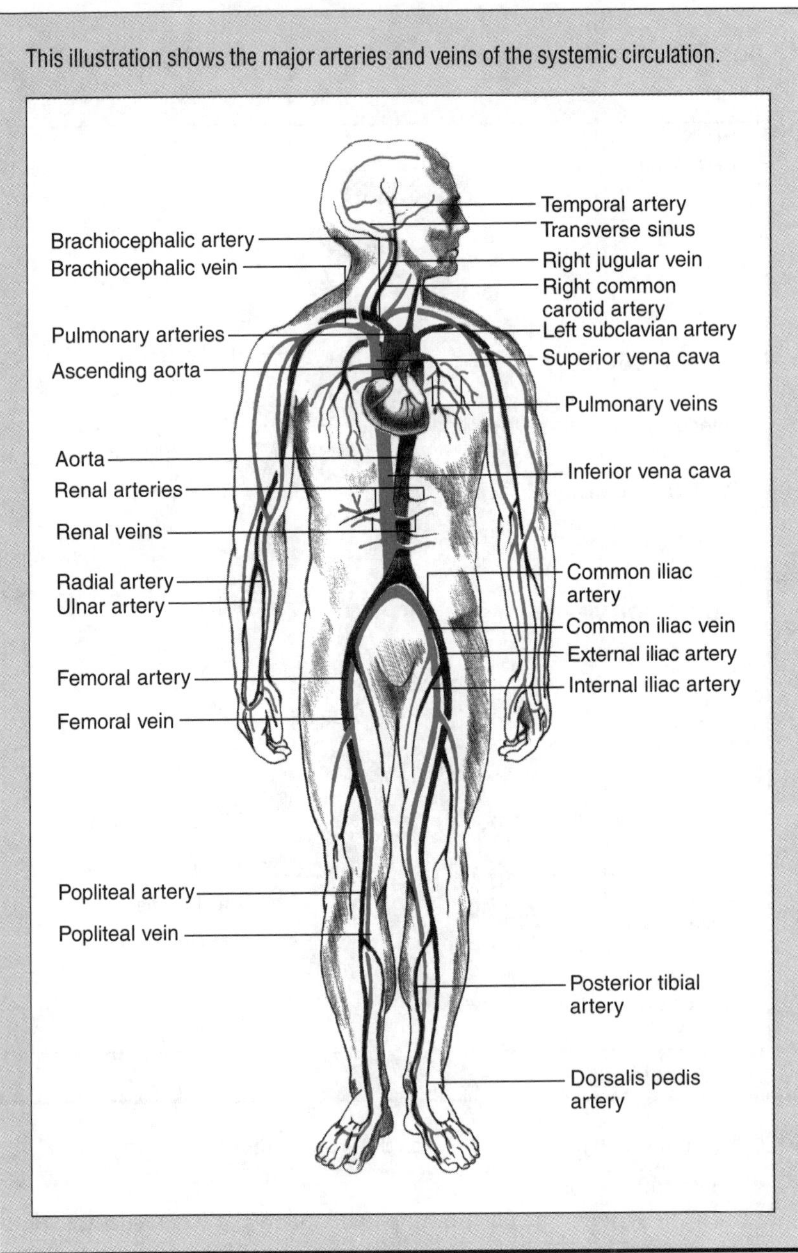

   a. The brachiocephalic (innominate) artery branches to the right side of the heart
   b. The left common carotid artery and left subclavian artery branch to the left side of the heart
4. The descending aorta becomes the thoracic aorta, which has four visceral and two parietal branches
5. As the thoracic aorta continues through the body, it becomes the abdominal aorta
   a. The abdominal aorta has several visceral and parietal branches
   b. Ultimately, it bifurcates to form the right and left iliac arteries
6. Small end-arteries (arteries that do not connect with other arteries) join arterioles and capillary beds, which in turn join venules and progressively larger veins that carry venous blood to the superior or inferior vena cava

E. Hepatic circulation
   1. The hepatic circulation (also called the hepatic portal system) circulates blood through the liver
   2. Veins from the digestive viscera empty blood into the hepatic portal vein
   3. This venous blood then passes through the liver before entering the systemic circulation via hepatic veins

F. Fetal circulation
   1. Fetal circulation is a special adaptation of the circulatory system required for fetal development
   2. It includes the umbilical vessels and three vascular shunts — ductus venosus, foramen ovale, and ductus arteriosus
   3. The umbilical vein carries oxygenated blood from the placenta to the liver of the fetus
   4. Blood flows from the liver via the ductus venosus or hepatic veins to the inferior vena cava
      a. The *ductus venosus* is a shunt that allows most blood to bypass the liver
      b. It is necessary because the fetal liver does not process blood
   5. From the inferior vena cava, blood enters the right atrium of the heart
      a. Some blood entering the right atrium flows directly into the left atrium via the *foramen ovale,* a shunt in the interatrial septum
      b. Blood entering the right ventricle is pumped out through the pulmonary artery
   6. Much of the blood in the pulmonary trunk passes through the ductus arteriosus
      a. The *ductus arteriosus* is a vessel that connects the pulmonary artery directly to the descending aorta
      b. Thus, it shunts blood away from the pulmonary circulation

7. Blood flowing through the aorta passes through the internal iliac arteries into the umbilical arteries and back to the placenta
8. At birth, the two umbilical arteries, the umbilical vein, and the three shunts are occluded (closed off)

♦ VII. Blood pressure

A. General information
1. The pressure of blood in the pulmonary and systemic arteries varies with the phase of the cardiac cycle
2. Pressure is highest when the blood is ejected during systole (systolic pressure) and lowest during diastole immediately before the next cardiac contraction (diastolic pressure)
3. *Blood pressure* refers to the pressure of blood in the systemic circulation, which is about six times higher than the pressure of blood in the pulmonary circulation
4. A sphygmomanometer and stethoscope can be used to measure systolic and diastolic blood pressure
5. Blood pressure varies rhythmically with the heart beat
    a. The pressure is the highest during ventricular systole when blood is ejected from the ventricles; this represents systolic blood pressure
    b. The pressure is lowest during ventricular diastole when blood is flowing through the arteries into the capillaries; this represents diastolic blood pressure
6. Systolic blood pressure depends primarily on CARDIAC OUTPUT (the force and volume of blood ejected from the ventricles during systole); diastolic pressure depends on PERIPHERAL RESISTANCE (degree of impedance to blood flow, which may be increased by vasoconstriction)
7. Blood pressure also is influenced to a lesser degree by blood volume, blood viscosity, and arterial elasticity
8. Systolic pressure is a measure primarily of the force of ventricular contraction; diastolic pressure is a measure of the peripheral resistance caused by arteriolar vasoconstriction
9. Blood pressure does not drop precipitously during diastole; it declines slowly as blood is released gradually into the capillaries by the arterioles, helping to maintain a fairly constant blood pressure
10. A relatively constant blood pressure is necessary to maintain blood flow to tissues and prevent organ damage

ALERT

11. Sustained high blood pressure (hypertension) can lead to congestive heart failure and other disorders (for teaching tips, see *Patient with hypertension*)

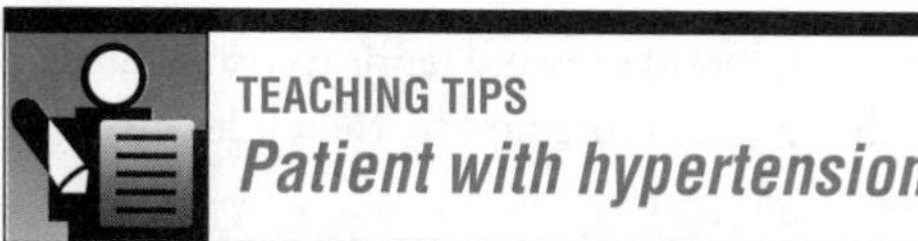

TEACHING TIPS

Patient with hypertension

Be sure to include the following topics when teaching a patient with hypertension.

- Factors that affect blood pressure
- Definition of hypertension and patient's type of hypertension
- Complications and the need for compliance with regimen
- Diagnostic tests
- Exercise program and precautions
- Dietary restrictions, such as increased potassium intake, decreased salt intake, and decreased calories (if needed for weight loss)
- Use of antihypertensives, diuretics, or other drugs
- Home blood pressure monitoring
- Other measures to prevent complications, such as stress reduction and smoking cessation
- Sources of information and support

B. Cardiac output

1. *Cardiac output* refers to the amount of blood ejected per minute from a ventricle
2. This amount equals the STROKE VOLUME (volume of blood ejected from a single ventricle at each contraction) multiplied by the heart rate in beats per minute
3. The basal (resting) stroke volume is about 70 ml; the basal heart rate is about 72 beats per minute
   a. Therefore, cardiac output is about 5 L per minute (70 x 72 = 5,040 ml)
   b. This amount also equals an individual's total blood volume (approximately 5,000 ml)
4. The END-DIASTOLIC VOLUME (EDV) (total blood volume in each ventricle before ventricular systole) is about 120 ml
5. The ventricles are not emptied completely of blood during systole
   a. Each ventricle ejects only about 70 ml of blood
   b. The END-SYSTOLIC VOLUME (unejected blood remaining in each ventricle) is about 50 ml (120 - 70 = 50 ml)
   c. The EJECTION FRACTION is the amount of blood ejected during each ventricular contraction in relation to the EDV
   d. In this example, 70 ml (stroke volume) is divided by 120 ml (EDV), which equals an ejection fraction of 0.58, or 58%
6. The heart can increase its rate and stroke volume as needed to increase cardiac output above the basal level
   a. This increase can be fourfold, if necessary
   b. Trained athletes can increase their cardiac output even more

c. If cardiac output increases, blood pressure tends to rise because blood is delivered to the arteries more rapidly than it leaves through the arterioles

C. Peripheral resistance

1. The degree of peripheral resistance is determined by the degree of arteriolar vasoconstriction
2. Arterioles restrict blood flow from the arteries into the capillaries
   a. If arteriolar constriction and peripheral resistance increase, blood pressure rises because blood flow from the arteries into the capillaries is impeded
   b. If the arterioles relax and peripheral resistance decreases, blood flows more rapidly into the capillaries and arterial pressure drops

D. Blood volume

1. Blood pressure tends to vary directly with the total blood volume in the cardiovascular system

ALERT

2. Blood pressure tends to rise if blood volume increases (which occurs in some diseases) and tends to drop if blood volume falls below normal (which occurs in severe hemorrhage)

E. Blood viscosity

1. The greater the viscosity of a fluid, the slower it flows through a narrow orifice; the reverse also is true

ALERT

2. In some diseases, blood viscosity rises as a result of an increase in proteins in the blood or in the number of erythrocytes
   a. These conditions restrict blood flow through arterioles into capillaries
   b. As a result, blood pressure tends to rise

F. Arterial elasticity

1. Blood pressure changes if the elasticity of the large arteries changes
   a. Normally, large artery distention absorbs some of the force of the blood ejected during systole
   b. Distention prevents excessive elevation of systolic pressure during each ventricular contraction
   c. The arteries recoil during diastole and propel the blood forward

ALERT

2. In some diseases, the aorta and large arteries gradually lose their elasticity and become more rigid
   a. Then they cannot distend and absorb the impact of the ejected blood
   b. As a result, systolic pressure tends to rise

♦ VIII. Regulation of cardiac output and blood pressure

A. General information
   1. Adequate cardiac output and stable blood pressure are essential for proper performance of major body organs
   2. Cardiac output normally varies in response to the body's requirements; blood pressure normally remains within a specific range
   3. Several mechanisms control cardiac output and blood pressure
      a. The heart exerts control over its stroke volume, as described by STARLING'S LAW
      b. The autonomic nervous system (ANS) controls nerve impulse discharge based on information relayed to the brain from baroreceptors and chemoreceptors in major arteries
      c. The kidneys secrete hormones that affect the heart

B. Starling's law
   1. According to Starling's law, the amount of stretching of cardiac muscle fibers helps regulate stroke volume and maintain equal output from both ventricles
   2. Muscle stretching commonly occurs in two ways
      a. If venous return to the ventricle increases, the ventricle becomes overdistended and its muscles become stretched
      b. If the diastolic pressure rises, the heart must eject blood against a higher peripheral resistance; when this occurs, the ventricle tends to empty less completely and becomes overdistended, stretching the cardiac muscles
   3. Stretching of the fibers causes the ventricle to contract more forcefully to expel the additional blood
   4. The more forceful ventricular contractions maintain normal cardiac output and supply adequate blood to the tissues despite increased peripheral resistance

C. Regulation by baroreceptors
   1. The ANS controls the heart and blood vessels
   2. A diffuse network of interconnecting neurons in the medulla regulate the discharge of autonomic nerve impulses, primarily in response to impulses from *baroreceptors* (specialized pressure-sensitive receptors in the carotid artery and walls of the aortic arch)
   3. This medullary control center exerts opposing effects
      a. Its cardioacceleratory portion controls nerve impulse discharge from the sympathetic division of the ANS, which speeds the heart rate
      b. Its cardioinhibitory portion controls nerve impulse discharge from the parasympathetic division, which slows the heart rate

c. The net effect of the ANS on the heart and blood vessels reflects the combined response of the two portions of the medullary control center

4. In response to input from baroreceptors, the medullary centers also send regulatory impulses to the heart and blood vessels, which maintain a stable cardiac output and blood pressure
   a. If the intravascular pressure rises, baroreceptors send impulses to the medullary center
      (1) These impulses initiate discharge of parasympathetic impulses in the vagal nerve to slow the heart rate and reduce the force of ventricular contraction, which reduces cardiac output, and to reduce arteriolar vasoconstriction, which reduces intravascular pressure
      (2) Impulses simultaneously inhibit sympathetic output from the cardioacceleratory portion of the center
   b. If the intravascular pressure falls, baroreceptors relay fewer impulses to the medullary center
      (1) The medullary center responds by discharging sympathetic nerve impulses to increase the heart rate and force of ventricular contraction, which increases cardiac output, and to constrict the arterioles, which raises intravascular pressure
      (2) Impulses simultaneously inhibit parasympathetic output from the cardioinhibitory portion of the center

D. Regulation by chemoreceptors
1. Chemoreceptors (chemical-sensitive receptors in the aortic arch and carotid sinus) respond to decreases in blood oxygen concentration and pH; they also respond to increases in blood carbon dioxide concentration
2. The medullary center initiates impulses via the ANS that increase heart rate and blood pressure
3. Chemoreceptors do not play a major role in heart rate and blood pressure regulation under normal physiologic conditions; however, they respond to extreme arterial PO_2 and blood pH decreases and extreme arterial PCO_2 increases
4. They transmit impulses to the medullary control center via the same pathways that transmit impulses from baroreceptors

E. Hormonal regulation
1. In the kidneys, the hormones resin, angiotensin, and aldosterone help regulate blood pressure; the RENIN-ANGIOTENSIN-ALDOSTERONE MECHANISM responds more slowly to blood pressure changes than the reflex mechanisms
2. A sustained fall in blood pressure causes the kidneys to release resin, which is converted to angiotensin in the circulation

3. Angiotensin raises blood pressure by causing arteriolar constriction; it also stimulates the adrenal gland to release the steroid hormone aldosterone
4. Aldosterone promotes sodium and water retention by the kidneys; this retention increases blood volume and leads to a corresponding increase in blood pressure

♦ IX. Capillary and interstitial circulation

A. General information
1. Capillary blood and cells exchange such substances as oxygen, nutrients, and cellular waste products
2. These substances must pass in solution through the loose connective tissue (interstitial space) in which the cells are dispersed
3. The interstitial space is filled with a semisolid matrix containing connective tissue fibers and a small amount of interstitial fluid that has filtered through the capillaries
4. At the arterial end of the capillary, the HYDROSTATIC PRESSURE (which pushes fluid out) is higher than the osmotic pressure (which pulls fluid back), causing interstitial fluid to filter through the endothelium of the capillary into the interstitial space
5. At the venous end of the capillary, the hydrostatic pressure is lower than the osmotic pressure, causing fluid to diffuse back into the capillary

ALERT

6. *Edema* (excess fluid in the interstitial space) may result from any disturbance in fluid transfer between the capillaries and interstitial tissue

B. Fluid movement
1. The cyclic flow of fluid from the interstitial space to the capillaries and back into the interstitial space depends on capillary hydrostatic pressure, capillary permeability, osmotic pressure, and open lymphatic channels
2. Blood in the capillaries exerts capillary hydrostatic pressure
   a. This pressure tends to force fluid out from the blood through the capillary endothelium and into the interstitial fluid
   b. This pressure is much lower than that in the larger arteries because arteriolar constriction restricts blood flow into the capillaries, functioning like a pressure reduction valve
   c. As a result, the mean arterial pressure in larger arteries falls from about 85 mm Hg to about 35 mm Hg at the arterial end of the capillary and drops to a low of 15 mm Hg at the venous end of the capillary
3. Capillary permeability determines the ease with which fluid can pass through the capillary endothelium

4. The osmotic pressure exerted by the blood proteins (called the colloid osmotic pressure) tends to attract interstitial fluid back into the capillaries
5. Open lymphatic channels collect some fluid forced out into the interstitial tissues and return it to the circulation; this occurs because the pressure in the lymphatic channels is lower than that in the interstitial tissues

ALERT

6. Edema may result from any disturbance in the factors that regulate fluid transfer in the capillary-interstitial tissue-capillary cycle; causes of such disturbance include inflammation, decreased colloid osmotic pressure, increased capillary hydrostatic pressure, and lymphatic channel obstruction

Points to remember

- The heart is a physiologic pump that moves blood to and from the lungs (pulmonary circulation) and to and from the tissues (systemic circulation). Its upper chambers (atria) communicate with its lower chambers (ventricles) by AV valves.
- Events that occur during a single systole (contraction) and diastole (relaxation) of the atria and ventricles make up the cardiac cycle. They also produce heart sounds and a pulse.
- The cardiac conduction system controls the heartbeat. It consists of the SA node and internodal tracts, AV node, bundle of His, and Purkinje fibers.
- Blood vessels convey blood through out the body. Types of vessels include arteries, arterioles, veins, venules, and capillaries.
- The cardiovascular system includes the cardiac, pulmonary, systemic, hepatic, and (in pregnant women) fetal circulations.
- Blood pressure refers to the pressure of blood in the systemic circulation. Pressure is highest when the blood is ejected during systole (systolic pressure) and lowest during diastole (diastolic pressure).
- Cardiac output and blood pressure are controlled by Starling's law, baroreceptors and chemoreceptors in major arteries, and hormone secretion by the kidneys.
- The cyclic flow of fluid from the interstitial space to the capillaries and back into the interstitial space depends on capillary hydrostatic pressure, capillary permeability, osmotic pressure, and open lymphatic channels.

STUDY QUESTIONS

To evaluate your understanding of this chapter, answer the following questions in the space provided. Then compare your responses with the correct answers in Appendix B, page 331.

1. Which part of the heart acts as a pulmonary pump? As a systemic pump?
____
____

2. How does blood flow through the heart during the cardiac cycle? ________
____
____

3. What is the heart's pacemaker and where is it located? ________
____
____

4. How do arteries differ from veins? ________
____
____

5. What do the systolic and diastolic blood pressures measure? ________
____
____

CRITICAL THINKING AND APPLICATION EXERCISES

1. On a three-dimensional model of the heart, show where blood flows during each part of the cardiac cycle.
2. On an ECG strip, relate segments of the ECG tracing to cardiac conduction events.
3. Draw a schematic of blood flow in the pulmonary and systemic circulations.
4. Take a partner's blood pressure, accurately noting the systolic and diastolic pressures. Discuss the difference between these two measurements.
5. Write a one-page paper summarizing the factors that regulate cardiac output and blood pressure.

CHAPTER

11

Hematologic System

LEARNING OBJECTIVES

After studying this chapter, you should be able to:

- ♦ List the eight functions of blood.
- ♦ Describe the major characteristics of formed elements.
- ♦ Describe the basic functions of the formed elements and plasma.
- ♦ Discuss red blood cell maturation, including the hemoglobin synthesis.
- ♦ Discuss the structure and function of iron and hemoglobin.
- ♦ Compare the different types of hemoglobin.
- ♦ Contrast the process of blood coagulation and fibrinolysis.
- ♦ Describe the role of genetics, antigens, and antibodies in the ABO and Rh blood group systems.

CHAPTER OVERVIEW

Through the cardiovascular system, the hematologic system performs most of its functions. In this system, the blood acts as the body's major transport mechanism, bringing oxygen, nutrients, and hormones to the cells and carrying away cellular wastes. These and other functions make the hematologic system a principle factor in maintenance of homeostasis. Because the blood can provide clues to many hematologic and other disorders, the health care professional should be familiar with structures and normal functions.

♦ I. Blood composition and functions

A. General information

1. Blood is a specialized type of connective tissue; it consists of formed elements suspended in a viscous fluid called blood PLASMA
   a. The formed elements in blood are *red blood cells (RBCs* or *erythrocytes), white blood cells (WBCs* or *leukocytes),* and *platelets* (or *thrombocytes)*
   b. Plasma is a liquid containing dissolved substances
2. Blood is slightly alkaline (pH 7.35 to 7.45); its red color comes from its rich oxygen content
3. Blood accounts for about 8% of total body weight; the body of an average adult contains about 5 L (5 qt) of blood
4. Blood has eight functions that are generally classified as transportation, regulation, and protection
   a. It delivers oxygen to body cells from the lungs and delivers nutrients to body cells from the gastrointestinal tract
   b. It transports carbon dioxide to the lungs and nitrogenous wastes to the kidneys for elimination
   c. It transports hormones from endocrine glands to their target tissues
   d. It maintains body temperature by absorbing and distributing body heat
   e. It maintains acid-base balance
      (1) Blood proteins and other solutes act as buffers to prevent sudden changes in blood pH
      (2) Blood also stores bicarbonate atoms (an important component of the blood-buffer system needed to maintain normal blood pH)
   f. It maintains adequate fluid volume; salts (such as sodium chloride) and proteins (such as albumin) in the blood prevent excessive fluid loss
   g. It helps prevent blood loss through HEMOSTASIS, a mechanism that involves a vascular spasm, platelet plug formation, and coagulation
   h. It helps prevent infection through the action of the antibodies, complement proteins, and WBCs it contains

B. Plasma

1. Plasma accounts for about 55% of the total blood volume; it contains about 7% proteins and about 93% water with dissolved minerals, nutrients (such as glucose and amino acids), and cellular wastes
2. Plasma proteins consist of *albumin, globulins,* and *fibrinogen*
   a. Albumin comprises about half the total plasma proteins

   (1) It is essential in maintaining the colloid osmotic pressure of the blood
   (2) This pressure plays a major role in regulating fluid flow between the capillaries and interstitial tissues (for more information, see Chapter 10, Cardiovascular System)
  b. Globulins are divided into alpha, beta, and gamma globulins based on their physical and chemical characteristics; each type of globulin has a specific function
   (1) Some alpha and beta globulins are concerned with blood coagulation; others transport enzymes, hormones, vitamins, and other substances
   (2) Gamma globulins act as antibodies, defending the body against infection
  c. Fibrinogen plays a major role in blood coagulation; it is converted to fibrin when the blood coagulates
 3. SERUM is the fluid expressed from a clot
  a. Like plasma, serum contains no formed elements
  b. Unlike plasma, serum lacks fibrinogen and other proteins that are depleted by blood coagulation

C. Formed elements
 1. Formed elements of blood consist of RBCs, WBCs, and platelets
 2. Each type of cell has a characteristic structure and staining reaction when examined microscopically
 3. All formed elements develop from a common precursor cell, the stem cell, which is found in the red bone marrow of certain bones
  a. Stem cells transform into immature versions of each formed element, which then mature
  b. This process, called HEMATOPOIESIS, produces the various types of blood cells (see *Physiologic process: Hematopoiesis*)
 4. The quantity of each type of blood cell in circulation is maintained within narrow limits, which vary with the individual's age and physical demands
  a. Blood normally contains 4.5 to 5.5 million RBCs per mm^3
  b. Blood normally contains 5,000 to 10,000 WBCs per mm^3
  c. Blood normally contains 150,000 to 350,000 platelets per mm^3

♦ II. Red blood cells

A. General information
 1. RBCs are the most numerous formed element in the blood, averaging about 5 million per mm^3 and accounting for about 45% of total blood volume (measurement of their percentage in the blood is called the HEMATOCRIT)

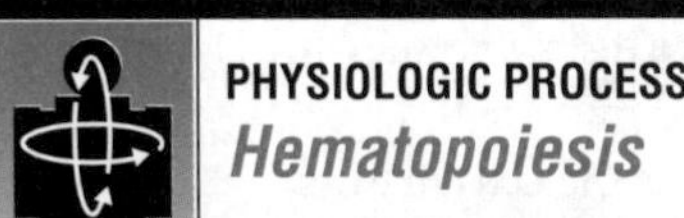

PHYSIOLOGIC PROCESS

Hematopoiesis

From one stem cell, hematopoiesis produces all seven types of blood cells.

Stem cell

Proerythoblast
Myeloblast
Lymphoblast
Monoblast
Megakaryoblast

Basophilic erythroblast
Progranulocyte

Polychromatic erythroblast
Basophilic myelocyte
Eosinophilic myelocyte
Neutrophilic myelocyte

Megakaryocyte

Orthochromic erythroblast (normoblast)

Megakaryocyte breakup

Basophilic band cell
Eosinophilic band cell
Neutrophilic band cell

Reticulocyte

Red blood cells

Basophil
Eosinophil
Neutrophil
Lymphocyte
Monocyte
White blood cells

Platelets

a. These cells are flexible, biconcave disks that measure about 7 microns in diameter (1 mm = 1,000 microns)
b. They lack nuclei, which are lost as the cells mature

2. RBC maturation requires HEMOGLOBIN formation
3. A protein vital to RBC function, hemoglobin is composed of *heme* and *globin*
   a. Heme is an iron-containing porphyrin compound
   b. Globin is a protein composed of amino acids
4. The mature RBC consists of a hemoglobin solution enclosed in a protein framework and surrounded by a lipoprotein cell membrane
   a. The mature RBC circulates through the cardiovascular system, carrying oxygen to tissues and removing carbon dioxide
   b. It contains enzymes that allow it to perform essential metabolic functions
5. RBCs lack mitochondria and cannot obtain energy from mitochondrial enzyme systems like other cells; instead, they derive energy from glucose breakdown via other enzyme pathways
6. The mature RBC cannot synthesize proteins because it lacks a nucleus; therefore, it cannot make new enzymes to replace those that wear out
7. RBC aging results in part from progressive deterioration of its enzyme systems
   a. After about 4 months, cells can no longer function
   b. In the spleen, the mononuclear phagocyte (reticuloendothelial) system removes aged RBCs from the circulation and breaks them down into components that are recycled or discarded
      (1) Globin chains are broken down and their component amino acids are used to make other proteins
      (2) Iron is extracted and recycled to make new hemoglobin
      (3) In the heme molecule, the porphyrin ring cannot be salvaged; instead, it is broken down and transported to the liver, where it is excreted as bile pigment (bilirubin)

B. Functions

1. RBCs transport oxygen to body tissues
   a. The hemoglobin in RBCs combines with oxygen from the lungs, forming oxyhemoglobin
   b. When the RBCs reach the body tissues, the hemoglobin releases the oxygen, which then diffuses into tissue cells
   c. The RBC's shape and flexibility facilitate this process
      (1) The biconcave shape gives the RBC a relatively large surface area for oxygen diffusion

ALERT

(2) The RBC's flexibility lets it squeeze through narrow capillaries

(3) Sickle cell anemia forces RBCs to take a sickle shape, which makes them more rigid; this causes them to become stuck in small capillaries, which can lead to a painful sickle cell crisis

2. RBCs transport carbon dioxide to the lungs
   a. In the capillaries, the hemoglobin in RBCs combines with carbon dioxide to form carbaminohemoglobin
   b. When the RBCs reach the lungs, the hemoglobin releases the carbon dioxide, which is exhaled
3. RBCs also contribute to blood viscosity
   a. As they increase in number, blood becomes more viscous
   b. As they decrease in number, blood becomes less viscous

C. RBC production and maturation

1. RBC production is called ERYTHROPOIESIS; it occurs in the bone marrow of certain bones and is regulated by the oxygen content of the arterial blood
   a. If the number of circulating RBCs falls below normal, the blood delivers less oxygen to the tissues; the marrow responds to this oxygen decrease by increasing RBC output
   b. The kidneys mediate this marrow response
      (1) Specialized kidney cells respond to low oxygen tension by liberating the enzyme *renal erythropoietic factor,* which acts on blood protein to form erythropoietin
      (2) Erythropoietin stimulates the stem cells in the bone marrow to produce erythroblasts
2. Erythroblasts develop over several stages
3. As each erythroblast matures, hemoglobin accumulates in the cytoplasm, and the nuclear chromatin condenses; normal RBC maturation is called *normoblastic erythropoiesis* to differentiate it from abnormal maturation, or megablastic erythropoiesis
   a. When the cell has synthesized most of its hemoglobin, it extrudes its nucleus and becomes a reticulocyte
   b. Then the reticulocyte enters one of the sinusoids in the bone marrow and is carried into the circulatory system
      (1) In a microscopic examination of stained blood, the reticulocyte appears slightly larger than a mature RBC and has a faint blue color because it contains less red-staining hemoglobin than an RBC
      (2) The reticulocyte also can be distinguished by using special stains that precipitate and clump the mitochondria and other organelles within the cytoplasm and cause them to appear as a meshwork (reticulum) of irregular blue-staining strands and granules in the cytoplasm; the name reticulocyte is derived from this meshwork

4. Final cell maturation occurs in the circulation
   a. After losing its nucleus, the cell retains its organelles and continues to synthesize additional hemoglobin for the next 24 hours
   b. The reticulocyte matures into an RBC over the next 24 hours; the cell gradually decreases in size and loses its blue tinge as more hemoglobin is synthesized
5. The proportion of reticulocytes serves as a useful index of RBC production
   a. Because RBCs survive in the circulation for about 100 days (actually 120 days, but considered as 100 days to simplify calculations), approximately 1% of the body's RBCs must be produced each day to replace those that wear out and are eliminated from the circulation
   b. The normal reticulocyte percentage in the circulation, therefore, is approximately 1%

ALERT

   c. RBC production increases to compensate for increased blood loss (such as after blood donation) or reduced RBC survival (as in some types of anemia); the percentage of circulating reticulocytes also increases correspondingly

D. Iron structure and formation
1. Iron forms an essential part of hemoglobin and also appears in *myoglobin,* a similar compound in muscle
2. The body contains about 4 grams of iron; hemoglobin contains about 75% of this amount
3. Additional iron is stored with the protein *apoferritin* in the bone marrow, liver, and spleen, forming two different iron-protein complexes
   a. Ferritin is about 20% iron
   b. Hemosiderin is about 25% iron
4. Small amounts of iron circulate in the plasma with the iron-binding transport protein transferrin; this protein transports iron from the intestinal tract (where iron is absorbed) and from mononuclear phagocytes (where iron is recovered from RBC breakdown) to the bone marrow, liver, and spleen (where extra iron is stored as ferritin and hemosiderin)
5. Only small amounts of iron are absorbed and excreted; intestinal mucosal cells closely control the body's iron absorption to ensure an adequate — but not excessive — iron supply
   a. Dietary iron absorption occurs principally in the duodenum; it is regulated by the iron content of the intestinal mucosal cells
   b. When iron stores are abundant, the mucosal cells contain ferritin, which inhibits their uptake of additional iron
   c. When iron stores are low, the mucosal cells absorb more iron, which enters the plasma and is carried by transferrin to the bone marrow and storage sites until it is needed for hemoglobin synthesis

6. The usual diet provides about 10 to 20 mg of iron daily
   a. Men absorb about 1 mg per day
   b. Women and children absorb slightly more

ALERT

      (1) Women require more iron to compensate for blood loss during menstruation and for fetal needs during pregnancy
      (2) Children require extra iron to synthesize hemoglobin during periods of growth when blood volume increases
7. Pregnancy, childhood growth, or chronic or excessive blood loss may deplete iron stores; because dietary iron intake may not be sufficient to compensate for this depletion, iron-deficiency anemia may result
8. Normally, iron from RBC breakdown is recycled to make new hemoglobin
9. One ml of blood contains approximately 0.5 mg of iron

E. Hemoglobin structure and formation
1. Hemoglobin is the oxygen-carrying protein formed in the cytoplasm of developing RBCs
2. It is composed of four monomers fitted together to form a tetramer, like the sections of an apple cut into quarters
3. Each monomer is a complex composed of the iron-containing compound heme and the protein globin
   a. Heme is constructed from four nitrogen-containing ring compounds called pyrrole rings
   b. These rings are joined to form a more complex ring structure called a porphyrin ring
4. An atom of iron, with six binding sites, occupies the central position of the porphyrin ring
   a. Nitrogen atoms bind to four of the sites on the porphyrin ring
   b. The amino acid histidine binds the globin chain to the iron at the fifth site
   c. The sixth binding site is available for reversible combination with oxygen
5. Globin forms the largest part of the hemoglobin monomer
   a. It is composed of an amino acid chain joined together to form a coiled polypeptide chain
   b. The heme is tucked into one of the bends in the globin coil and held there by the bond between the iron atom and histidine in the globin chain
6. Heme and globin are synthesized in different locations in the cell
   a. Transferrin brings iron to the erythroblast
   b. Once inside the mitochondria, iron is incorporated into the porphyrin ring to form heme (nearby reticuloendothelial cells remove excess iron that is not used in heme synthesis)

   c. At the same time, ribosomes in the cytoplasm produce globin chains
   d. The globin chains and heme join to form a hemoglobin monomer
   e. The four monomers aggregate to form the complete hemoglobin tetramer

F. Globin chains
1. The five types of globin chains — alpha, beta, gamma, delta, and epsilon — have different amino acid compositions
2. Globin chains are produced at different times and in different proportions, beginning in the embryonic period and extending into adult life
3. In most hemoglobin tetramers, two of the subunits contain one type of globin chain, and the other two subunits have a different globin chain
   a. Each of the four chains is combined with heme to form a hemoglobin monomer
   b. Four monomers aggregate to form a tetramer
4. Adults produce two types of hemoglobin
   a. In adults, about 98% of the hemoglobin consists of tetramers in which two subunits contain alpha chains and the other two contain beta chains; this is hemoglobin A, or adult hemoglobin
   b. The other 2% of hemoglobin consists of tetramers with alpha and delta chains; this is *hemoglobin* A_2
5. The embryo and fetus produce different hemoglobins
   a. The embryo initially produces hemoglobin that contains only epsilon chains
   b. The fetus soon replaces this tetramer with production of a tetramer that contains alpha and gamma chains; this is *hemoglobin F*, or fetal hemoglobin, which is the predominant hemoglobin in the fetus
   c. Late in the fetal period, the beta chains of adult hemoglobin are produced in small quantities
6. Fetal hemoglobin can take up and release oxygen at lower oxygen tensions than hemoglobin A; this is advantageous because the oxygen tension in the fetal blood is relatively low
7. After birth, hemoglobin production is characterized by declining gamma-chain synthesis and increasing beta-chain synthesis
   a. Hemoglobin F in the RBCs gradually declines
   b. Hemoglobin A rises correspondingly

ALERT

8. Genes control the globin chain structure by directing the order in which amino acids are incorporated into the chains; mutation of these genes can alter the amino acid sequence, causing hemoglobin abnormalities, such as sickle cell anemia

♦ III. White blood cells

A. General information
1. WBCs (leukocytes) are nucleated cells; they are less numerous than RBCs
2. Based on their structure, they are classified as granulocytes or agranulocytes
   a. *Granulocytes* contain cytoplasmic granules; they are subdivided into *neutrophils, eosinophils,* and *basophils*
   b. *Agranulocytes* lack cytoplasmic granules; they are subdivided into *lymphocytes* and *monocytes*
3. Normally, the WBC differential count (a percentage count of WBCs) is 40% to 60% neutrophils, 0% to 1% basophils, 1% to 3% eosinophils, 20% to 40% lymphocytes, and 4% to 8% monocytes
4. WBCs undergo maturation in the bone marrow
   a. WBC maturation is characterized by condensation of nuclear chromatins and an increase in cytoplasm
   b. Several types of WBCs develop different kinds of cytoplasmic granules and multilobed nuclei
5. Most WBCs have a short life span
   a. They circulate about 4 to 8 hours after they are released from the bone marrow; then they leave the circulation and enter the tissues
   b. They live another 4 to 5 days in various tissues
   c. The total life span may decrease to a few hours in an individual with a severe infection

B. Functions
1. Each type of WBC has specific functions (for details, see sections C through G)
2. Generally, WBCs participate in the inflammatory and immune responses
   a. They defend the body against viruses, bacteria, and other foreign particles

ALERT

   b. A WBC count above 11,000 per mm^3 signals viral or bacterial infection
3. WBCs use an amoeboid motion to move in and out of blood vessels and through tissue spaces

C. Neutrophils
1. Neutrophils (polymorphonuclear WBCs) have a segmented nucleus and a cytoplasm containing fine granules
2. Neutrophils are the most numerous WBCs, comprising about 65% of all WBCs; they are twice as large as RBCs

3. These cells are phagocytic and can destroy bacteria, viruses, and other foreign substances
4. Their numbers increase in response to infections

D. Eosinophils
1. Eosinophils contain large, bright red-staining (eosinophilic) granules
2. Eosinophils account for about 2% of all WBCs
3. Their major function is phagocytosis of antigen-antibody complexes; these complexes form in allergic reactions when antibodies combine with the antigens that triggered their release

ALERT

4. The number of eosinophils increases in many allergic conditions and in response to some parasitic infections

E. Basophils
1. Basophils contain dark purple (basophilic) granules
2. The least abundant type, they account for less than 1% of all WBCs; they are slightly larger than RBCs

ALERT

3. Basophils play an essential role in some allergic reactions
4. In a sensitized individual, specific antigens, such as penicillin and bee venom, cause basophils to rupture
   a. Basophil rupture releases large quantities of histamine, bradykinin, heparin, and some lysosomal enzymes
   b. These substances produce the tissue and vascular reactions that cause allergy signs and symptoms

F. Lymphocytes
1. Lymphocytes are small, mononuclear, nonphagocytic WBCs; they have a deep-staining nucleus that contains dense chromatin and a pale blue-staining cytoplasm
2. The second most abundant type of WBC, lymphocytes normally comprise about 30% of WBCs; however, they are more common in lymphoid tissues than in blood
3. Lymphocytes play a major role in the body's immune response (for details, see Chapter 12, Lymphatic System)
   a. *T lymphocytes* (thymus-dependent lymphocytes) act directly against infected cells and tumors
   b. *B lymphocytes* (bursa-dependent lymphocytes) give rise to plasma cells, which produce humoral antibodies called immunoglobulins
4. Lymphocytes can be divided into two groups based on their survival length
   a. One group has a short survival comparable to other WBCs
   b. The other lymphocyte group survives for several years; the cells in this group are known as memory cells

ALERT

5. Lymphocytes increase in number in response to some infections

G. Monocytes
   1. Monocytes are phagocytic cells that form part of the mononuclear phagocyte system
      a. They have a single, U-shaped nucleus
      b. They differentiate into macrophages, phagocytic cells that serve as the first line of defense against viruses, certain bacteria, and some chronic infections
   2. The largest WBCs, they account for about 3% of all WBCs
   3. They leave the blood stream and function as scavenger cells, cleaning up the debris after acute inflammation
   4. Monocytes also function as the body's chief defense against some chronic diseases, such as tuberculosis, and some systemic fungal infections
   5. They participate along with the lymphocytes in the body's immune response (for details, see Chapter 12, Lymphatic System)

♦ IV. Platelets

A. General information
   1. Named for their resemblance to small plates, platelets (thrombocytes) are small anucleated cells, about one-third the size of RBCs
   2. Like RBCs, platelets have no nucleus

B. Functions
   1. Platelets play an essential role in blood clotting and in plugging blood vessel breaks (for details, see "Hemostasis," below)

ALERT

   2. Inadequate platelet quantity or function can cause serious bleeding problems

C. Platelet life cycle
   1. Platelets are formed from large, multinucleated cells called *megakaryocytes* in the bone marrow
      a. Megakaryocytes are extremely large cells that develop from stem cells
      b. On the surface of megakaryocytes, platelets form as buds that pinch off to enter the circulation
      c. Blood normally contains 150,000 to 350,000 platelets per mm^3
   2. Platelets are motile and can store and release biochemicals and change shape
   3. Their life span is about 10 to 14 days

♦ V. Hemostasis

A. General information
   1. Hemostasis refers to stoppage of bleeding; the body arrests all bleeding as quickly as possible to prevent life-threatening hemorrhage

TEACHING TIPS

Patient with thrombocytopenia

Be sure to include the following topics when teaching a patient with thrombocytopenia.

- Explanation of platelets and their role in clotting
- Possible causes of thrombocytopenia
- Severity of thrombocytopenia
- Reportable signs and symptoms of bleeding and complications
- Platelet counts and other diagnostic tests
- Treatments, such as platelet infusion, immunosuppressive agents, and splenectomy
- Bleeding precautions and activity restrictions
- Sources of information and support

2. Blood vessels, platelets, and coagulation factors help blood to clot, which stops the bleeding
3. After the blood vessel has healed and the clot no longer is needed, it must be lysed (dissolved)
4. The body normally maintains a balance between clotting and clot FIBRINOLYSIS, which is controlled largely by substances that inhibit and activate clotting and lysis

B. Role of blood vessels and platelets

1. Blood vessels and platelets function together to prevent bleeding
2. Injury to a blood vessel causes it to constrict, narrowing its diameter and facilitating closure by a blood clot
3. Vessel injury also disrupts the endothelium and exposes the underlying connective tissue, stimulating platelets and coagulation factors to react
4. Platelets aggregate and adhere to the injury site
   a. They release vasoconstrictors, causing vessels to constrict further
   b. These platelets also release platelet phospholipid that initiates COAGULATION
5. Platelets also play an important role in preventing bleeding from capillaries
   a. Small breaks in capillaries occur frequently, but are sealed promptly by formation of a platelet plug rather than a blood clot

ALERT

   b. If the number of platelets is inadequate (thrombocytopenia) or if platelets do not function properly, pinpoint areas of bleeding (petechiae) develop in the skin and internal organs and may be followed by more serious bleeding (for teaching tips, see *Patient with thrombocytopenia*)

C. Coagulation factors
1. Coagulation factors are designated by name and Roman numeral (see *Coagulation factors,* page 180)
2. They circulate as precursor compounds and are activated during coagulation
3. Coagulation is a chain reaction in which each coagulation factor is activated in sequence and in turn activates the next coagulation factor in the chain

ALERT

4. Several coagulation factors are manufactured in the liver and require vitamin K for their synthesis; vitamin K deficiency can inhibit their synthesis and disrupt normal coagulation
5. All phases of coagulation require calcium ions; however, coagulation disturbances do not result from abnormally low blood calcium levels because a calcium level low enough to affect coagulation would be incompatible with life

D. Coagulation factor activation
1. Although the coagulation cascade is a continuous sequence, it can be divided into three phases for discussion purposes (see *Physiologic Process: Coagulation cascade,* page 181)
2. In phase 1, prothrombin activator forms
   a. Prothrombin activator is produced by two different mechanisms — the intrinsic system and the extrinsic system
   b. The intrinsic system is so named because all of its components come from the blood
      (1) Platelets accumulate at the injury site and release phospholipids, which interact with coagulation factors
      (2) The factors are activated in sequence to yield prothrombin activator
   c. In the extrinsic system, tissue injury liberates thromboplastin (factor III), which interacts with coagulation factors to produce factor X_a
      (1) The extrinsic system is so named because prothrombin activator is derived primarily from injured tissue rather than blood
      (2) This system requires about half the number of coagulation factors as the intrinsic system; it requires no platelets
3. Phase 2 involves conversion of prothrombin (factor II) to thrombin by prothrombin activator, which was formed in phase 1
   a. Prothrombin is a protein made in the liver
   b. Prothrombin activator splits prothrombin into fragments
   c. Fragmentation produces thrombin, a protein-digesting enzyme

Text continues on page 182.

Coagulation factors

Various factors perform vital functions in the coagulation process, as described in the chart below.

FACTOR NUMBER AND NAME	DESCRIPTION AND FUNCTION
I (fibrinogen)	High-molecular-weight protein synthesized in liver; converted to fibrin in phase 3 (a common phase)
II (prothrombin)	Protein synthesized in liver (requires vitamin K); converted to thrombin in phase 2 (a common phase)
III (tissue thromboplastin)	Factor released from damaged tissue; required in phase 1 of the extrinsic system
IV (calcium ions)	Factor required throughout the entire clotting sequence
V (proaccelerin, or labile factor)	Protein synthesized in liver; functions in phases 1 and 2 of the intrinsic and extrinsic systems
VII (serum prothrombin conversion accelerator, stable factor, or proconvertin)	Protein synthesized in liver (requires vitamin K); functions in phase 1 of the extrinsic system
VIII (antihemophilic factor, or antihemophilic globulin)	Protein synthesized in liver; required in phase 1 of the intrinsic system
IX (plasma thromboplastin component)	Protein synthesized in liver (requires vitamin K); required in phase 1 of the intrinsic system
X (Stuart factor or Stuart-Prower factor)	Protein synthesized in liver (requires vitamin K); required in phase 1 of the intrinsic and extrinsic systems
XI (plasma thromboplastin antecedent)	Protein synthesized in liver; required in phase 1 of the intrinsic system
XII (Hageman factor)	Protein required in phase 1 of the intrinsic system
XIII (fibrin stabilizing factor)	Protein required to stabilize the fibrin strands in phase 3

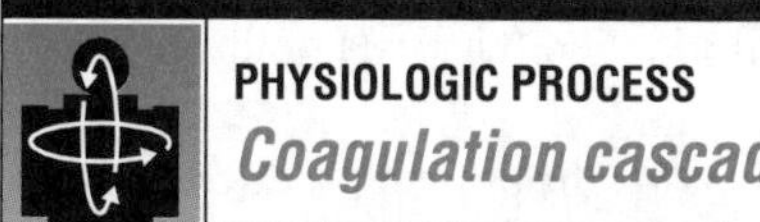

PHYSIOLOGIC PROCESS

Coagulation cascade

Via the intrinsic and extrinic systems, various factors interact and lead to coagulation. The role of calcium ions and platelets, also essential in the coagulation process, is not illustrated in this diagram.

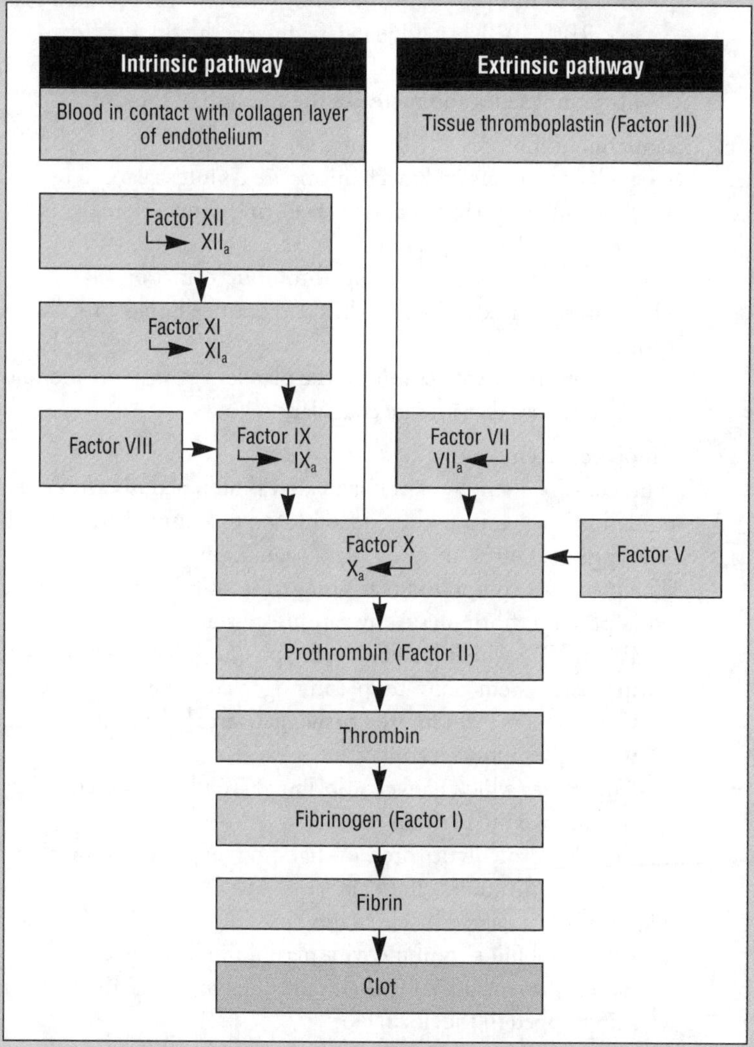

Intrinsic pathway

Blood in contact with collagen layer of endothelium

Factor XII → XII_a

Factor XI → XI_a

Factor VIII → Factor IX → IX_a

Extrinsic pathway

Tissue thromboplastin (Factor III)

Factor VII → VII_a

Factor X → X_a ← Factor V

Prothrombin (Factor II)

Thrombin

Fibrinogen (Factor I)

Fibrin

Clot

Adapted from Baer, C., and Williams, B. *Clinical Pharmacology and Nursing,* 3rd ed. Springhouse, Pa.: Springhouse Corp., 1996.

4. Phase 3 involves conversion of fibrinogen (factor 1) to fibrin by thrombin
   a. Fibrinogen is a high-molecular-weight protein produced by the liver
   b. Thrombin cleaves part of the fibrinogen molecule to form a smaller molecule, called a fibrin monomer
   c. Then fibrin monomers join end-to-end and cross link from side-to-side to form a meshwork of fibrin threads that contain plasma, RBCs, WBCs, and platelets; this meshwork is a clot
   d. Another plasma factor (XIII) strengthens the bonds between the fibrin molecules and increases the strength of the clot

E. Coagulation inhibition
   1. Coagulation factors and mechanisms are counterbalanced by inhibitors and anticoagulants that retard clotting, which prevents excessive intravascular coagulation
   2. Antithrombin in plasma inhibits thrombin formation
   3. Heparin, which exists in basophils and mast cells, has anticoagulant properties
   4. Prostaglandin derivatives inhibit the platelet aggregation and phospholipid release that initiate coagulation

F. Fibrinolytic system
   1. This clot-dissolving system is activated simultaneously with the coagulation mechanism; it restricts clotting to a limited area, thereby preventing excessive intravascular coagulation
   2. The precursor compound plasminogen (profibrinolysin) is converted to plasmin (fibrinolysin) by various substances
      a. Factor XII_a, which formed during phase 1 of coagulation by the intrinsic system, activates plasminogen conversion
      b. Components from injured tissues activate the extrinsic system as well as plasminogen conversion
      c. Thrombin, which converts fibrinogen to fibrin, also converts plasminogen to plasmin
   3. Plasmin is a proteolytic (protein-digesting) enzyme that breaks down the fibrin strands in the clot
   4. Plasmin is inactivated by circulating inhibitors called alpha globulins
      a. Alpha globulins combine with plasmin to form inactive complexes; this prevents unwanted clot breakdown by inactivating plasmin trapped in the fibrin clot
      b. These inhibitors also inactivate plasmin that diffuses from the coagulation sites; this prevents plasmin from attacking and degrading other clotting factors

♦ VI. Blood groups

A. General information
   1. The surface of RBCs contains antigens or agglutinogens (glycoproteins) that are inherited through Mendelian patterns; an *antigen* is a substance that stimulates formation of antibodies that can combine with the antigen
   2. When exposed to certain antibodies, these antigens cause reactions that are the basis for classifying blood groups (blood typing)
   3. Many different blood group systems have been described; the ABO and Rh systems are the most important

B. ABO blood group system
   1. The ABO group is identified by testing for A and B antigens on the RBC surface; each person's blood belongs to one of four groups — A, B, O, or AB
   2. RBCs are classified primarily by the presence or absence of A and B antigens on their surfaces and secondarily by the presence or absence of anti-A and anti-B antibodies in the serum
   3. Individuals normally have antibodies directed against antigens their RBCs lack
      a. Group A individuals (41% of the population) have A antigen on the RBCs and anti-B antibody in the serum
      b. Group B individuals (10% of the population) have B antigen on the RBCs and anti-A antibody in the serum
      c. Group O individuals (45% of the population) have no A or B antigens on the RBCs; they have anti-A and anti-B antibodies in the serum
         (1) Type O is the most common blood type among white Americans
         (2) Individuals with type O blood are called universal donors because their blood may be given to persons with any other ABO type
      d. Group AB individuals (4% of the population) have both A and B antigens on the RBCs and no anti-A or anti-B antibodies in the serum
         (1) AB is the rarest blood type
         (2) Individuals with type AB blood are called universal recipients because they may receive blood of any other ABO type
   4. ABO blood group (blood type) is determined by identifying the ABO antigens on the RBCs and the anti-A and anti-B antibodies in the serum
   5. Antigens are identified by mixing a sample of the RBCs with anti-A typing serum and another sample with anti-B typing serum; this ABO antigen typing is known as *direct typing*

  a. RBC clumping (AGGLUTINATION) in the typing serum determines the antigens
  b. For example, if the cells agglutinate with anti-A typing serum, but not anti-B typing serum, then the individual's RBCs contain the A antigen
6. Serum antibodies are determined by mixing one serum sample with a suspension of known group A test cells and another sample with a suspension of known group B test cells; this antibody typing is known as *reverse typing* and is used to confirm direct typing
  a. Test cell agglutination indicates the corresponding antibody in the serum
  b. For example, if the serum sample agglutinates group B test cells but not group A test cells, the serum contains only anti-B antibody
7. ABO antigens are determined genetically
  a. The gene locus on each chromosome may be occupied by an A, B, or O gene; these genes are transmitted to offspring by Mendelian inheritance patterns
    (1) An individual is homozygous for ABO genes if the alleles are the same on both chromosomes (AA, BB, or OO)
    (2) An individual is heterozygous if the genes are different (AO, BO, AB)
  b. The gene combination on the chromosomes determines the ABO *genotype*
  c. The blood type obtained by testing RBCs with anti-A and anti-B typing serum determines the ABO *phenotype*
    (1) A phenotype may include more than one genotype
    (2) For example, the phenotype B may represent genotype BB (homozygous) or BO (heterozygous)
  d. Because parents may transmit either allele to their offspring, an infant may not have the same ABO genotype or phenotype as either parent
    (1) For example, two heterozygous type A (AO) parents may produce a homozygous type A (AA), heterozygous type A (AO), or type O (OO) infant; the same pattern is true for two heterozygous type B (BO) parents
    (2) Two type AB parents may produce a homozygous type A (AA), homozygous type B (BB), or type AB infant
    (3) A heterozygous type A (AO) parent and a type AB parent can produce a homozygous type A (AA), heterozygous type A (AO), heterozygous type B (BO), or type AB infant

C. Rh blood group system
   1. In the Rh system, RBCs are classified according to a group of inherited antigens on their surface
   2. Scientists performed the original Rh studies by immunizing rabbits and guinea pigs with blood from rhesus monkeys
      a. The immunized animals formed anti-Rhesus antibodies that reacted not only with the rhesus monkey RBCs but with the RBCs of about 85% of white individuals and 95% of black individuals; those whose RBCs were agglutinated by the anti-Rhesus antibodies were called Rhesus-positive or simply Rh-positive
      b. Those whose RBCs did not react with the anti-Rhesus antibodies were called Rhesus-negative or Rh-negative

ALERT

   3. When exposed to Rh-positive blood by blood transfusion or pregnancy with an Rh-positive fetus, an Rh-negative individual may form anti-Rh antibodies
      a. Subsequent transfusion of Rh-positive blood to this individual leads to rapid destruction of the transfused cells (transfusion reaction)
      b. If a woman whose blood contains anti-Rh antibodies becomes pregnant with an Rh-positive fetus, the anti-Rh antibodies cross the placenta and destroy fetal RBCs, causing hemolytic disease of the newborn
   4. Although many genes and RBC antigens are involved in the Rh system, the Rh antigen described first is the most important clinically; it is called the D antigen or the Rh_o antigen (the subscript o stands for *original*)
      a. Of the eight types of Rh antigens, only C, D, and E are common
      b. Normally, blood contains the Rh antigen (in other words, it is Rh-positive and lacks anti-Rh antibodies)
   5. The gene D and its allele d determine the presence of D antigen on RBCs
   6. Individuals whose RBCs contain the D antigen (genotype DD or Dd) are considered Rh-positive (regardless of other Rh antigens on the RBCs); individuals who lack the D antigen (genotype dd) are considered Rh-negative
   7. An Rh-positive individual may be homozygous (DD) or heterozygous (Dd); the latter is more common
   8. Because each parent transmits one of two alleles to offspring, an infant may not have the same Rh genotype or phenotype as either parent
      a. Two heterozygous Rh-positive (Dd) parents may produce a homozygous Rh-positive (DD), heterozygous Rh-positive (Dd), or Rh-negative (dd) infant

b. A homozygous Rh-positive (DD) parent and a heterozygous Rh-positive (Dd) parent may produce a homozygous Rh-positive (DD) or heterozygous Rh-positive (Dd) infant
c. A heterozygous Rh-positive (Dd) parent and an Rh-negative (dd) parent may produce an Rh-positive (Dd) or Rh-negative (dd) infant

POINTS TO REMEMBER

- A type of connective tissue, blood consists of formed elements (RBCs, WBCs, and platelets) suspended in a viscous fluid called blood plasma.
- Blood performs transportation, regulation, and protection functions.
- In RBCs, hemoglobin carries oxygen to body tissues and brings carbon dioxide to the lungs for exhalation.
- Based on their structure, WBCs are classified as granulocytes (neutrophils, eosinophils, and basophils) and agranulocytes (lymphocytes and monocytes). Neutrophils are the most numerous WBCs, are phagocytic, and increase in number in response to infection. Lymphocytes also play a major role in the body's immune response.
- Blood vessels, platelets, and coagulation factors help blood to clot, which stops the bleeding. When the clot no longer is needed, it must be lysed (dissolved), which is done by fibrinolysis.
- The surface of RBCs contains antigens that cause reactions when exposed to certain antibodies. These reactions are the basis for typing blood in the ABO and Rh blood group systems.

STUDY QUESTIONS

To evaluate your understanding of this chapter, answer the following questions in the space provided. Then compare your responses with the correct answers in Appendix B, pages 331 and 332.

1. What are the eight functions of blood? ______________________

____

____

2. How are granulocytes different from agranulocytes? ______________________

____

____

3. Which process is responsible for producing seven types of blood cells?

____

____

4. What roles do hemoglobin and iron play in RBCs? ______________________

____

____

5. What are the general functions of the WBCs? ______________________

____

____

6. What role do platelets play in hemostasis? ______________________

____

____

7. How are the ABO and Rh blood groups similar? ______________________

____

____

Critical Thinking and Application Exercises

1. Write a one-page paper that explains the functions of blood.
2. Trace the process of hematopoiesis from one stem cell to all seven of the body's blood cells.
3. Prepare a chart that compares the five different types of WBCs.
4. Examine each type of blood cell under a microscope. Discuss your findings.
5. Contrast the factors that activate coagulation with those that inhibit it.
6. Review a case study of a transfusion reaction. Try to determine if the ABO or Rh blood group incompatibility was involved.

CHAPTER

12

Lymphatic System

Learning objectives

After studying this chapter, you should be able to:

- Name the tissue found in lymphatic system.
- Describe the functions, formation, and flow of lymph.
- Identify the lymphatic vessels and describe their functions.
- Discuss the formation of the T and B lymphocytes.
- Discuss the major mechanisms of nonspecific response to disease.
- Contrast nonspecific resistance and acquired immunity.
- Compare cell-mediated immunity and humoral immunity.
- Differentiate among the five types of immunoglobulins.

Chapter overview

The lymphatic system parallels the circulatory system, returning excess fluid and protein from interstitial fluid to the circulatory system. Perhaps more importantly, the lymphatic system provides several lines of defense against disease. Without a properly functioning lymphatic system, an injury as mild as a paper cut could be life-threatening. Because this system is so vital to homeostasis and immunity, the health care professional should be aware of its basic structures and functions.

♦ I. Lymph tissue

A. General information
   1. The *lymphatic system* consists of lymphocyte-containing (lymphoid) tissues, lymph, and a network of lymphatic vessels
   2. Lymph tissues are concentrated in the lymph nodes, spleen, and thymus; they also are present in the mucous membranes of the respiratory and gastrointestinal tracts
   3. All lymphoid tissues consist of reticular connective tissue and free cells (lymphocytes and macrophages)
   4. The lymphatic system provides circulatory and immune functions for the body

B. Function
   1. The lymphatic system functions as a second circulatory system
      a. Lymphatic vessels drain excess fluid from interstitial spaces and return it to the blood (for details, see Chapter 10, Cardiovascular System)
      b. Lymphatic vessels absorb fats from the gastrointestinal tract and transport them into the bloodstream
   2. Lymphatic tissue forms the cornerstone of the immune system

C. Lymph nodes
   1. *Lymph nodes* are small, bean-shaped structures composed of reticular connective tissue, lymphocytes, and sinuses
   2. The body contains hundreds of lymph nodes
      a. Many lymph nodes appear along the surface of the gastrointestinal tract
      b. Large clusters are found in the inguinal, axillary, and cervical regions
   3. Lymph nodes are located along lymphatic vessels, where they act as filters
   4. Each lymph node consists of a mass of lymphocytes supported by a meshwork of reticular fibers; it is enclosed by a fibrous capsule and divided into an outer cortex and inner medulla
      a. The outer cortex divides into the superficial and deep cortex
         (1) The superficial cortex contains follicles composed predominantly of B cells; in an immune response, the follicles expand and develop clusters of proliferating cells, called germinal centers
         (2) The interfollicular areas and deep cortex contain mostly T cells
      b. The inner medulla contains loosely arranged lymphocytes and scattered groups of mononuclear phagocytes derived from monocytes (for details on blood cell development, see Chapter 11, Hematologic System)

5. Lymph flows into the lymph node through afferent lymphatic vessels into a subcapsular sinus at the periphery of the node; lymph filters slowly through the node and is collected into efferent lymphatic channels, which drain from an indentation on the concave side (hilus) of the node
   a. As lymph flows through the node, mononuclear phagocytes filter out and destroy foreign substances
   b. They also interact with lymphocytes to generate an immune response

D. Spleen
1. The *spleen* is a dark red, ovoid, fist-sized structure in the left upper abdominal quadrant, located posterior and inferior to the stomach
2. The spleen filters antigens and other particles from the blood
3. It is surrounded by a dense fibrous capsule from which bands of connective tissue extend into its interior, which is called the splenic pulp
4. The pulp is divided into white pulp and red pulp
   a. White pulp is composed of compact masses of lymphocytes that surround branches of the splenic artery
   b. Red pulp consists of a network of blood-filled sinusoids, which are supported by a framework of reticular fibers and star-shaped mononuclear phagocytes; lymphocytes, plasma cells, and monocytes also appear in the framework
      (1) In the red pulp, pulp cords surround and separate the sinusoids
      (2) Long, narrow endothelial cells line the splenic sinusoids; they lie parallel to the long axis of the sinusoids and are supported by a fenestrated basement membrane
5. Blood enters the spleen in two ways
   a. Splenic blood flows from branches of the splenic arteries; some of it flows directly into the splenic sinusoids
   b. Most of it is discharged from branches of the splenic arteries directly into the pulp cords
      (1) Blood cells pass from the meshwork of cells and fibers between the pulp cords into the sinusoid lumens by squeezing through the long, slitlike openings between adjacent endothelial cells
      (2) This forces the blood to flow through the framework of reticular fibers, macrophages, and other cells before entering the sinusoids
6. The spleen performs several functions
   a. Splenic phagocytes engulf and break down worn-out red blood cells (RBCs); this action releases hemoglobin, which is broken

down into its components (for details, see Chapter 11, Hematologic System)

b. Splenic phagocytes also selectively retain and destroy damaged or abnormal RBCs and cells with a large amount of abnormal hemoglobin

c. The spleen filters out bacteria and other foreign substances that enter the blood stream; splenic phagocytes promptly remove these substances

d. Phagocytes also interact with lymphocytes to initiate an immune response

ALERT

7. Injury or disease may require spleen removal, which affects the body's defense mechanisms
   a. Bacteria elimination and antibody production are less efficient
   b. Consequently, the individual becomes susceptible to serious blood infections caused by various pathogenic organisms

E. Thymus
   1. The *thymus* is a double-lobed mass of lymphoid tissue located over the base of the heart in the mediastinum
   2. This organ helps develop T lymphocytes in the fetus and in the infant for a few months after birth; it has no function in the body's immune defenses after this time
   3. The thymus is a large structure in infants but gradually undergoes atrophy when its function is no longer required; only a remnant persists in adults

F. Other lymph tissues
   1. Other lymph tissues include the tonsils, adenoids, appendix, and Peyer's patches in the intestines
   2. These tissues are distributed in mucous membranes where they can intercept invading organisms or toxins before they can spread widely
      a. Tissues in the throat and pharynx (tonsils and adenoids) can intercept antigens that enter by the upper respiratory tract
      b. Tissues in the gastrointestinal tract (the appendix and Peyer's patches) can intercept antigens that attempt to enter via the gut

♦ II. Lymph

A. General information
   1. *Lymphatic fluid* or *lymph* is a transparent, colorless, alkaline fluid; it contains lymphocytes, interstitial fluid, and plasma proteins
   2. Lymph travels through lymphatic vessels to large ducts, where it empties into the subclavian vein

3. The osmotic pressure of lymph slightly exceeds that of plasma; consequently, fluid moves from blood into the interstitial space and ultimately into the lymphatic system

B. Functions
1. Lymph helps maintain homeostasis by conveying foreign substances (such as viruses and bacteria) that have entered the tissue fluids to the lymph nodes, where lymphocytes act on them
2. Lymph maintains the osmotic pressure of interstitial fluid by transporting protein that has leaked from the arteriolar ends of capillaries back to the bloodstream and plasma
3. Lymph also transports nutrients, such as fats, that are absorbed from the digestive tract

C. Formation and flow
1. More fluid seeps out of capillaries into interstitial fluid than is absorbed by the capillaries; the excess fluid, which totals about 3 L daily, forms lymph
2. Lymph flows from the lymphatic capillaries to lymphatic vessels to the thoracic duct or right lymphatic duct to the subclavian veins
3. Several mechanisms keep lymph flowing properly
   a. Skeletal muscle contractions compress lymphatic vessels, moving the lymph through them
   b. Lymphatic vessels use one-way valves to prevent lymph from flowing backward
   c. Respiratory movements produce a pressure gradient in the lymphatic system, forcing lymph to flow from the abdominal area to the thoracic area

♦ III. Lymphatic vessels

A. General information
1. Lymph tissues are connected by a complex network of lymphatic vessels, which are thin-walled drainage channels similar to veins
2. These vessels collect lymph and return it to the circulation
3. Small lymphatic channels converge to form larger vessels with valves that prevent reflex

B. Function
1. Lymphatic vessels carry lymph toward the heart, eventually emptying into the right or left subclavian vein
2. Beginning from the tiny lymphatic capillaries, lymph flows through progressively larger vessels until it reaches the thoracic duct (on the left side of the body) or the right lymphatic duct (on the right side of the body)
   a. The right lymphatic duct empties lymph from the upper right part of the body into the right subclavian vein; the duct joins

the venous circulation at the junction of the internal jugular vein and subclavian vein on the right side

b. The thoracic duct empties lymph from the rest of the body into the left subclavian vein; this duct joins the venous circulation at the junction of the internal jugular vein and subclavian vein on the left side

C. Lymphatic capillaries

1. Lymphatic capillaries are located throughout most of the body; they are not found in avascular tissue, bone marrow, central nervous system structures, or splenic pulp
2. Wider than blood capillaries, lymphatic capillaries allow interstitial fluid to flow in, but not out
   a. When interstitial fluid pressure exceeds the pressure in the lymphatic capillaries, their cells separate slightly to let fluid enter
   b. When their fluid pressure exceeds the interstitial fluid pressure, their cells cling together to prevent fluid from leaving the lymphatic capillaries
3. Anchoring filaments attach the lymphatic endothelium to surrounding tissues

ALERT

4. In edema, excess interstitial fluid causes the tissues to swell, which pulls on the anchoring filaments; this separates the lymphatic capillary cells further, allowing more fluid to enter the capillaries

♦ IV. Lymphocytes

A. General information

1. Lymphocytes are a type of white blood cell (WBC or leukocyte)
2. They develop from stem cells in the bone marrow, which differentiate into lymphocyte precursor cells (for details, see Chapter 11, Hematologic System)
3. The precursor cells develop into two types of lymphocytes — T lymphocytes and B lymphocytes; both types perform specific immune functions

B. Types

1. *T (thymus-dependent) lymphocytes* arise from precursor cells that migrate from the bone marrow to the thymus, where they undergo further differentiation
2. *B (bone marrow-dependent) lymphocytes* arise from precursor cells that continue to differentiate in the bone marrow
3. T and B lymphocytes migrate into the lymph nodes, spleen, and other lymph tissues, where they proliferate to form the mature lymphocytes that populate these lymph tissues

a. These lymphocytes do not remain permanently in a specific lymphatic organ; they continually recirculate between the blood and various lymphatic tissues and organs
b. About 70% of these circulating cells are T lymphocytes; most of the remainder are B lymphocytes
4. A small proportion of lymphocytes are called *null cells*
a. Null cells cannot be classified as B or T lymphocytes
b. They are hematopoietic stem cells and may include B- and T-lymphocyte precursors and precursor, myeloid, and platelet cells
c. Null cells can destroy tumor cells spontaneously or through an antibody-dependent cellular cytotoxic mechanism

C. Functions
1. B lymphocytes have distinct initial and ultimate functions
a. Initially, they synthesize and insert antibodies on their surface
b. When mature, B lymphocytes produce humoral immunity
(1) Their plasma cells secrete antibodies
(2) Their memory cells become plasma cells during subsequent exposure to an antigen
2. T lymphocytes also have initial and ultimate functions
a. Initially, they seek, recognize, and attach to antigens that fit their surface receptors
b. Later, they produce cell-mediated immunity

♦ V. Nonspecific resistance to disease

A. General information
1. The body has two mechanisms to protect itself against microorganisms and other potentially harmful substances
2. The first is a group of general protective mechanisms that function without prior exposure to harmful agents; these mechanisms provide *nonspecific resistance*
a. Resistance refers to the body's ability to fend off disease; susceptibility refers to lack of resistance
b. Nonspecific resistance wards off a wide range of pathogens, using a variety of physiologic responses
c. It includes factors in the skin and mucous membranes, antimicrobial substances, phagocytosis, inflammation, and fever
3. The second mechanism depends on the lymphatic system and provides acquired IMMUNITY

B. Skin and mucous membranes
1. The skin and mucous membranes provide mechanical and chemical protection from invading organisms
2. Mechanical protection occurs in several ways

   a. Intact skin resists invasion by organisms by preventing their attachment; skin desquamation and low pH further impede bacterial colonization
   b. Mucus in the respiratory and other tracts traps bacteria and other foreign substances
   c. Body fluids, such as tears, saliva, urine, and vaginal secretions, help wash away or dilute microorganisms
3. Chemical protection typically results from body secretions
   a. Gastric acid secretions and digestive enzymes destroy organisms swallowed into the stomach
   b. Chemical compounds in the blood attach to and destroy foreign substances or toxins
      (1) The enzyme lysozyme, which is present in tears, nasal secretions, perspiration, and saliva, acts as an antibacterial agent
      (2) Basic polypeptides inactivate certain gram-positive bacteria
      (3) The serum protein properdin destroys gram-negative bacteria
   c. Sebaceous gland secretions, which are slightly acidic, discourage bacterial growth

C. Antimicrobial substances
1. Antimicrobial substances include interferon and the COMPLEMENT SYSTEM, which provide a second line of defense when organisms penetrate the skin and mucous membranes.
2. In response to viral infection, lymphocytes, macrophages, and fibroblasts produce proteins called interferons
   a. Interferons bind to surface receptors on uninfected neighboring cells
   b. This causes the uninfected cells to synthesize antiviral proteins, which inhibit viral replication
3. The complement system is a group of about 20 proteins in blood plasma and on cell membranes
   a. Normally, these proteins are inactive
   b. When activated, they enhance certain immune, allergic, and inflammatory reactions

D. Phagocytosis
1. Phagocytosis refers to the ingestion of organisms or foreign substances by cells called phagocytes
2. Granulocytes (neutrophils, eosinophils, and basophils) and macrophages perform phagocytosis
3. Phagocytosis occurs in three phases: chemotaxis, adherence, and ingestion
   a. During CHEMOTAXIS (movement toward a chemical stimulus), phagocytes are attracted to the invasion site by chemicals, such as microbial products and activated complement proteins

b. During adherence, the phagocyte's cell membrane attaches to the organism's surface
c. During ingestion, the phagocyte's cell membrane extends projections, called pseudopods, that engulf the organism; then the pseudopods fuse and surround it in a phagocytic vesicle

4. After ingestion, the phagocyte releases chemicals that kill organisms

E. Inflammation

1. The *inflammatory response* (a nonspecific reaction to any harmful agent) mobilizes WBCs to engulf and destroy bacteria and other foreign substances
   a. After organisms invade, tissue injury leads to release of histamine, kinins, and prostaglandins, which cause vasodilation and increased capillary permeability
   b. This increases blood flow to the affected tissues, where fluid collects
   c. Neutrophils and other WBCs are attracted to the invasion site
   d. These cells engulf and destroy the organisms, foreign substances, and debris

ALERT

2. Inflammation usually causes redness, pain, heat, and swelling; it also may produce loss of function in the affected area, depending on the site and degree of the damage
3. Inflammation helps remove organisms, toxins, and foreign substances from the affected site; inhibits their spread; and prepares the site for tissue repair

F. Fever

1. Fever intensifies the effects of interferons
2. It also prevents the growth of some organisms and hastens tissue repair

♦ VI. Immunity

A. General information

1. The lymphatic system provides acquired immunity
2. Acquired immunity consists of specific immune responses directed against specific organisms or toxins
3. These responses usually require previous exposure to a foreign substance and cause antibody formation or lymphatic activation

B. Types of immunity

1. Two types of acquired immunity exist — cell-mediated immunity and humoral immunity
2. Both types provide immunity against specific invading agents, such as viruses, bacteria, toxins, and other foreign substances
   a. Cell-mediated immune functions are carried out by T lymphocytes

(1) They require formation of large numbers of sensitized lymphocytes

(2) After phagocytic cells (macrophages) present processed antigens to the lymphocytes, the T lymphocytes are sensitized by the antigens and become capable of destroying them on subsequent exposure

b. Humoral immune functions are carried out by B lymphocytes

(1) They require formation of *antibodies* (immunoglobulins formed in response to a specific antigen)

(2) After macrophages present processed antigens to the lymphocytes, the B lymphocytes differentiate into plasma cells that produce antibodies

c. Both types of immunity interact to protect the body against invading antigens

(1) Some B and T lymphocytes retain a memory of the sensitizing antigen, which they pass on to succeeding generations of lymphocytes

(2) Later contact with this antigen leads to rapid proliferation of sensitized lymphocytes or antibody-forming plasma cells

C. Antigens and antibodies

1. Acquired immunity develops after the first invasion by a foreign organism or first contact with a toxin

a. Each toxin or type of organism contains specific chemical compounds that make it different from all other substances

b. These compounds, called *antigens,* cause acquired immunity; they usually are high-molecular-weight proteins, polysaccharides, or lipids

2. The initial phase of the immune response involves macrophage and lymphocyte interaction; both types of cells are distributed widely throughout the body and can respond to a foreign substance wherever they encounter it (see *Physiologic process: Immune response,* page 198)

a. Macrophages ingest the foreign material, process its antigens, and present the processed material the lymphocytes

b. The lymphocytes respond and transform into antibody-forming plasma cells and sensitized lymphocytes, respectively, which proliferate rapidly to perform immune functions

3. After initial contact with an antigen, several weeks are required for macrophages to process the antigen and for lymphocytes to respond

4. Once the body has reacted to the antigen, some lymphocytes (called *memory cells)* retain the ability to respond promptly to the same antigen on subsequent exposure; successive generations of lymphocytes derived from these memory cells also retain this ability

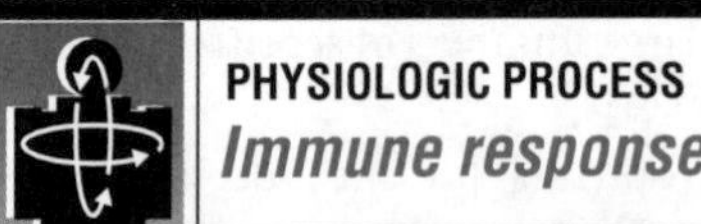

PHYSIOLOGIC PROCESS
Immune response

When foreign substances invade the body, humoral and cell-mediated immunity can come to the body's defense. Both types of immunity involve lymphocytes that share a common origin in stem cells of the bone marrow. These lymphocytes undergo differential development to become B cells and T cells. The following chart shows how these cells evolve to perform their immune functions.

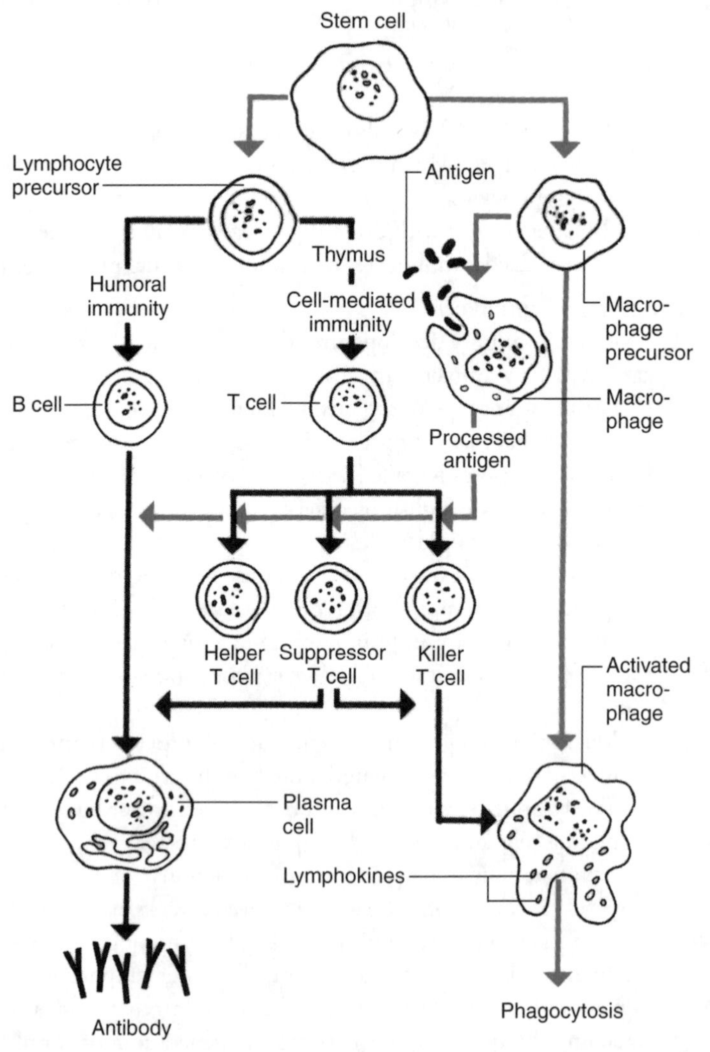

Stem cell
Lymphocyte precursor
Antigen
Thymus
Humoral immunity
Cell-mediated immunity
Macrophage precursor
B cell
T cell
Macrophage
Processed antigen
Helper T cell
Suppressor T cell
Killer T cell
Activated macrophage
Plasma cell
Lymphokines
Antibody
Phagocytosis

a. Subsequent contact with the sensitizing antigen provokes a renewed immune response
b. This response is rapid because earlier exposure to the antigen has primed the immune system

5. The ability to generate an immune response is controlled genetically; immune-response genes regulate T- and B-lymphocyte proliferation

♦ VII. Cell-mediated immunity

A. General information

1. Cell-mediated immunity results from the function of sensitized T lymphocytes
2. Cell-mediated immunity is the main defense against viruses, fungi, parasites, and some bacteria

ALERT

3. Cell-mediated immunity also eliminates abnormal cells that may arise during cell division; these cells can develop into tumors if not destroyed
4. This mechanism also causes organ transplant rejection
5. Cell-mediated immunity commonly is associated with hypersensitivity to bacterial antigens or other foreign substances; this reaction is characterized by an intense inflammatory reaction at the site of contact with the foreign substance

B. Cell-mediated immune response

1. Three types of sensitized T lymphocytes perform specific functions in cell-mediated immune response: *cytotoxic T cells, helper T cells,* and *suppressor T cells*
2. Also called killer cells, cytotoxic T cells directly kill organisms or other invading cells
   a. Cytotoxic T cells bind tightly to the invading cell, swell, and release cytotoxic substances directly into the attacked cell
   b. These cells can attack and kill many organisms in succession, without being harmed
3. Helper T cells interact with other T and B lymphocytes to enhance the immune response
   a. When activated, helper T cells secrete lymphokines, which increase activation of B cells, cytotoxic T cells, and suppressor T cells by antigens
   b. They attract macrophages and promote more efficient phagocytosis
4. Suppressor T cells inhibit the immune response
   a. They suppress the actions of cytotoxic and helper T cells
   b. This regulates the other T cells, preventing them from causing excessive immune reactions and severe tissue damage

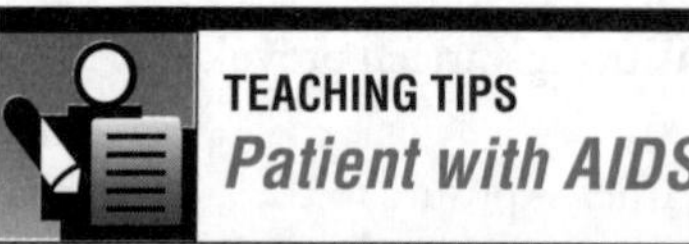

TEACHING TIPS

Patient with AIDS

Be sure to include the following topics when teaching a patient with acquired immunodeficiency syndrome (AIDS).

- Effects of human immunodeficiency virus on the immune response
- Opportunistic infections, cancer, and other disorders associated with AIDS
- Diagnostic criteria for AIDS
- Diagnostic tests, such as Western blot and helper T-cell count
- Activity modifications, include adequate rest and moderate exercise
- Adequate nutrition to prevent opportunistic infections
- Techniques for preventing infection
- Drug therapy, such as zidovudine, cotrimoxazole, and pentamidine
- Safe sex practices, including condom use
- Sources of information and support

5. Sensitized T lymphocytes are classified into two major groups according to specific antigens on their membranes
   a. One group, the CD4 lymphocytes, are the helper T cells; they account for about 70% of the T cells
   b. The other group, the CD8 lymphocytes, consists of the suppressor and cytotoxic T cells; they account for about 30% of all T cells
   c. A normal ratio of CD4 to CD8 lymphocytes (which reflects the normal proportions of helper to suppressor and cytotoxic T cells) is essential for proper immune function

ALERT

   (1) Loss or destruction of helper T cells (as in acquired immunodeficiency syndrome [AIDS]) leads to a relative excess of suppressor T cells, inhibiting the immune response and increasing susceptibility to infection (for teaching tips, see *Patient with AIDS*)
   (2) A relative lack of suppressor T cells allows the immune system to respond unchecked, increasing the likelihood of autoimmune disease in which the immune defenses attack the body's own cells and tissues

♦ VIII. Humoral immunity

A. General information
   1. Humoral immunity results from B lymphocyte function
   2. Humoral immunity forms the major defense against many bacteria and bacterial toxins

3. In response to antigen stimulation, B lymphocytes differentiate into plasma cells; these plasma cells produce antibodies (immunoglobulins) that can combine with and eliminate the foreign substance

B. Antibody mechanisms of action
1. Antibodies act by direct attack on the invader or by activating the complement system, which destroys the invader
2. Antibodies can directly inactivate an invader in one of four ways
   a. Through *agglutination,* antibodies can cause clumping of multiple large structures with antigens on their surfaces, such as red blood cells or bacteria
   b. Through *precipitation,* antibodies produce an antigen-antibody complex so large that it is insoluble and precipitates; tetanus toxin is a soluble antigen that is susceptible to precipitation
   c. Through *neutralization,* antibodies cover the toxic sites on an antigen
   d. Through *lysis,* potent antibodies attack the cell membrane of an antigen, causing it to rupture; this process requires complement activation
3. The complement system augments the effects of the direct actions of antibodies
   a. Exposure to an antigen activates the complement system, triggering a complex cascade of sequential reactions
   b. The cascade ultimately produces many end-products
   c. Some of the end-products help prevent antigen-induced damage by causing certain effects
      (1) Some end-products increase phagocytosis through OPSONIZATION, which can increase bacteria destruction by many hundredfold
      (2) The end-product, called lytic complex, directly causes cell *lysis* by rupturing the membrane of bacteria and other organisms
      (3) Some end-products cause invading organisms to adhere to each other by altering their surfaces; this produces agglutination
      (4) Enzymes and other end-products can neutralize viruses by attacking their structures
      (5) By causing chemotaxis, one end-product attracts many neutrophils and macrophages to the area affected by the antigen

C. Immunoglobulins
1. Immunoglobulins are proteins produced by the plasma cells derived from B lymphocytes
2. Immunoglobulins differ in chemical composition, molecular weight, and size, but they all have the same basic structure: two

matched pairs of polypeptide (protein) chains bound together by chemical bonds

3. The chains are arranged to resemble a fork with four tines
   a. The two central chains, called heavy chains, form the handle and inner tines of the fork
   b. The two outer chains, called light chains, form the outer tines of the fork
   c. The open end of each tine is different for each immunoglobulin; this variable part gives the immunoglobulin its specificity (ability to respond to a particular antigen)
   d. The handle end is the constant part of the immunoglobulin; it is the same in every immunoglobulin
   e. The constant part does not combine with an antigen; however, it determines other properties of the immunoglobulin, such as its ability to activate complement and attach to the surface of an antigen's cell membrane
4. All immunoglobulins are composed of the same basic four-chain units, but some aggregate to form clusters of two, three, or five units
5. Five types of antibodies exist: immunoglobulin M (IgM), immunoglobulin G (IgG), immunoglobulin A (IgA), immunoglobulin D (IgD), and immunoglobulin E (IgE)
   a. IgM is the largest antibody molecule
      (1) Each molecule is an aggregate of five basic immunoglobulin units
      (2) It commonly is called a macroglobulin because of its large size and high molecular weight
      (3) It is particularly efficient in combining with large particulate antigens
   b. IgG is the principal immunoglobulin molecule formed in response to most infectious agents
      (1) Each molecule is composed of a single basic immunoglobulin unit
      (2) It combines with antigens and activates complement
   c. IgA is produced by antibody-forming cells in the respiratory system, gastrointestinal tract, and other mucous membranes
      (1) It appears in secretions
      (2) IgA is an aggregate of two basic immunoglobulin units
      (3) It combines with potentially harmful ingested or inhaled antigens, preventing their absorption
   d. IgD coats the surface of B lymphocytes
      (1) It is composed of one basic immunoglobulin unit
      (2) Its prongs (antigen-binding sites) can attach antigens to the surface of B lymphocytes, stimulating them to produce antibodies

TEACHING TIPS
Patient with anaphylaxis

Be sure to include the following topics when teaching a patient with anaphylaxis.
- Causes, signs, and symptoms of anaphylaxis
- Complications of anaphylaxis, include respiratory failure and cardiovascular collapse
- Skin testing and elimination diet to identify allergens
- Importance of immediate treatment after reexposure to allergen
- Use of an anaphylaxis kit
- Application of a tourniquet
- Avoidance of known allergens
- Use of medical identification, such as a bracelet
- Sources of information and support

e. IgE usually is present in small amounts in the blood of most persons; it is composed of a single immunoglobulin unit and appears in much larger amounts in the blood of allergic individuals

ALERT

D. Allergic reaction

1. Some individuals form specific IgE antibodies (become allergic) to ragweed, plant pollens, and other substances that do not affect most people (see *Physiologic process: Allergic response,* page 204)
   a. The allergy-prone individual is called atopic
   b. The sensitizing antigen is called an allergen
2. The primary response begins with the initial exposure to an antigen; it ends with sensitization of mast cells
   a. The handle end of IgE attaches to the membrane of mast cells and basophils
   b. The tine ends project from the cell membrane
3. The secondary response begins with reexposure to the sensitizing antigen
   a. Reexposure causes the antigen to fix to the antigen-combining sites on the projecting ends of the IgE molecules
   b. This event triggers basophil and mast cell granules to release histamine and other chemicals; because these chemicals incite an inflammatory reaction, they are called mediators of inflammation

ALERT

4. Histamine and other chemicals typically produce allergic manifestations, such as sneezing, stuffy nose, and itchy eyes
5. A more severe allergic reaction, called *anaphylaxis*, can be life-threatening, causing acute respiratory failure and vascular collapse (for teaching tips, see *Patient with anaphylaxis*)

PHYSIOLOGIC PROCESS

Allergic response

An allergen is an antigen that triggers an allergic response. The first exposure to an allergen causes lymphocytes and plasma cells to produce specific immunoglobulin E (IgE) antibodies, which bind to mast cells and basophils. Subsequent exposure to this allergen leads to antigen-antibody interaction, causing mast cells and basophils to release histamine and other mediators. These mediators produce allergic manifestations.

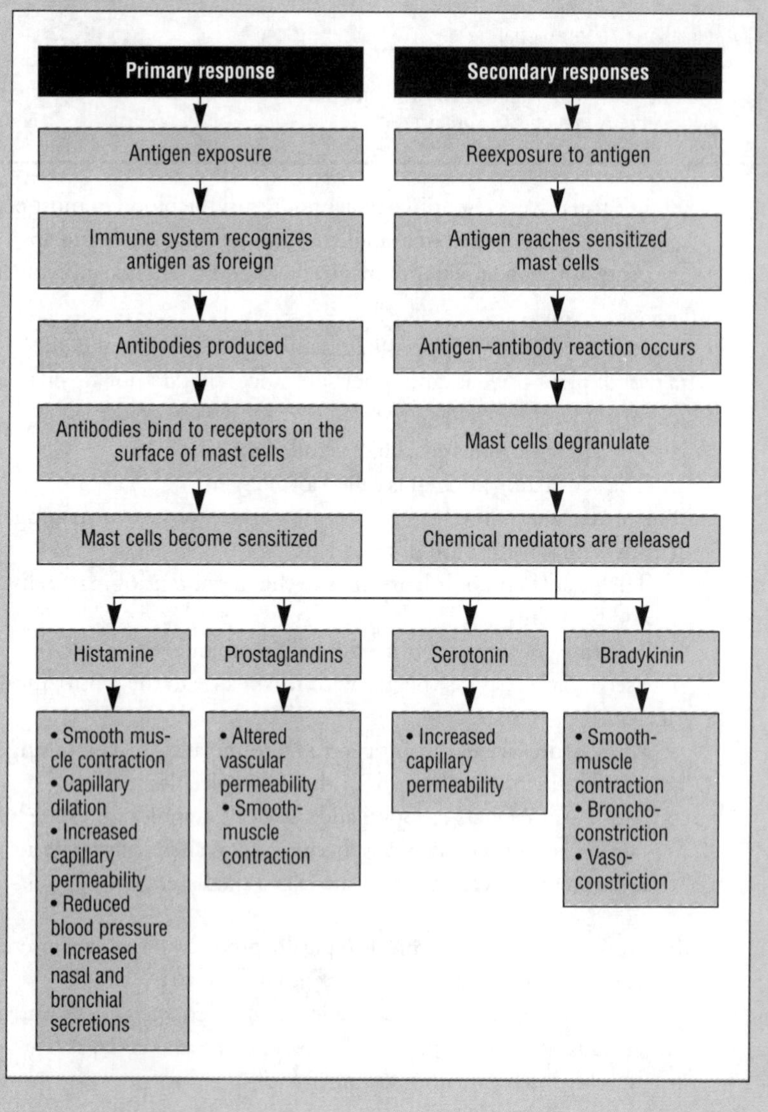

POINTS TO REMEMBER

- Lymph tissues include the lymph nodes, spleen, thymus, tonsils, adenoids, appendix, and Peyer's patches.
- Lymph carries foreign substances that have entered the tissue fluids to the lymph nodes, where lymphocytes act on them.
- Lymphatic vessels collect lymph and return it to the circulation. Beginning from the tiny lymphatic capillaries, lymph flows through progressively larger vessels until it reaches the subclavian vein.
- The two types of lymphocytes — T lymphocytes and B lymphocytes — perform specific immune functions.
- Nonspecific resistance provides general protection against harmful agents, without prior exposure to them. It occurs through factors in the skin and mucous membranes, antimicrobial substances, phagocytosis, inflammation, and fever.
- Acquired immunity consists of specific immune responses directed against specific organisms or toxins. These responses usually require previous exposure to a foreign substance and cause antibody formation (humoral immunity) or lymphatic activation (cell-mediated immunity).
- Cell-mediated immunity, which relies on sensitized T lymphocytes, is the main defense against viruses, fungi, parasites, and some bacteria.
- Humoral immunity, which relies on B lymphocyte function, forms the major defense against many bacteria and bacterial toxins.

STUDY QUESTIONS

To evaluate your understanding of this chapter, answer the following questions in the space provided. Then compare your responses with the correct answers in Appendix B, page 332.

1. What are the major lymph tissues? ______________________________

____

____

2. What are the functions of lymph? ______________________________

____

____

3. Where are T and B lymphocytes formed? ______________________

____

____

4. Through what mechanisms does the body maintain nonspecific resistance?

____

____

5. How does the body obtain acquired immunity?______________________

____

____

6. What role do T lymphocytes play in cell-mediated immunity?___________

____

____

7. What are the causes and effects of an allergic response? ______________

____

____

CRITICAL THINKING AND APPLICATION EXERCISES

1. On an illustration, locate the lymph tissues and explain their functions.
2. On a poster of the circulatory and lymphatic systems, trace the flow of lymph from the capillaries to the subclavian vein.
3. Observe T lymphocytes and B lymphocytes under a microscope and describe your findings.
4. Diagram the process of phagocytosis.
5. Prepare a chart that compares cell-mediated immunity to humoral immunity.

CHAPTER

13

Respiratory System

Learning objectives

After studying this chapter, you should be able to:

- ♦ Describe the structures and functions of the respiratory system.
- ♦ Discuss the importance of negative intrapleural pressure.
- ♦ Contrast the various pulmonary volumes and capacities.
- ♦ Explain how the partial pressure of a gas relates to its concentration in a gas mixture.
- ♦ Compare the concentrations of oxygen and carbon dioxide in inspired (atmospheric), alveolar, and expired air.
- ♦ Explain how oxygen is transferred from the lungs to the tissues and how carbon dioxide is transferred from the tissues to the lungs.

Chapter overview

Working with the cardiovascular system, the respiratory system ensures that tissues receive sufficient oxygen and that carbon dioxide is removed promptly. To maintain homeostasis, it must perform this gas exchange under widely varying external conditions and internal demands. Every body cell needs oxygen. Without it, death would occur within minutes. Therefore, the health care professional must be familiar with the respiratory system and be prepared to maintain it as needed.

♦ I. Airway

A. General information
   1. The chief function of the respiratory system is to supply body tissues with oxygen and eliminate carbon dioxide
   2. The respiratory system consists of upper and lower airways and the lungs (see *Structures of the respiratory tract*)
      a. *Upper airways* include the nose, pharynx, and larynx
      b. *Lower airways* include the trachea and bronchi, which lead to the lungs
   3. *Respiration* consists of two processes
      a. VENTILATION refers to air movement through the respiratory passages to and from the lungs
      b. GAS EXCHANGE refers to oxygen and carbon dioxide transport between the pulmonary alveoli and the blood in the pulmonary capillaries
      c. Both processes must function properly to achieve adequate tissue oxygenation and efficient carbon dioxide elimination

B. Nose
   1. The *nose* is formed superiorly by the nasal and frontal bones, laterally by the maxillary bones, and inferiorly by movable plates of HYALINE CARTILAGE (lateral and alar plates)
   2. It is the usual site of inspiration (inhalation) and expiration (exhalation)
   3. The nose filters, warms, and moistens air inspired through the nostrils; it connects to the pharynx
   4. The nose has two *nasal cavities,* which open on the face through the anterior nasal apertures (nares); the nasal septum separates the cavities
      a. The anterior portion of the nasal septum is composed of hyaline cartilage
      b. The posterior portion is composed of a flat bone called the vomer and the perpendicular plate of the ethmoid bone
   5. Posteriorly, the nasal cavities join the pharynx through the internal nares (choanae)
   6. Each nasal cavity has three mucosa-covered passageways, called the superior, middle, and inferior conchae
   7. The nasal cavities are lined with hairs that trap dust and foreign particles before they reach the lungs
      a. Epithelial cells lining the nasal cavities secrete mucus, which collects foreign particles
      b. Ciliated cells of the nasal mucosa move mucus toward the pharynx, where it can be removed by swallowing, sneezing, or spitting

Structures of the respiratory tract

This illustration shows the main structures of the respiratory tract.

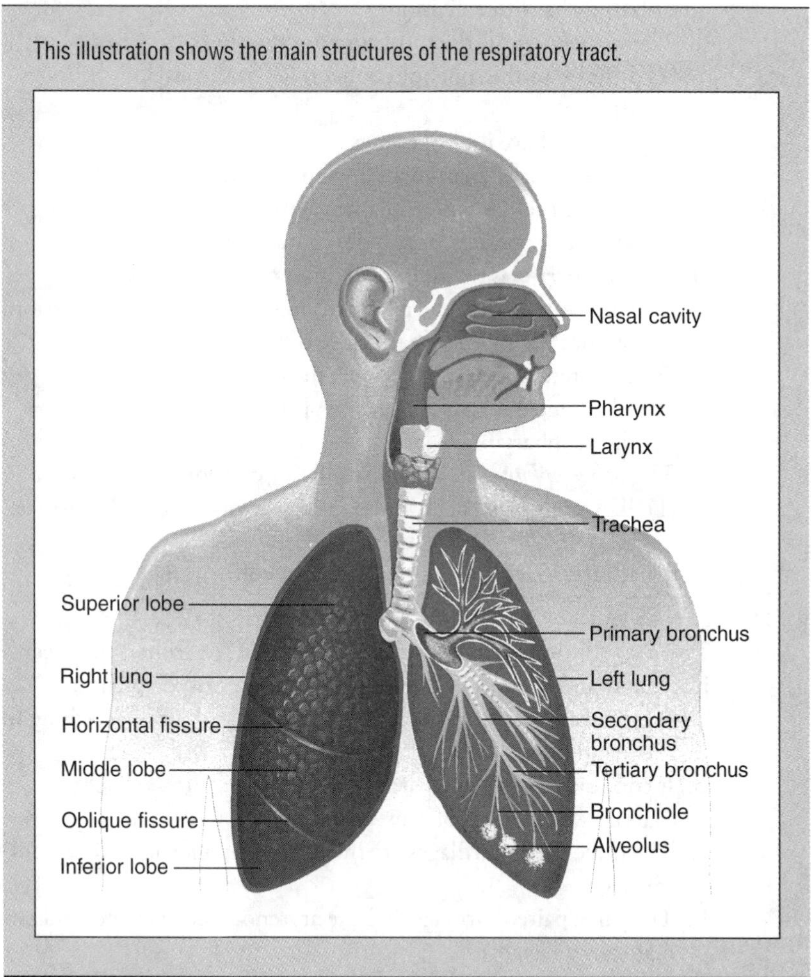

8. The *paranasal sinuses,* which surround and drain into the nasal cavities, are located in the frontal, sphenoid, and maxillary bones

C. Pharynx

1. The *pharynx* is a cavity that extends from the base of the skull to the esophagus (at the sixth cervical vertebra)
2. It acts as a passageway for air entering the nose and for food entering the gastrointestinal tract; it also functions in speech, changing shape to allow phonation of vowel sounds
3. It extends down from the juncture of the nasal and oral cavities and splits into the larynx and the esophagus

4. The entire pharynx is composed of striated muscle and lined with mucous membrane
5. The pharynx has three divisions
   a. The *nasopharynx* is the most superior division
      (1) Inferior to the sphenoid bone, it lies at the level of the soft palate
      (2) Its walls have four openings
         (a) The eustachian tubes open out of the lateral walls to enter the middle ear (tympanic cavity)
         (b) Two openings lead to the posterior nares
   b. The *oropharynx* is the middle division of the pharynx
      (1) Continuous with the posterior oral cavity, it extends inferiorly from the soft palate to the hyoid bone
      (2) Its anterolateral walls support the palatine tonsils
      (3) The lingual tonsils at the base of the tongue protrude into the oropharynx
   c. The *laryngopharynx* is the most inferior division of the pharynx
      (1) It extends from the hyoid bone to the opening of the esophagus
      (2) It is lined with stratified squamous epithelium

D. Larynx

1. The *larynx* (voice box) is a triangular organ in the front of the neck, just below and in front of the most inferior part of the pharynx
   a. It extends from the fourth to sixth cervical vertebrae, attaching to the hyoid bone
   b. It connects the inferior part of the pharynx with the trachea
2. The larynx is composed of muscle and numerous cartilages
   a. The three single cartilages are the cricoid, epiglottic, and thyroid cartilages
   b. The three paired cartilages are the arytenoid, corniculate, and cuneiform cartilages
   c. Ligaments connect all the cartilages
3. The *true vocal cords* are a pair of horizontal folds that project into the laryngeal cavity; they are separated by a space called the *glottis*
4. The main function of the larynx is to provide a permanent airway to the lungs
   a. The epiglottis, which overhangs the larynx, prevents food from entering the lungs
   b. The glottis and vocal cords serve as the phonation apparatus; vibration of the vocal cords by expired air causes the sounds made in phonation

E. Trachea

1. The *trachea* (windpipe) is a membranous tube that measures 4" to 5" (10 to 12.5 cm) long; located anterior to the esophagus, it extends from the larynx at the level of the sixth cervical vertebra to the upper border of the fifth thoracic vertebra
   a. On entering the MEDIASTINUM, the trachea branches into the right and left main bronchi at the fifth thoracic vertebrae
   b. Dorsally, the trachea contacts the esophagus
2. The trachea serves as an open passageway through which air enters the lungs
3. A series of C-shaped cartilage rings strengthens the trachea and prevents it from collapsing during inspiration
4. The trachea is lined with ciliated PSEUDOSTRATIFIED COLUMNAR EPITHELIUM containing mucus-secreting goblet cells, which trap and propel inhaled debris upward to the pharynx for removal through coughing

F. Bronchi

1. The right and left *primary bronchi* are the two larger air passages of the lungs; they branch from the trachea
2. The *secondary bronchi* are smaller passageways that branch from the primary bronchi
   a. The right primary bronchus divides into three secondary bronchi
   b. The left primary bronchus divides into two secondary bronchi
3. The secondary bronchi branch into *tertiary bronchi,* which, in turn, branch into increasingly smaller *bronchioles* (see *Bronchioles and alveoli,* page 212)
4. Along with the trachea, the bronchi and their branches constitute the *bronchial tree*

ALERT

5. The main function of the bronchi is to distribute air to the lungs
   a. Some disorders, such as asthma, cause bronchoconstriction (partial or complete closure of bronchi and bronchioles), which typically produces dyspnea, wheezing, and coughing (for teaching tips, see *Patient with asthma,* page 213)
   b. Bronchitis (inflammation of the bronchi) can result from a cold or other respiratory tract infection

♦ II. Lungs

A. General information

1. The *lungs* are paired, cone-shaped organs that fill the pleural divisions of the thoracic cavity; they extend from the root of the neck to the diaphragm
2. The lungs are the main component of the respiratory system, distributing air and exchanging gases

Bronchioles and alveoli

This illustration shows the bronchioles branching into progressively smaller tubes that eventually become alveolar ducts. These ducts terminate in clusters called alveoli. The alveoli are the basic functional units of the respiratory system and the site of gas exchange (exchange of oxygen and carbon dioxide) between the lungs and the bronchi.

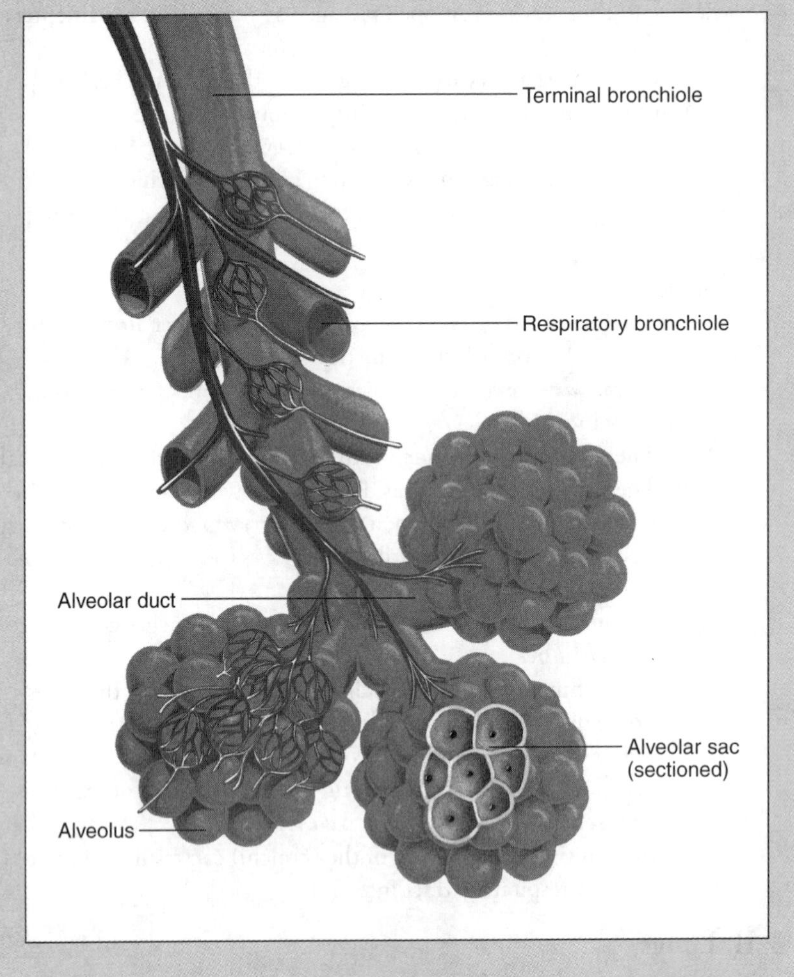

3. The right and left lungs are separated by the mediastinum, which contains the heart, blood vessels, and other midline structures; fissures divide each lung into lobes
4. Each primary bronchus enters its respective lung at the *hilus,* an indentation on the mediastinal surface; the bronchi and pulmonary

TEACHING TIPS
Patient with asthma

Be sure to include the following topics when teaching a patient with asthma.

- Process by which asthma causes bronchoconstriction, airway edema, and mucus production
- Possible complications, such as status asthmaticus
- Diagnostic tests, such as arterial blood gas analysis and pulmonary function tests
- Dietary changes, including increased fluid intake
- Prevention methods for—and warning signs of—respiratory infections
- Theophylline or other drug use
- Use of prescribed inhaler
- Identification and avoidance of asthma triggers
- Methods of controlling an asthma attack
- Sources of information and support

blood vessels are bound together by connective tissue to form the root of the lung

a. The *base,* the inferior surface of the lung, rests on the diaphragm

b. The *apex,* the most superior portion of the lung, projects above the clavicle

5. Each lung is enclosed in a PLEURA, a protective, double-layered serous membrane

a. The *visceral pleura* covers the lungs and dips into the fissures

b. At the hilus, the visceral pleura folds back to form the *parietal pleura,* which lines the chest wall and covers the diaphragm

c. The space between the lungs and chest wall is called the pleural cavity

(1) This space usually contains a small amount of fluid, which lubricates the lungs as they expand and contract

ALERT

(2) Pleurisy (inflammation of the parietal and visceral pleura) may result from pneumonia or another disorder and may lead to respiratory failure

d. When fully expanded, the lungs completely fill the pleural cavity, and the parietal and visceral pleurae come in contact

B. Lobes

1. The lungs are divided by fissures into lobes

a. The right lung is separated into three lobes (superior, middle, and inferior) by the horizontal and oblique fissures

b. The left lung, smaller than the right, is separated into two lobes (upper and lower) by the oblique fissure; it contains a concavity (cardiac notch), which is molded to accommodate the heart

2. Functionally, each lobe is divided into *bronchopulmonary segments*
   a. The right lung has 10 bronchopulmonary segments
   b. The left lung has 8 bronchopulmonary segments

C. Bronchioles
1. The *bronchioles* are flexible tubes that extend from bronchi; air travels through them to gas-exchange sites in the lungs
   a. Like bronchi, bronchioles branch repeatedly, becoming progressively smaller; unlike bronchi, they contain no cartilage in their walls
      (1) Bronchioles progress to form terminal bronchioles (smallest bronchioles that conduct air only)
      (2) They also form respiratory bronchioles (tubes distal to the terminal bronchioles that conduct air and participate in gas exchange)
   b. The diameter of the bronchioles varies with the respiratory phase; they increase slightly during inspiration and decrease slightly during expiration
2. Eventually, bronchioles branch into alveolar ducts, which terminate in clusters called ALVEOLI

D. Alveoli
1. *Alveoli* are tiny, grapelike clusters of air sacs at the ends of bronchioles
2. Alveoli are surrounded by an extensive network of capillaries, with which they exchange oxygen and carbon dioxide by diffusion
3. Alveoli are separated by thin vascular partitions called alveolar septa, which are lined by flat squamous cells and small numbers of secretory cells
4. The secretory cells produce surfactant
   a. The lipoprotein surfactant reduces surface tension, allowing the fluid that lines the alveoli to spread as a thin film rather than coalescing into droplets
   b. Surfactant reduces the cohesive surface tension of water molecules in the alveoli, allowing the alveoli to expand uniformly during inspiration

ALERT

      (1) Without surfactant, surface tension could restrict alveolar expansion or cause alveolar collapse during expiration
      (2) This condition commonly occurs in neonates born before 28 weeks' gestation, producing respiratory distress syndrome of the newborn; decreased surfactant in adults also causes alveolar collapse and adult respiratory distress syndrome

E. Blood supply
1. Blood circulates through the lungs via the pulmonary and systemic circulatory systems

2. In the pulmonary circulation, pulmonary arteries branch profusely into the pulmonary capillaries, which surround the alveoli
   a. Pulmonary arteries carry deoxygenated blood to the lungs
   b. Pulmonary veins return oxygenated blood from the lungs to the heart
3. The systemic circulation supplies blood directly to lung tissues
   a. This blood travels through the bronchial arteries (one artery on the right and two on the left)
   b. Venous blood returns via the bronchial veins

F. Pressures
1. The lungs remain expanded in the pleural cavity because the INTRAPLEURAL PRESSURE (pressure in the pleural cavity) is less than the INTRAPULMONARY PRESSURE (air pressure in the lungs)
2. These pressure differences develop at birth when the thoracic cavity enlarges and respiration begins
3. As the lungs expand and fill with air at atmospheric pressure, the elastic tissue of the lungs stretches
4. The stretched lungs tend to pull away from the chest wall and return to their original state; this creates a slight vacuum in the pleural cavity and makes the intrapleural pressure slightly less than atmospheric pressure
5. Because the intrapleural pressure is slightly less than atmospheric pressure, it commonly is called negative or subatmospheric pressure; without this pressure to hold the lungs in the expanded position, the elastic tissue would contract and the lungs would collapse

♦ III. Ventilation

A. General information
1. The diaphragm and intercostal muscles produce the normal inspiratory and expiratory movement of the lungs and ribs; this movement allows ventilation
2. During respiration, the intrapulmonary and intrapleural pressures change from their levels at rest, which are 760 and 756 mm Hg, respectively; the atmospheric pressure remains constant at about 760 mm Hg
3. The volume of air in the lungs varies during the phases of respiration, inspiration (air movement into the lungs) and *expiration* (air movement out of the lungs)
4. Pulmonary volume (amount of air in the lungs) varies greatly between normal inspiration and expiration; it varies even more with forced inspiration and expiration

B. Inspiration
   1. Stimulated by the central nervous system (CNS), the diaphragm contracts and descends, pulling down the lower surfaces of the lungs
   2. At the same time, the external intercostal muscles contract and raise the rib cage; this expands the lungs by lifting the sternum up and forward
   3. Thoracic expansion lowers the intrapleural pressure to 754 mm Hg, and the lungs expand to fill the enlarged thoracic cavity
   4. The intrapulmonary pressure decreases to 758 mm Hg; the intrapulmonary-atmospheric pressure gradient pulls air into the lungs

C. Expiration
   1. Normally, expiration is a passive process
   2. As CNS impulses cease after inspiration, the diaphragm slowly relaxes and moves up
   3. The external intercostal muscles relax and the rib cage descends
   4. These actions allow the lungs and thorax to return to their resting size and position
   5. Lung and thorax relaxation causes the intrapulmonary pressure to rise above the atmospheric pressure to 763 mm Hg; the intrapleural pressure rises to 756 mm Hg
   6. The intrapulmonary-atmospheric pressure gradient forces air out of the lungs until the two pressures are equal
   7. During vigorous exertion, the lungs can expel air more actively
      a. Contraction of the internal intercostal muscles actively forces down the ribs
      b. Abdominal muscle contraction pushes the abdominal contents up against the bottom of the diaphragm, expelling air more rapidly than is possible with normal diaphragm and intercostal muscle relaxation

D. Pulmonary volumes and capacities
   1. Pulmonary volumes and capacities vary with the individual's size, which influences the size of the lungs and thorax
   2. During normal quiet breathing, the average adult inspires and expires about 500 ml of air with each breath, which is called the TIDAL VOLUME
   3. At the end of a normal tidal inspiration, an adult can forcefully inhale an additional 3,000 ml of air, which is called the INSPIRATORY RESERVE VOLUME
   4. At the end of a normal tidal expiration, an adult can forcefully exhale about 1,300 ml of air, which is called the EXPIRATORY RESERVE VOLUME

5. Even if the expiratory reserve volume is expelled from the lungs, an additional 1,200 ml of air remains; this remaining air is called the RESIDUAL VOLUME
6. The maximum amount of air that can be moved out of the lungs after a maximum inspiration and expiration, called the VITAL CAPACITY, is about 4,800 ml (500 ml + 3,000 ml + 1,300 ml)
7. The *total lung capacity* is approximately 6,000 ml
8. Although the tidal volume is 500 ml, about 150 ml of this air never reaches the alveoli; it fills the upper respiratory passages and is exhaled with the next breath
   a. The upper airway containing air that does not enter the alveoli is called the *dead space;* the volume of air it contains is called the *dead space volume*
   b. Because of this dead space, only about 350 ml of air actually enters the alveoli with each breath and mixes with the 2,500 ml of air already in the lungs (expiratory reserve volume plus the residual volume)
   c. Consequently, less than 15% of alveolar air is replaced by new atmospheric air with each breath
   d. This slow replacement of alveolar air has several advantages
      (1) The slow admixture of atmospheric air with alveolar air prevents wide fluctuations in oxygen and carbon dioxide concentration in alveolar air, which could produce adverse effects
      (2) Because oxygen and carbon dioxide in the blood are in equilibrium with their gas forms in the alveolar air, stable concentrations of alveolar oxygen and carbon dioxide promote stable concentrations of these gases in the arterial blood

♦ IV. Gas exchange

A. General information
   1. Oxygen and carbon dioxide diffusion (exchange) between the alveoli, blood, and tissues depends on the concentrations and pressures of these gases
   2. In a mixture of gases, the pressure exerted by each gas (PARTIAL PRESSURE) is independent of that of the other gases and directly corresponds to the percentage (concentration) it represents of the total mixture
      a. For example, air exerts a total pressure of 760 mm Hg (atmospheric pressure) at sea level
      b. Air contains about 21% oxygen; consequently, the partial pressure of oxygen (PO_2) is 21% of the atmospheric pressure: 0.21 x 760 = 159.6 mm Hg

3. Oxygen and carbon dioxide exist in three physiologically important areas: in the atmosphere and pulmonary alveoli as gases, and in the blood in solution

B. Gas concentrations in inspired air

1. Most air inspired from the atmosphere (almost 79%) consists of the inert gas nitrogen; air contains only about 21% oxygen
2. The rest is a mixture of small amounts of water vapor (about 0.5%) and carbon dioxide (about 0.04%)

C. Gas concentrations in alveolar air

1. Alveolar air contains more water vapor (about 6.2%) than inspired air because of the moist secretions in the respiratory passages
2. The oxygen content (about 13.6%) is lower than that of inspired air because red blood cells (RBCs) take up oxygen as they pass through the pulmonary capillaries
3. The carbon dioxide concentration (about 5.3%) is higher than that of inspired air because the gas diffuses continually from the pulmonary capillaries into the alveolar air
4. Nitrogen accounts for about 74.9% of alveolar air

D. Gas concentrations in expired air

1. Expired air contains about the same amount of water vapor as alveolar air (about 6.2%)
2. Expired air contains more oxygen (about 15.7%) and less carbon dioxide (about 3.6%) than alveolar air because it is a mixture of alveolar air and atmospheric air from the dead space
3. Nitrogen accounts for about 74.5% of expired air

E. Gas diffusion

1. *Diffusion* refers to the exchange of gases — particularly oxygen and carbon dioxide — between the alveoli and capillaries and between body cells and RBCs
2. In diffusion, substances move from an area of higher concentration to one of lower concentration; a gas diffuses from an area with a high partial pressure of the gas to one with a low partial pressure
3. Inspired air has a PO_2 of 158 mm Hg and a PCO_2 of 0.3 mm Hg
4. When blood returns to the heart, the right ventricle pumps it to the lungs, where it passes through the pulmonary capillaries
5. The PO_2 in venous blood, which is returned to the heart by the vena cavae, is 40 mm Hg; the PCO_2 is 47 mm Hg
6. Because alveolar air has a higher PO_2 (100 mm Hg) and a lower PCO_2 (40 mm Hg) than the blood in the pulmonary capillaries, oxygen diffuses from alveolar air into the pulmonary capillaries, and carbon dioxide diffuses in the opposite direction

TEACHING TIPS

Patient with pneumonia

Be sure to include the following topics when teaching a patient with pneumonia.

- Respiratory defense mechanisms and process by which pneumonia develops
- Classifications, risk factors, and symptoms of pneumonia
- Diagnostic tests, such as chest X-ray and sputum analysis
- Treatments, including activity restrictions, drug therapy, breathing and coughing exercises, chest physiotherapy, hydration, and oxygen therapy
- Methods for preventing pneumonia, such as influenza vaccinations, and for preventing its spread, such as proper hand washing and tissue disposal
- Sources of information and support

7. As a result, arterial blood has a PO_2 of 97 mm Hg, which is almost the same as the alveolar PO_2; it also has a PCO_2 of 40 mm Hg, which is the same as the alveolar PCO_2
8. In the tissues, the PO_2 is lower (40 mm Hg) and the PCO_2 is higher (about 60 mm Hg) than in arterial blood
9. Therefore, oxygen diffuses into the tissues from the arterial blood, and carbon dioxide diffuses in the opposite direction, from the tissues into the blood

ALERT

10. In pneumonia, inflammatory exudate accumulates in the alveoli and causes consolidation, filling one or more lobes with mucus, pus, and other substances (for teaching tips, see *Patient with pneumonia*)

♦ V. Oxygen and carbon dioxide transport

A. General information
   1. Once diffusion occurs, arterial blood transports oxygen to the tissues in two ways: physically dissolved in plasma and chemically bound to hemoglobin
   2. The tissues release carbon dioxide into the bloodstream, where it travels to the lungs in three forms: dissolved in plasma, combined with hemoglobin, and combined with water as carbonic acid and its component ions
   3. In the lungs, oxygen and carbon dioxide transport is the reverse of that in the tissues

B. Oxygen transport in blood
   1. Only about 3% of oxygen is dissolved in blood plasma
   2. The remaining 97% is chemically bound with hemoglobin in a ratio of 1 g of hemoglobin to approximately 1.34 cc of oxygen

   a. 100 ml of blood contains about 15 g of hemoglobin; therefore, 100 ml of blood should combine with about 20 cc of oxygen (15 x 1.34 = 20.1)
   b. However, oxygenated blood normally carries slightly less than the predicted 20 cc of oxygen because it is only about 97% oxygen-saturated; in other words, the hemoglobin does not carry its full complement of oxygen
3. The tissues remove about 5 cc of oxygen from each 100 ml of blood; blood returning to the heart contains about 15 cc of oxygen per 100 ml of blood (75% oxygen saturation)
4. During vigorous exercise, muscles remove more oxygen from the blood, and the rate of blood flow to the tissues increases greatly, which increases the amount of oxygen available to the tissues
5. Oxygen uptake by hemoglobin is most efficient in the lungs, where the oxygen concentration is high; oxygen release occurs most readily in the tissues, where the oxygen concentration is low
6. The lower acidity (pH) and higher temperature of actively metabolizing tissue, which may occur during vigorous exercise, also enhances oxygen release from hemoglobin

C. Carbon dioxide transport in blood
1. Carbon dioxide is transported in several forms in the blood
   a. A small amount is dissolved in plasma
   b. Some is loosely combined with amino groups in the hemoglobin molecule
   c. Most of the carbon dioxide is converted in RBCs to bicarbonate by the enzyme carbonic anhydrase
      (1) Conversion occurs when oxygen is liberated from hemoglobin
      (2) Bicarbonate combines with sodium and is transported in the plasma as sodium bicarbonate
2. RBC uptake of carbon dioxide begins in the capillaries
   a. In the RBCs, hemoglobin liberates oxygen to supply the tissues
   b. Simultaneously, carbon dioxide diffuses from the tissues into RBCs, where carbonic anhydrase rapidly catalyzes carbonic acid formation by combining with carbon dioxide and water
   c. Then carbonic acid dissociates into hydrogen ions (H^+) and bicarbonate ions (HCO_3)
   d. During oxygen release to the tissues, hemoglobin molecules take up hydrogen ions; after releasing oxygen, the molecule is reduced and has an increased capacity to combine with hydrogen ions
   e. The remaining bicarbonate ions accumulate until their concentration in RBCs exceeds that in plasma; then bicarbonate ions diffuse from RBCs into plasma

   f. Simultaneously, chloride ions diffuse into RBCs to replace the bicarbonate ions; this exchange is called the *chloride shift*
3. Then the bicarbonate ions combine with plasma sodium ions to form sodium bicarbonate

D. Gas transport in the lungs
1. In the lungs, the carbon dioxide-oxygen exchanges are the reverse of those in the tissues
2. Reduced hemoglobin takes up oxygen, decreasing the hemoglobin's capacity to combine with hydrogen ions
   a. Then hemoglobin releases hydrogen ions
   b. Simultaneously, bicarbonate ions diffuse into RBCs and chloride ions diffuse out
   c. As bicarbonate ions move into RBCs, they combine with hydrogen ions liberated from hemoglobin to form carbonic acid
   d. Carbonic acid rapidly decomposes, liberating carbon dioxide
   e. Carbon dioxide diffuses from RBCs into plasma
   f. Some carbon dioxide travels to the alveoli and is excreted by the lungs
   g. Most remains in plasma as part of bicarbonate ions, which play an essential role in maintaining the acid-base balance of the blood

♦ VI. Control of respirations

A. General information
1. A control center in the brain stem, called the RESPIRATORY CENTER, regulates the rate and depth of respiration
2. This center discharges impulses to neurons that innervate the diaphragm and intercostal muscles
3. The impulse discharge rate from the respiratory center is influenced by the chemical composition of arterial blood and by nerve impulses sent to the respiratory center

B. Arterial blood concentration
1. Neurons in the respiratory center are stimulated directly by increased arterial concentrations of carbon dioxide and hydrogen ions
2. Normally, the respiratory center is regulated primarily by arterial PCO_2; it adjusts respirations automatically to variations in this level
3. During exercise, more carbon dioxide is produced and arterial PCO_2 rises
   a. This stimulates the respiratory center to increase respiratory rate and depth
   b. This eliminates carbon dioxide more rapidly by the lungs, allowing arterial PCO_2 to decrease to normal

4. Chemoreceptors in the aortic arch and carotid sinus also convey impulses to the respiratory center
5. These chemoreceptors respond to arterial blood changes in PCO_2, hydrogen ion concentration (acidity), and PO_2; they signal the respiratory center to adjust the respiratory rate and depth as needed

C. Nervous system control
1. The cranial nerves control functions related to breathing; the pulmonary plexus, a network of nerves comprised of tributaries from the vagus nerve (cranial nerve X), innervates the lungs
2. The phrenic and intercostal nerves regulate the muscles of respiration
   a. Innervated by the phrenic nerve, the *diaphragm* is the chief muscle of respiration; this dome-shaped muscle separates the thoracic and abdominopelvic cavities
   b. Innervated by the intercostal nerves, the intercostal muscles connect the ribs
      (1) When these muscles contract, they pull the rib cage upward and outward, expanding the lungs and pulling air into them
      (2) They work in concert (synergistically) with the diaphragm
   c. In forced expiration, the scalene and sternocleidomastoid muscles lift the ribs and the quadratus and lumborum muscles of the abdominal wall aid expiration
3. The respiratory center controls respiratory rate and depth and regulates smooth transitions from inspiration to expiration
4. Nerve impulses from the lungs, cerebral cortex, and sensory nerve endings affect the rate of impulse discharge from the respiratory center
   a. Receptors in the lungs respond to stretching as the lungs inflate, sending impulses to the respiratory center to inhibit further inspiration
      (1) When the lungs deflate (expiration), the stretch receptors are no longer stimulated
      (2) Inhibitory impulses are no longer transmitted to the respiratory center
      (3) Inspiration follows automatically
      (4) This pulmonary reflex mechanism prevents lung overinflation and helps maintain normal respiratory rhythm
   b. The cerebral cortex sends impulses to the respiratory center in response to strong emotions, such as anxiety, fear, and anger; these impulses increase the respiratory rate
   c. Some sensory stimuli, such as irritating vapors in the upper respiratory passages, may cause reflex inhibition of respiration

POINTS TO REMEMBER

- The respiratory system performs tissue oxygenation and carbon dioxide removal. It consists of upper airways (nose, pharynx, and larynx), lower airways (trachea and bronchi) and the lungs.
- The lungs have lobes, bronchioles, alveoli, and a dedicated blood supply. The alveoli are surrounded by capillaries, with which they exchange oxygen and carbon dioxide.
- The diaphragm and intercostal muscles produce the normal inspiratory and expiratory movement of the lungs and ribs, which allows ventilation.
- Oxygen and carbon dioxide diffusion (exchange) between the alveoli, blood, and tissues depends on the concentrations and pressures of these gases. They diffuse from an area with a high partial pressure of the gas to one with a low partial pressure.
- Arteries transport oxygen to the tissues physically dissolved in plasma and chemically bound to hemoglobin. Veins transport carbon dioxide to the lungs dissolved in plasma, combined with hemoglobin, and combined with water as carbonic acid and its component ions. In the lungs, oxygen and carbon dioxide transport is the reverse of that in the tissues.
- In the brain, the respiratory center regulates the rate and depth of respiration. It is influenced by the chemical composition of arterial blood and by nerve impulses sent to the respiratory center.

STUDY QUESTIONS

To evaluate your understanding of this chapter, answer the following questions in the space provided. Then compare your responses with the correct answers in Appendix B, page 332.

1. What structures comprise the upper and lower airways? ______________

____

____

2. Where does gas exchange take place? ______________________

____

____

3. What keeps the lungs expanded in the pleural cavity? ____

4. How is the inspiratory reserve volume different from the expiratory reserve volume? ____

5. In which direction do gases move during diffusion? ____

6. How does carbon dioxide travel to the lungs? ____

7. Which blood gas is the primary regulator of the respiratory center? ____

CRITICAL THINKING AND APPLICATION EXERCISES

1. Using a model, identify the structures of the respiratory system.
2. On an illustration, diagram the mechanics of ventilation, noting intrapulmonary and intrapleural pressure changes.
3. Using a spirometer, measure and record your tidal volume, expiratory reserve capacity, and vital capacity.
4. Make a chart that compares gas concentrations in inspired, alveolar, and expired air.
5. Write a one-page paper that describes the exchange of oxygen and carbon dioxide between the alveoli and capillaries and between body cells and RBCs.

CHAPTER

14

Gastrointestinal System

Learning objectives

After studying this chapter, you should be able to:

- Identify the six organs of the gastrointestinal (GI) tract.
- Describe the five main functions of the GI system.
- Describe the structure and functions of the liver, pancreas, and gallbladder.
- Explain how carbohydrates, proteins, and lipids are broken down, absorbed, and metabolized.
- Describe the three processes by which glucose is broken down to yield energy.
- Explain the purpose of deamination and transamination in protein metabolism.
- Describe the significance of ketone bodies in lipid metabolism.
- Compare the functions of the six hormones that regulate metabolic processes.

Chapter overview

Through the GI system, the body obtains and processes almost all of the nutrients it needs. The GI system supplies all of the energy and building materials required by the body for daily activities, growth, and repair. For these reasons, the health care professional should recognize GI structures and understand the processes of digestion, absorption, and metabolism.

♦ I. Gastrointestinal Tract

A. General information
   1. The *GI system* (also called the digestive system) consists of the structures that ingest, digest, and absorb food
   2. It includes the organs of the GI tract and the accessory GI organs (see *Structures of the gastrointestinal system*)
   3. The GI tract (or ALIMENTARY CANAL) is a continuous tube open at both ends; it extends through the ventral cavities from the mouth to the anus
   4. It consists of the oral cavity, pharynx, esophagus, stomach, and small and large intestines; it is surrounded by the peritoneum

B. Functions
   1. The overall purpose of the GI system is to modify and prepare food chemically and physically for use by body cells
   2. It accomplishes this purpose through five main functions
      a. It ingests food (via the oral cavity)
      b. It propels food through the pharynx and esophagus into the stomach
      c. It digests food mechanically and chemically
      d. It absorbs food molecules
      e. It eliminates indigestible materials from the body (via defecation)

C. Oral cavity
   1. The *oral cavity* is bounded by the lips, cheeks, palate, and tongue; it also contains the salivary glands and 32 permanent teeth
   2. It joins the pharynx at a junction called the fauces
   3. The oral cavity prepares food for swallowing and begins DIGESTION
      a. The teeth cut and grind food into small particles
      b. The salivary glands pour saliva into the mouth
         (1) The food mixes with saliva to form a pliable mass (bolus) for swallowing
         (2) Saliva contains amylase, an enzyme that begins starch digestion

D. Pharynx
   1. The *pharynx* is a cavity that extends from the base of the skull to the esophagus (about the level of the sixth vertebra); it is lined with mucous membrane
   2. The pharynx aids swallowing by grasping food and moving it toward the esophagus

Structures of the gastrointestinal system

This illustration shows the organs of the GI tract (mouth, pharynx, esophagus, stomach, small intestine, and large intestine) and several accessory GI organs (liver, gallbladder, and pancreas).

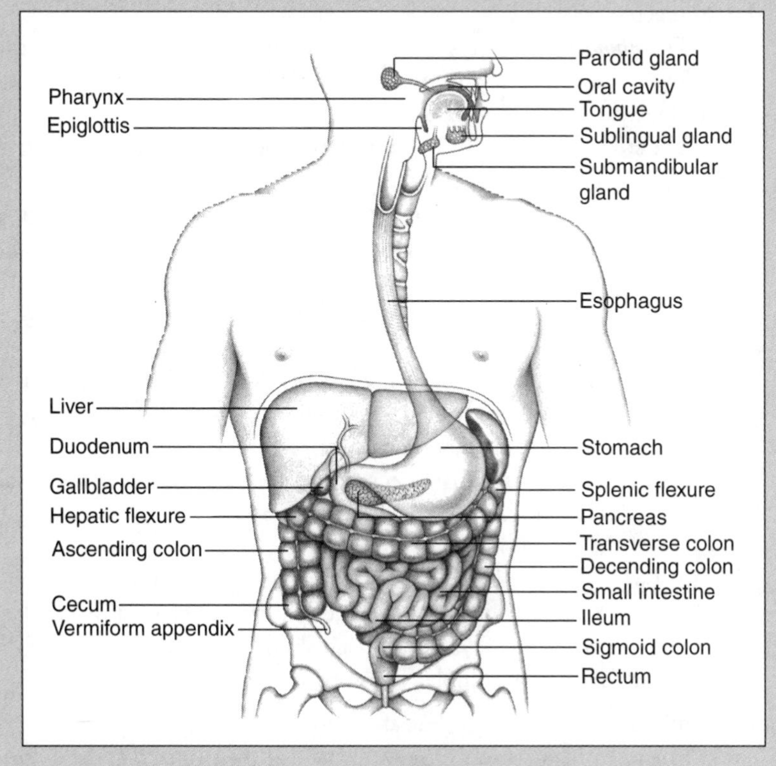

   a. Food leaving the mouth is propelled into the oropharynx and laryngopharynx (the middle and inferior portions of the pharynx, respectively)
   b. Normally, food does not pass through the nasopharynx (the superior portion of the pharynx), which connects the oral cavity to the nasal cavities

E. Esophagus
   1. The *esophagus* is a collapsible, muscular tube that extends from the laryngopharynx through the mediastinum to the stomach
   2. It conducts food from the pharynx to the stomach
      a. Swallowing triggers food passage from the laryngopharynx into the esophagus

ALERT

b. PERISTALSIS — rhythmic contraction of smooth muscle — propels liquids and solids through the esophagus into the stomach

c. Normally, the lower esophageal sphincter closes after food enters the stomach; if it fails to close or remain closed, gastric juices can flow backward into the esophagus, causing gastroesophageal reflux

F. Stomach

1. The *stomach* is a collapsible, pouchlike structure that attaches to the lower end of the esophagus and is immediately inferior to the diaphragm
2. The stomach serves as a temporary storage area for food, which remains there until it is digested partially
3. The stomach churns the ingested food and mixes it with gastric juices; this results in a thick, acidic fluid called *chyme*
   a. GI hormones, such as gastrin, gastric inhibitory peptides, secretin, and cholecystokinin (CCK), regulate gastric secretion and motility
   b. Stimulation of gastric acid secretion occurs during two phases
      (1) In the cephalic phase, secretion is stimulated by the sight, smell, or anticipation of food
      (2) In the gastric phase, secretion is stimulated by *gastrin,* the GI hormone released in response to food in the stomach and duodenum
   c. Gastric acid activates the gastric enzyme precursor pepsinogen to form pepsin, which digests proteins by breaking peptide bonds
   d. Intrinsic factor (IF) in gastric acid combines with vitamin B_{12}; the vitamin B_{12}-IF complex is absorbed later in the small intestine

G. Small intestine

1. The *small intestine* joins to the PYLORUS of the stomach at the pyloric sphincter
2. The longest organ of the GI tract, the small intestine has three major divisions — the duodenum, jejunum, and ileum
3. Its main function is to complete food digestion; the stomach expels chyme through the pylorus into the upper part of the small intestine (duodenum)
   a. Segmenting contractions (alternating contractions and relaxations of adjacent segments of the small intestine) mix the contents of the small intestine

ALERT

      (1) The small intestine's contents are propelled by peristalsis
      (2) Abnormal peristalsis can lead to constipation, diarrhea, or both — as in irritable bowel syndrome (for teaching tips, see *Patient with irritable bowel syndrome*)

TEACHING TIPS

Patient with irritable bowel syndrome

Be sure to include the following topics when teaching a patient with irritable bowel syndrome.

- Explanation of the disorder (including excessive peristalsis and spasms) factors that promote exacerbations
- Preparation for tests, such as barium enema, that may be done to rule out other disorders
- Dietary changes to minimize pain, bloating, constipation, and diarrhea
- Use of prescribed drugs, such as antispasmodics, laxatives, antidiarrheals, and tranquilizers
- Self-care measures, such as stress-reduction techniques and smoking cessation

b. Most of the nutrients, water, and electrolytes in foods are digested and absorbed during the 6- to 8-hour passage through the small intestine

c. Intestinal glands secrete enzymes that further digest various nutrients

d. The intestinal hormones CCK and secretin also regulate gallbladder function and pancreatic fluid and bile secretion

e. Bile and pancreatic fluid mix with intestinal contents to continue digestion, as discussed in the next section

4. After digestion, food molecules are absorbed through the wall of the small intestine into the circulatory system for delivery to body cells

H. Large intestine

1. The large intestine extends from the ILEOCECAL VALVE of the small intestine to the anus
2. The large intestine has five segments — the cecum, vermiform appendix, ascending colon, transverse colon, descending colon, and sigmoid colon
3. The rectum is the last several inches of the large intestine; it extends to the anus, which allows passage of feces
4. The large intestine's main function is to absorb water and eliminate digestive waste products

a. Peristalsis and segmenting contractions move the intestinal contents slowly; water and minerals are absorbed from the contents, leaving a residue of fecal material

(1) Intestinal bacteria act on the residue, releasing decomposition products and intestinal gases

(2) These bacteria also synthesize vitamin K and some B vitamins, which are absorbed in the colon

b. Peristalsis propels fecal material into the rectum; this causes reflex contraction of rectal smooth muscle and relaxation of the internal anal sphincter (defecation reflex)
c. Voluntary relaxation of the external anal sphincter combined with bearing-down efforts results in evacuation of rectal contents

I. Peritoneum
1. The *peritoneum* is a strong, colorless membrane that completely lines the walls of the abdominal cavity; it includes the parietal peritoneum and VISCERAL PERITONEUM
a. The *parietal peritoneum* lines the abdominal and pelvic walls and the underside of the diaphragm
b. The *visceral peritoneum,* a continuation of the parietal peritoneum, covers the external surfaces of most abdominal organs, including the stomach, spleen, and liver
2. Folds of peritoneum called *mesenteries* hold the intestines and other GI organs in place; they contain blood vessels, lymphatic vessels, and nerves
3. Other peritoneal folds, called *omenta,* attach to the stomach
4. Additional peritoneal folds form the *ligaments* of the liver, spleen, and stomach

♦ II. Accessory Organs

A. General information
1. Accessory organs of the GI tract include gastrin and intestinal glands as well as the liver, gallbladder, and pancreas
2. The liver, gallbladder, and pancreas lie outside the GI tract
3. Most accessory organs produce or store secretions needed for digestion

B. Gastrin glands and intestinal glands
1. Gastrin glands are located in the mucosal lining of the stomach; they produce the hormone gastrin when stimulated by partially digested proteins
a. They secrete gastrin directly into capillaries in the stomach
b. Circulating gastrin stimulates secretion of gastric juice, which has a high content of pepsin and hydrochloric acid
2. Intestinal glands include intestinal crypts and Brunner's glands
a. Intestinal crypts, found in the intestinal mucosa, secrete intestinal juice (a mixture of digestive enzymes, mucus, and hormones)
b. Brunner's glands, found in the duodenal submucosa, secrete an alkaline mucus that helps neutralize the acidic chyme entering the duodenum from the stomach

C. Liver
1. The liver is the largest gland in the body; it is located immediately inferior to the diaphragm and partially anterior to the stomach

2. The liver consists of a right lobe, left lobe, caudate lobe (behind the right lobe), and quadrate lobe (below the left lobe)
3. A fold of peritoneum called the *lesser omentum* covers most of the liver; the hepatic artery and hepatic portal vein (which enter the liver) and the COMMON BILE DUCT and hepatic veins (which leave the liver) all pass through the lesser omentum
4. A specialized accessory organ, the liver has digestive, metabolic, and regulatory functions; its chief digestive function is production of bile, which acts as a fat emulsifier in the small intestine
5. The liver receives the products of digestion through the portal vein
   a. It can convert the absorbed hexoses, amino acids, and lipid digestion products into whatever nutrient mixture the body needs for metabolic processes
   b. The liver also forms ketone bodies from products of lipid metabolism
   c. The liver produces blood proteins (such as albumin and globulin), lipoproteins, and proteins involved with blood coagulation; it stores a small reserve of fat and glycogen, iron, and vitamins A, B_{12}, D, E, and K
   d. The liver secretes 500 to 1,000 ml of bile daily to promote fat digestion (see *Functions of digestive secretions,* page 232)
      (1) Bile is a complex secretion composed of cholesterol, lecithin (a phospholipid), bile salts (composed of cholesterol and amino acid derivatives), minerals, bile pigments (derived from hemoglobin breakdown), and water
      (2) Bile emulsifies fats into small globules for more efficient digestion; bile salts promote the absorption of fats and fat-soluble vitamins
   e. The liver detoxifies or excretes many wastes and toxins
      (1) It converts potentially toxic compounds, such as ammonia, to nontoxic compounds
      (2) It inactivates such substances as drugs, antibiotics, and steroid hormones
      (3) It excretes bilirubin derived from red blood cell breakdown; in the colon, intestinal bacteria break down bilirubin into various compounds that produce the normal color of feces
      (4) The liver also excretes cholesterol and other inactivated or detoxified products

D. Gallbladder
1. The *gallbladder* is a muscular sac located on the ventral surface of the liver, between the right and quadrate lobes; it is covered by visceral peritoneum
2. The cystic duct joins the gallbladder to the common bile duct
3. The gallbladder stores and concentrates the bile secreted by the liver

Functions of digestive secretions

Most digestive secretions contain enzymes that have specific digestive functions, as shown below. Only one secretion (bile) performs its functions without enzymes.

DIGESTIVE SECRETION	ENZYME	FUNCTION
Saliva	• Amylase	• Digests starch
Gastric acid	• Pepsin	• Digests protein
	• Intrinsic factor	• Promotes vitamin B_{12} absorption
Small intestine secretions	• Disaccharidases (such as maltase, sucrase, and lactase)	• Digest carbohydrates
	• Peptidases	• Digest proteins
	• Amylase	• Digests starch further
	• Lipase	• Digests fats
	• Enterokinase	• Activates pancreatic trypsinogen to form trypsin, which continues protein digestion
Bile	• None	• Emulsifies fats and other lipids
Pancreatic secretions	• Trypsin, chymotrypsin, and carboxypeptidase	• Digest protein
	• Ribonuclease and deoxyribonuclease	• Digest nucleic acids
	• Amylase	• Digests starch further
	• Lipase	• Digests fats and other lipids
	• Cholesterol esterase	• Splits cholesterol esters to cholesterol and fatty acids

a. Bile travels through the cystic duct and enters the gallbladder, where it is stored and concentrated tenfold through water absorption
b. Bile can enter the duodenum only when the ampullary Oddi's sphincter is open, during digestion
c. A fatty meal induces CCK release
   (1) This stimulates gallbladder contraction

(2) Simultaneously, the ampullary sphincter relaxes, permitting bile to enter the small intestine

d. Various factors regulate cholesterol solubility in bile

(1) Micelles formed from bile salts have a lipid-soluble center and a water-soluble periphery

(2) Cholesterol remains in solution in bile by dissolving in the lipid-soluble centers of the micelles

ALERT

(3) Cholesterol may precipitate from bile and form gallstones if the cholesterol concentration in bile exceeds the capacity of the micelles to hold cholesterol in solution

E. Pancreas

1. The *pancreas* is an elongated, triangular gland located transversely behind the stomach, between the spleen and duodenum

2. The exocrine pancreas contains cells that secrete digestive enzymes into the duodenum through the pancreatic duct; the endocrine pancreas contains cells that secrete hormones directly into the bloodstream

a. The exocrine pancreas secretes about 1,500 ml of alkaline pancreatic fluid into the duodenum daily

(1) Pancreatic fluid contains potent digestive enzymes

(a) Amylase digests starch

(b) Trypsin, chymotrypsin, and carboxypeptidase digest proteins

(c) Lipase digests certain lipids

(d) Cholesterol esterase digests cholesterol esters

(e) Ribonuclease and deoxyribonuclease digest nucleic acids

(2) The pancreas secretes proteolytic (protein-digesting) enzymes as inactive precursors

(a) The intestinal enzyme enterokinase activates trypsinogen to trypsin

(b) In turn, trypsin activates chymotrypsinogen and procarboxypeptidase to form chymotrypsin and carboxypeptidase

(3) The small intestine releases the hormone secretin when acidic chyme is expelled into the duodenum; this hormone stimulates the pancreas to secrete a large volume of pancreatic fluid that is low in enzymes

(4) The small intestine also releases CCK when lipids and proteins enter the duodenum; this stimulates secretion of pancreatic fluid, which is rich in digestive enzymes, and stimulates gallbladder contraction

ALERT

(5) In chronic pancreatitis, the duct through which enzymes leave the pancreas becomes blocked; this can cause enzymes to back up into the pancreas and destroy pancreatic tissue

b. The endocrine pancreas consists of about 1 million small clusters of endocrine cells (islets of Langerhans), each composed of three major cell types
   (1) Alpha cells secrete glucagon to increase blood glucose in response to decreased blood glucose levels

ALERT

   (2) Beta cells secrete insulin to lower blood glucose in response to increased blood glucose levels; these cells are absent or defective in individuals with diabetes mellitus, resulting in elevated blood glucose
   (3) Delta cells secrete somatostatin (growth hormone inhibitory hormone), which inhibits glucagon and insulin secretion (see Chapter 17, Endocrine System, for details about the endocrine pancreas)

♦ III. Nutrient digestion and absorption

A. General information
1. The body needs a continual supply of water and various nutrients to maintain its functions; virtually all nutrients come from digested food
2. The three major types of nutrients the body needs are *carbohydrates, proteins,* and *lipids*
   a. When nutrients are used to yield energy, the energy is measured in kilocalories (kcal), or calories, per gram of nutrient
   b. Adults require approximately 2,000 kcal daily
3. All major nutrients must be digested in the GI tract by enzymes that hydrolyze (split) large units into smaller ones; then these smaller units are absorbed from the small intestine and transported to the liver through the portal venous system
4. The body also needs vitamins (biologically active organic compounds essential to normal metabolism and growth and development); vitamins may be water-soluble or fat-soluble
   a. Water-soluble vitamins include the B complex and C vitamins
   b. Fat-soluble vitamins include vitamins A, D, E, and K
5. The body also needs minerals (inorganic substances required for enzyme metabolism, membrane transfer of essential compounds, maintenance of acid-base balance and osmotic pressure, nerve impulse transmission, muscle contractility, and growth)
   a. Major minerals include calcium, chloride, magnesium, phosphorus, potassium, sodium, and sulfur
   b. Trace minerals include chromium, cobalt, copper, fluorine, iodine, iron, manganese, molybdenum, selenium, and zinc

B. Carbohydrate digestion and absorption
1. Enzymes break down complex carbohydrates into hexoses by hydrolyzing the glycoside bonds; HYDROLYSIS restores the water molecules that were released when the bonds were formed
2. Salivary amylase begins starch hydrolysis into disaccharides in the oral cavity; pancreatic amylase continues this process in the small intestine
3. Intestinal mucosal disaccharidases hydrolyze disaccharides into monosaccharides
   a. Lactase hydrolyzes lactose to glucose and galactose
   b. Sucrase splits sucrose into glucose and fructose
4. Monosaccharides, such as glucose, fructose, and galactose, are absorbed through the intestinal mucosa by diffusion and active transport and are transported to the liver through the portal venous system
   a. Enzymes in the liver convert fructose and galactose to glucose
   b. Ribonucleases and deoxyribonucleases break down nucleotides from deoxyribonucleic acid (DNA) and ribonucleic acid (RNA) into pentoses and nitrogen-containing compounds (nitrogen bases), which are absorbed through the intestinal mucosa like glucose

C. Protein digestion and absorption
1. Enzymes digest proteins by hydrolyzing peptide bonds
   a. These bonds link the amino acids that make up the protein chains
   b. This process restores water molecules that were released when the peptide bonds were formed
2. Gastric pepsin breaks proteins into polypeptides
3. Pancreatic trypsin, chymotrypsin, and carboxypeptidase convert polypeptides to peptides
4. Intestinal mucosal peptidases break peptides into their constituent amino acids
   a. These amino acids are absorbed through the intestinal mucosa by active transport mechanisms
   b. Then they are carried through the portal venous system to the liver, which converts amino acids not needed for protein synthesis into glucose

D. Lipid digestion and absorption
1. Bile from the liver emulsifies fats and other lipids into small droplets for more efficient digestion and eventual absorption in the small intestine
2. Pancreatic lipase breaks fats and phospholipids into a mixture of glycerol, short- and long-chain fatty acids, and monoglycerides

(fats composed of one molecule of a fatty acid and one molecule of glycerol); these substances are transported to the liver via the portal venous system

a. Lipase hydrolyzes the bonds between glycerol and fatty acids
b. This process restores water molecules that were released when the bonds were formed

3. Glycerol diffuses directly through the mucosa
4. Short-chain fatty acids diffuse into the intestinal epithelial cells and are transported to the liver via the portal venous system
5. Long-chain fatty acids and monoglycerides in the intestine dissolve in the bile salt micelles
   a. They diffuse from the micelles into the intestinal epithelial cells
   b. In the endothelial cells, lipase breaks down absorbed monoglycerides into glycerol and fatty acids
6. Fatty acids and glycerol are recombined to form fats in the smooth endoplasmic reticulum of the epithelial cells
7. Triglycerides (fats), along with a small amount of cholesterol and phospholipid, are coated with a thin layer of protein to form lipoprotein particles called *chylomicrons*
   a. Chylomicrons collect in the intestinal lacteals (lymphatic vessels) and are transported through lymphatic channels
   b. Then chylomicrons enter the circulation through the thoracic duct and are distributed to body cells
      (1) In the cells, fats are extracted from the chylomicrons and broken down into fatty acids and glycerol by enzymes
      (2) They are absorbed and recombined in fat cells to reform triglycerides (fat) for storage and later use

♦ IV. Carbohydrate metabolism

A. General information

1. Metabolism is the transformation of substances into energy or materials the body can use or store; it consists of two processes
   a. Anabolism is the synthesis of simple substances into complex ones
   b. Catabolism is the breakdown of complex substances into simpler ones or into energy
2. All ingested carbohydrates are converted to glucose, the body's main energy source
3. Glucose that is not needed for immediate energy requirements is stored as glycogen or converted to lipids
4. Energy from glucose catabolism is generated in three phases: GLYCOLYSIS, the CITRIC ACID CYCLE, (also called the Krebs, or tricarboxylic acid, cycle), and the ELECTRON TRANSPORT SYSTEM

a. Glycolysis, which occurs in the cell cytoplasm, does not require oxygen
b. The citric acid cycle and electron transport system, which occur in mitochondria, require oxygen

B. Glycolysis
1. During glycolysis, enzymes break down the six-carbon glucose molecule into two three-carbon pyruvic acid (pyruvate) molecules; this process yields energy in the form of adenosine triphosphate (ATP)
2. If the oxygen supply to the tissues is inadequate, pyruvic acid is reduced by cytoplasmic enzymes to lactic acid by the addition of two hydrogen atoms
3. When adequate oxygen becomes available, lactic acid is oxidized back to pyruvic acid

C. Citric acid cycle
1. The citric acid cycle is a pathway by which a molecule of acetyl coenzyme A (acetyl CoA) is oxidized enzymatically to yield energy
2. In this phase of carbohydrate metabolism, pyruvic acid releases a CO_2 molecule and is converted in the mitochondria to a two-carbon acetyl fragment, which combines with coenzyme A (a complex organic compound) to form acetyl CoA
3. Then the two-carbon acetyl fragments of acetyl CoA enter the citric acid cycle by combining with the four-carbon compound oxaloacetic acid to form citric acid, a six-carbon compound; in this process, the coenzyme A molecule is detached from the acetyl group and becomes available to form more acetyl-CoA molecules
4. Enzymes then convert citric acid into intermediate compounds and eventually convert it back into oxaloacetic acid, which is available to repeat the cycle
5. Each turn of the citric acid cycle releases hydrogen atoms, which are picked up by the coenzymes nicotinamide adenine dinucleotide (NAD) and flavin adenine dinucleotide (FAD); it also liberates carbon dioxide and generates energy

D. Electron transport system
1. In the electron transport system, carrier molecules on the inner mitochondrial membrane pick up electrons from the hydrogen atoms carried by NAD and FAD (each hydrogen atom consists of a hydrogen ion and an electron)
2. The carrier molecules transport the electrons through a series of enzyme-catalyzed oxidation-reduction reactions in the mitochondria
   a. During OXIDATION, a chemical compound loses electrons
   b. During REDUCTION, a compound gains electrons
3. These reactions release the energy contained in the electrons and generate ATP

4. After passing through the electron transport system, the hydrogen ions produced in the citric acid cycle combine with oxygen to form water

E. Role of the liver and muscle cells
   1. The liver plays an essential role in regulating blood glucose levels
      a. When the amount of glucose exceeds immediate needs, hormones stimulate the liver to convert glucose into glycogen or lipids
         (1) Glycogen is formed through GLYCOGENESIS
         (2) Lipids are formed through LIPOGENESIS
      b. When the blood glucose level is inadequate, the liver can form glucose by two processes
         (1) The liver can break down glycogen to glucose through GLYCOGENOLYSIS
         (2) It also can synthesize glucose from amino acids through GLUCONEOGENESIS
   2. Muscle cells can convert glucose to glycogen for storage, but they lack enzymes to convert glycogen back to glucose when needed
      a. During vigorous muscular activity, when oxygen demand exceeds the supply, muscle cells break down glycogen to yield lactic acid and energy
         (1) Lactic acid accumulates in the muscles, and muscle glycogen is depleted
         (2) Some lactic acid diffuses from muscle cells; it is transported to the liver and reconverted to glycogen
         (3) Then the liver converts the newly formed glycogen to glucose, which is transported through the bloodstream to the muscles and reformed into glycogen
      b. When muscular exertion ceases, part of the accumulated lactic acid is reconverted to pyruvic acid and then oxidized completely to yield energy by means of the citric acid cycle and electron transport system

♦ V. Protein metabolism

A. General information
   1. Proteins are absorbed as amino acids; they are transported by the portal venous system to the liver and then throughout the body by blood
   2. Absorbed amino acids mix with other amino acids in the body's amino acid pool; these other amino acids may be produced by protein breakdown or synthesized in the body from other substances, such as keto acids
   3. Amino acids cannot be stored; they are converted to protein or glucose or are catabolized to provide energy

4. For these changes to occur, amino acids must be transformed by DEAMINATION or TRANSAMINATION
   a. In deamination, an amino group (-NH_2) is removed and the amino residue is excreted as urea
   b. In transamination, an amino group is exchanged for a keto group in a keto acid, through the action of transaminase enzymes; the process converts the amino acid to a keto acid and the original keto acid to an amino acid

B. Amino acid synthesis
1. Body proteins are synthesized from 20 different amino acids selected from the body's amino acid pool
2. The body can synthesize 12 amino acids from carbohydrates, fats, or other amino acids; they are called nonessential amino acids
3. The body cannot synthesize the other eight amino acids and must obtain them through dietary intake; they are called essential amino acids

C. Amino acid conversion
1. Amino acids that are not used for protein synthesis can be converted to keto acids and metabolized by the citric acid cycle and electron transport system to yield energy
   a. Some keto acids can enter the citric acid cycle directly by combining with one of the intermediate compounds in the cycle
   b. Others must undergo one of two possible conversions
      (1) They may be converted to pyruvic acid and then to acetyl CoA, which combines with oxaloacetic acid to form citric acid
      (2) They may be converted directly to acetyl CoA, which combines with oxaloacetic acid to form citric acid
2. Amino acids can be converted to other nutrients
   a. They can be converted to fats
      (1) Amino acids that are not used for protein synthesis may be converted to pyruvic acid and then to acetyl CoA
      (2) The acetyl CoA fragments condense to form long-chain fatty acids; this process is the reverse of fatty acid breakdown
      (3) These fatty acids combine with glycerol to form fats
   b. Amino acids also can be converted to glucose
      (1) They are converted to pyruvic acid
      (2) Pyruvic acid then may be converted to glucose

♦ VI. Lipid metabolism

A. General information
1. Fats (lipids) are stored in adipose tissue within cells until required for energy

2. When required for energy, each fat molecule is hydrolyzed to glycerol and three molecules of fatty acids
3. Glycerol is converted to pyruvic acid and then to acetyl CoA, which enters the citric acid cycle to yield energy
4. Long-chain fatty acids are catabolized into two-carbon fragments, which combine with coenzyme A to form acetyl CoA fragments; the acetyl CoA then enters the citric acid cycle to yield energy

B. Ketone body formation

1. The liver normally forms ketone bodies from acetyl CoA fragments, which are derived primarily from fatty acid catabolism
2. Acetyl CoA molecules yield three types of ketone bodies: acetoacetic acid, betahydroxybutyric acid, and acetone
   a. Acetoacetic acid forms when two acetyl CoA molecules combine and coenzyme A is released from them
   b. Beta-hydroxybutyric acid forms when hydrogen is added to the oxygen atom in the acetoacetic acid molecule; the designation beta refers to the location of the carbon atom that contains the hydroxyl (OH) group
   c. Acetone forms when the carboxyl (COOH) group of acetoacetic acid releases CO_2

ALERT

3. Muscle, brain, and other tissues oxidize ketone bodies for energy
4. Certain conditions may cause production of more ketone bodies than the body can oxidize for energy
   a. Such conditions include fasting, starvation, and uncontrolled diabetes (in which the body cannot break down glucose)
   b. In all these conditions, the body must use fat, rather than glucose, as a primary energy source
   c. The resulting excess of ketone bodies disturbs the body's normal acid-base balance and homeostatic mechanisms, leading to ketosis

C. Lipid formation from proteins and carbohydrates

1. Excess amino acids can be converted to fat through keto acid–acetyl CoA conversion
2. Glucose may be converted to pyruvic acid and then to acetyl CoA, which is converted into fatty acids and then fat in the same way that amino acids are converted into fat

♦ VII. Hormonal regulation of metabolism

A. General information

1. Blood glucose levels must remain within a certain range for the body to maintain its normal functions
2. Various hormones are secreted in response to changes in blood glucose level

3. These hormones stimulate metabolic processes that return the blood glucose level to normal

B. Hormones that increase blood glucose level
1. Glucagon, epinephrine, growth hormone (GH), cortisol, and thyroxine can increase the blood glucose level
2. Glucagon promotes glycogen breakdown to glucose (glycogenolysis), amino acid conversion to glucose (gluconeogenesis), and lipid breakdown (lipolysis), which liberates free fatty acids and glycerol that can be converted to glucose
3. Epinephrine promotes glycogenolysis, gluconeogenesis, and lipolysis
4. GH has multiple effects
   a. It promotes protein synthesis by facilitating amino acid entry into cells
   b. It causes fat lipolysis from adipose tissue and promotes the use of fat rather than carbohydrate as an energy source
   c. It suppresses carbohydrate use for energy, causing blood glucose to rise as a result of reduced glucose use
   d. It promotes conversion of liver glycogen to glucose, which also tends to increase blood glucose level
5. Cortisol promotes protein hydrolysis to amino acids, which can be converted to glucose through gluconeogenesis
6. Thyroxine usually raises the blood glucose level by promoting gluconeogenesis and lipolysis

C. Hormones that decrease blood glucose level
1. Insulin is the only hormone that substantially lowers the blood glucose level
2. Insulin promotes cell uptake and use of glucose as an energy source
3. It promotes glucose storage as glycogen (glycogenesis) and lipids (lipogenesis)

POINTS TO REMEMBER

- The GI tract is a continuous tube open at both ends; it includes the oral cavity, pharynx, esophagus, stomach, and small and large intestines.
- Accessory GI organs include gastrin glands, intestinal glands, the liver, gallbladder, and pancreas. They produce or store secretions used in digestion.
- The major nutrients are carbohydrates, proteins, and lipids. They are digested in the GI tract by enzymes that hydrolyze them into smaller units that are absorbed from the small intestine.

- All ingested carbohydrates are converted to glucose. To supply energy, glucose is catabolized in three phases: glycolysis, the citric acid cycle, and the electron transport system.
- All ingested proteins are absorbed as amino acids. These acids must be converted to protein or glucose or catabolized for energy, which occurs by deamination and transamination.
- Lipids are stored in adipose tissue. When the body needs energy, lipid molecules are hydrolyzed.
- Glucagon, epinephrine, GH, cortisol, and thyroxine increase the blood glucose level. Insulin is the only hormone that lowers it.

STUDY QUESTIONS

To evaluate your understanding of this chapter, answer the following questions in the space provided. Then compare your responses with the correct answers in Appendix B, pages 332 and 333.

1. What is the general purpose of the GI system? ______________________

____

____

2. What is the main function of the large intestine? ____________________

____

____

3. What are the accessory organs and what is their overall function? ________

____

____

4. What hydrolyzes nutrients in the GI tract? _____________________

____

____

5. How are anabolism and catabolism alike? How are they different? _______

____

____

6. How is glycolysis different from the other phases of glucose catabolism?

____

____

7. What process converts excess amino acids to fat? ____________________

____

____

8. Which hormones promote glycogenolysis, gluconeogenesis, and lipolysis?

____

____

CRITICAL THINKING AND APPLICATION EXERCISES

1. On a poster, identify the major GI tract structures and describe their roles in digestion.
2. Using a three-dimensional model, trace the flow of bile.
3. In a one-page paper, contrast the digestion and absorption of carbohydrates, proteins, and lipids.
4. Using a molecular model, demonstrate deamination and transamination.
5. Create a chart that compares the processes by which hormones increase and decrease blood glucose levels.

CHAPTER

15

Urinary System

Learning objectives

After studying this chapter, you should be able to:

- Identify the main structures of the urinary system.
- Describe the functions of each of these structures.
- Discuss the role of glomerular filtration in urine production.
- Explain how hormones regulate urine volume and concentration.
- Describe how the countercurrent mechanism allows urine concentration.
- Explain how the kidneys regulate blood volume and blood pressure.
- Discuss the voiding reflex and urine elimination.

Chapter overview

Although metabolism of nutrients provides energy, it also creates toxic materials and excess essential materials. To maintain homeostasis, the body must eliminate both types of by-products. It does this through the urinary system as well as the lungs, skin, and GI tract. If these by-products are not continually eliminated, they quickly build up to fatal levels. Because of the urinary system's vital contribution to homeostasis, the health care professional must comprehend its basic structures and their functions.

♦ I. Kidneys

A. General information

1. The urinary system includes the kidneys, ureters, bladder, and urethra
2. The two *kidneys* are bean-shaped organs embedded in the dorsal part of the abdomen RETROPERITONEALLY, just behind the stomach and liver; the right kidney is situated slightly lower than the left
3. The kidneys have several functions
   a. The kidneys dispose of wastes and excess ions, in the form of urine
   b. They filter blood, regulating its volume and chemical makeup
   c. They maintain fluid, electrolyte, and acid-base balances
   d. They produce several hormones and enzymes
   e. They convert vitamin D to a more active form

B. Structure

1. The kidney has an outer region, called the renal cortex; a middle region, called the renal medulla; and an inner region, called the renal pelvis
   a. The *renal cortex* contains blood-filtering mechanisms
   b. The *renal medulla* consists of 8 to 12 triangular, striated wedges called *renal pyramids*
      (1) *Renal columns,* extensions of the renal cortex, jut inward among the renal pyramids
      (2) The APICES (tips, or papillae) of the renal pyramids project into the CALYCES (cavities) of the renal pelvis
   c. The funnel-shaped *renal pelvis* is an expansion of the upper end of the ureters
      (1) Urine is discharged at the apex of the renal pyramids into the calyces of the renal pelvis
      (2) From here, it flows into the ureters
2. The kidneys are encased in three layers of supportive and protective tissue — an inner renal capsule, a middle adipose capsule, and an outer renal FASCIA
3. The ureters, renal blood vessels, lymphatic vessels, and nerves enter or exit through the *hilus,* a notch on the inner, concave side of each kidney
4. On top of each kidney is an adrenal (suprarenal) gland, which functions separately from the kidney (for details, see Chapter 17, Endocrine System)

C. Nephron

1. The NEPHRON is the structural and functional unit of the kidney; each kidney contains more than 1 million nephrons

Internal structure of a nephron

Within each nephron's glomerular capsule are a renal tubule and a glomerulus. The long tubule has three portions: the proximal convoluted tubule, loop of Henle, and distal convoluted tubule. This illustration shows a nephron and its blood supply.

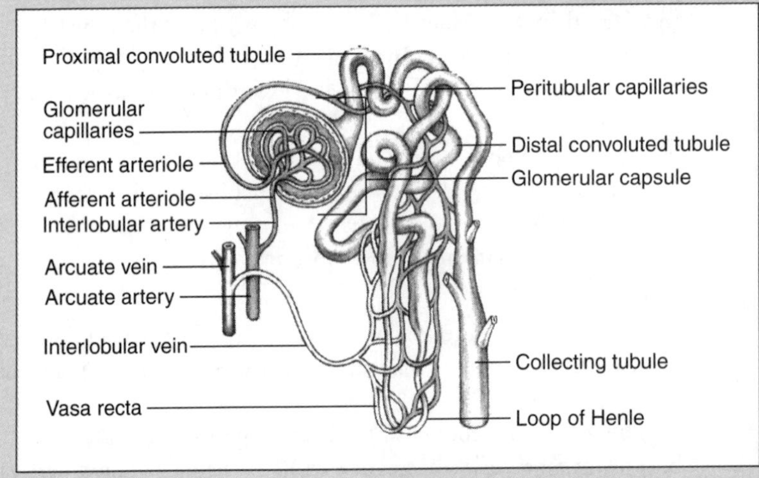

Illustration from *Illustrated Manual of Nursing Practice.* Springhouse, Pa.: Springhouse Corp., 1991.

2. Each nephron consists of a long tubule with a closed end, called the glomerular capsule, or Bowman's capsule (see *Internal structure of a nephron*)
   a. Each glomerular capsule contains a renal tubule and a GLOMERULUS, a structure consisting of a cluster of capillaries
      (1) The glomerular capsule and glomerulus comprise the *renal corpuscle*
      (2) The renal corpuscle is the main filtration site; it is highly porous
   b. The long tubule of the nephron is divided into three portions
      (1) The *proximal convoluted tubule* is the first portion, nearest to the glomerular capsule
      (2) The *loop of Henle* is the second portion, just beyond the proximal tubule; it has an ascending and a descending limb
      (3) The *distal convoluted tubule* is the third portion, most distal to the glomerular capsule
   c. The distal end of the tubule joins the distal ends of adjacent nephrons to form a larger *collecting tubule*

3. Reabsorption, secretion, and maintenance of an osmolality gradient within the interstitial fluid take place in different regions of the nephron
   a. In the proximal tubule, certain solutes are reabsorbed from the glomerular filtrate back into the blood
   b. In the descending tubule of the loop of Henle, water is removed from the filtrate (by osmosis) and returned to the interstitial fluid
   c. In the ascending limb of the loop of Henle, salts (sodium and chloride) are removed to maintain osmolality
   d. In the distal tubule, potassium and hydrogen ions are secreted and reabsorbed
   e. Some urea diffuses out of the collecting tubule and some returns to the nephron; however, most urea enters the interstitial fluid
4. The juxtaglomerular apparatus regulates blood flow through the glomerulus and regulates blood pressure by producing renin; it consists of juxtaglomerular cells and the macula densa
   a. Juxtaglomerular cells are specialized cells that contain renin granules; they are located in the wall of the afferent arteriole, where the tubule is in contact with the arteriole
   b. The macula densa is an area of compact, heavily nucleated cells in the distal convoluted tubule, where the tubule makes contact with the vascular pole of the glomerulus

D. Blood supply and innervation
1. Blood enters the kidney via large renal arteries, which branch from the abdominal aorta; these arteries deliver blood to the kidneys at a rate of about 1,200 ml/minute
   a. Each renal artery branches into five lobar (segmental) arteries
   b. Each lobar artery, in turn, branches into several interlobar arteries
   c. Each interlobar artery branches into ARCUATE ARTERIES at the junction of the renal medulla and renal cortex
   d. Afferent arterioles deliver blood to the glomerulus
2. Blood exits the kidneys via the arcuate, interlobar, lobar, and renal veins; from the glomeruli, efferent arterioles from the glomerular capsule form a capillary network (vasa recta) around the convoluted tubules and loop of Henle
3. The RENAL PLEXUS, a network of autonomic nerve fibers and ganglia, innervates the kidneys and ureters

♦ II. Ureters

A. General information
1. The two *ureters* are fibromuscular tubes that are extensions of the renal pelvis

a. Each ureter remains behind the peritoneum as it descends to the level of the bladder
b. Then it courses obliquely through the bladder wall before opening into the bladder

2. The ureters collect urine as it forms in the kidneys; then they convey it to the bladder

B. Structure

1. The walls of the ureters have three layers: the mucosa, the muscularis, and the fibrous coat
2. As the bladder fills, pressure constricts the ureters at their point of entry into the bladder

♦ III. Bladder

A. General information

1. The *bladder* is a freely movable, collapsible, muscular sac
2. It is located retroperitoneally, just posterior to the symphysis pubis
   a. In the male, the bladder lies anterior to the rectum; its neck is surrounded by the prostate gland at the urethral junction
   b. In the female, the bladder is located anterior to the uterus
3. The bladder stores urine until it is excreted; along with the urethra, it eliminates urine from the body
4. Folds of peritoneum hold the bladder in place
5. When empty, the bladder resembles a deflated balloon; as urine volume increases, it takes on a pear shape

B. Structure

1. A small, triangular area called the *trigone* lies at the base of the bladder
   a. The base of the trigone is formed by the openings of each ureter
   b. The apex of the trigone is formed by the opening of the urethra
2. The bladder wall has four layers
   a. The innermost mucosa consists of transitional epithelium
   b. The middle submucosa consists of connective tissue
   c. The third layer is muscular; the detrusor muscle in this layer contracts to expel urine
   d. The outermost layer consists of fibrous adventitia and parietal peritoneum

♦ IV. Urethra

A. General information

1. The urethra is a thin, muscular tube extending from the floor of the bladder to the surface of the body
2. The urethra drains urine from the bladder, then expels it from the body

3. The urethra has two sphincters
   a. The *internal urethral sphincter* is located at the junction with the bladder; it is composed of smooth (involuntary) muscle
   b. The *external urethral sphincter* is located at the pelvic floor; it is composed of skeletal (voluntary) muscle

B. Male urethra
1. The male urethra is approximately 8" (20 cm) long
2. It passes vertically through the prostate gland, then extends through the urogenital diaphragm and the penis
3. The male urethra has three regions
   a. The prostatic region connects to the bladder and passes through the prostate gland
   b. The membranous region passes through the urogenital diaphragm
   c. The penile region passes through the penis and terminates at the external urethral orifice
4. Besides expelling urine from the body, the male urethra serves as a passageway for semen discharge

C. Female urethra
1. The female urethra is approximately 1 to 1 1/2" (2.5 to 3.8 cm) long
2. Embedded in the anterior wall of the vagina behind the symphysis pubis, it connects the bladder with an external opening (urethral orifice or meatus)
3. It has three layers — an inner layer of mucous membrane, a middle layer of spongy tissue, and an outer layer of muscle

♦ V. Urine production

A. General information
1. The kidneys receive and filter a large volume of blood from the renal artery; tubular reabsorption and secretion converts glomerular filtrate into urine
2. Within the nephrons, glomeruli filter the blood; then the filtrate flows through the renal tubule
3. The tubules reabsorb and secrete various substances from the filtrate, changing its composition and concentration and ultimately producing urine
4. The glomerular filtration rate (GFR) depends on glomerular capillary permeability, blood pressure, and effective filtration rate

TEACHING TIPS

Patient with urinary tract infection

Be sure to include the following topics when teaching a patient with a urinary tract infection (UTI).

- Types of UTIs and their signs and symptoms
- Risk factors for UTIs
- Complications of UTIs, such as renal failure
- Diagnostic tests, such as urinalysis
- Treatments, such as antibiotic therapy
- Dietary guidelines, such as increased consumption of water and fruit juice (especially cranberry juice)
- Prevention techniques, such as perineal hygiene measures and frequent bladder emptying

5. The juxtaglomerular apparatus regulates glomerular filtration pressure by varying the glomerular filtration volume

ALERT

6. Urine and the urinary system normally are sterile; when bacteria enter through the urethra, a urinary tract infection (UTI) can occur (for teaching tips, see *Patient with urinary tract infection*)
   a. Lower UTIs include urethritis and cystitis, which affect the urethra and bladder respectively
   b. Upper UTIs include pyelonephritis, which affects the kidneys

B. Glomerular filtration
   1. The glomeruli filter about 125 ml of water and dissolved materials every minute from the blood as it flows through their capillary network

ALERT

   2. The GFR depends on three factors: permeability of the glomerular capillary walls, blood pressure, and effective filtration rate
      a. A change in any of these factors can alter the GFR significantly
      b. For example, decreased cardiac output and blood pressure can reduce renal blood flow and the GFR
   3. The juxtaglomerular apparatus helps maintain a stable GFR, despite wide variations in systemic arterial pressure
      a. A change in the GFR causes a change in filtration volume and sodium concentration of the filtrate
      b. The macula densa detects this change as the fluid flows into the distal convoluted tubule; it conveys the information to the juxtaglomerular cells in the walls of the adjacent afferent arterioles
      c. In response, the juxtaglomerular cells constrict or dilate the afferent arterioles and possibly the efferent arterioles to maintain a stable GFR

   d. The changes the glomerular filtration pressure (regulated by the juxtaglomerular apparatus) adjust the GFR of each nephron based on the character (volume and sodium concentration) of the glomerular filtrate

C. Tubular reabsorption and secretion
   1. As the filtrate passes through, the renal tubule selectively reabsorbs and secretes substances required by the body; reabsorption and secretion between tubular filtrate and peritubular blood occur via active and passive transport mechanisms
      a. Such substances as sodium, potassium, glucose, calcium, some phosphates, and amino acids undergo active transport, which requires energy
      b. Such substances as urea, water, chloride, some bicarbonates, and some phosphates undergo passive transport, which does not require energy
   2. Waste products and other unwanted substances are reabsorbed incompletely or not at all
   3. Most reabsorption occurs in the proximal convoluted tubule, which reabsorbs such substances as water, glucose, amino acids, sodium ions, chloride ions, and other electrolytes; the tubule also secretes hydrogen ions, foreign substances, and creatinine
   4. The proximal tubule also reabsorbs small amounts of protein that filter through the glomerular capillaries; the protein molecules are engulfed via pinocytosis, broken down by intracellular enzymes into amino acids, and reabsorbed
   5. The loop of Henle primarily reabsorbs sodium and chloride ions; it secretes sodium chloride
   6. The distal convoluted tubule reabsorbs sodium, chloride, and bicarbonate ions and water; it secretes such substances as hydrogen (H^+) and ammonium (NH_4^+) ions, which help maintain the normal hydrogen ion concentration (pH) of body fluids (for details, see Chapter 16, Fluid, Electrolyte, and Acid-Base Balance)
   7. The distal tubule also secretes potassium (K^+) ions in exchange for sodium (Na^+) ions, which are reabsorbed from the filtrate; this exchange is controlled by the adrenal cortical hormone aldosterone
      a. Potassium and hydrogen ions compete for secretion
      b. Increased hydrogen ion secretion reduces potassium excretion; decreased hydrogen ion secretion increases potassium excretion
   8. The collecting tubule can reabsorb or secrete sodium, potassium, hydrogen, and ammonium ions depending on the body's requirements; it also reabsorbs some water in the filtrate and secretes urea
   9. Because of reabsorption in the renal tubule and collecting tubule, only about 1% of the original filtrate volume is excreted as urine

♦ VI. Hormonal regulation of urine volume and concentration

A. General information

1. The hormones aldosterone and antidiuretic hormone (ADH) regulate urine volume and concentration
2. Aldosterone, a steroid hormone produced by the adrenal cortex, regulates the rate of sodium reabsorption from the tubules
3. ADH, a posterior pituitary hormone, is released in response to the solute concentration of blood flowing through the hypothalamus; it regulates water reabsorption from the collecting tubules

B. Aldosterone

1. This hormone acts primarily in the ascending limb of the loop of Henle and the distal tubule
2. It promotes sodium reabsorption and potassium secretion
3. Because chloride ions are absorbed along with sodium, aldosterone indirectly promotes chloride reabsorption
4. Aldosterone secretion depends primarily on the sodium and potassium concentration in body fluids
   a. A decreased sodium concentration in body fluids stimulates aldosterone secretion; this increases sodium reabsorption, raising the sodium concentration in body fluids
   b. An increased sodium concentration in body fluids reduces aldosterone secretion; this reduces sodium reabsorption, decreasing the sodium concentration in body fluids
   c. An increased potassium concentration in body fluids also stimulates aldosterone secretion; this increases sodium reabsorption and potassium secretion by the tubules, raising the sodium concentration and lowering the potassium concentration in body fluids
   d. A decreased potassium concentration in body fluids inhibits aldosterone release; this reduces potassium secretion, raising the potassium concentration in body fluids

C. ADH

1. ADH regulates water reabsorption from the collecting tubules
   a. The hormone increases collecting tubule permeability, which allows them to absorb more water from the filtrate; this makes urine more concentrated
   b. Without ADH, the collecting tubules are relatively impermeable to water; they reabsorb less water from the filtrate, and the urine remains dilute
2. Specialized cells in the hypothalamus, called *osmoreceptors,* regulate ADH release from the pituitary; these cells respond to osmotic pressure changes in the blood and body fluids

3. When body fluids are too concentrated (relatively low water and high solute content), osmotic pressure rises
   a. The pressure change stimulates osmoreceptors, which cause ADH secretion
   b. ADH causes more water to be reabsorbed from the tubules, diluting body fluids and lowering the osmotic pressure
4. When body fluids are too dilute (relatively high water and low solute content), osmotic pressure decreases
   a. ADH is not released, and water is not reabsorbed from the tubules
   b. The excess water is excreted in dilute urine
   c. Water excretion increases the relative concentration of substances dissolved in the blood, raising the osmotic pressure toward normal

♦ VII. Countercurrent mechanism

A. General information
1. The kidneys also can adjust body fluid concentrations
   a. When body fluids are too dilute, the kidneys eliminate excess water; this makes the fluids more concentrated
   b. When body fluids are too concentrated, the kidneys conserve water by excreting more concentrated urine; this makes the fluids more dilute
   c. The COUNTERCURRENT MECHANISM allows the kidneys to concentrate urine
2. Body fluid concentration is expressed in terms of fluid OSMOLARITY, which is a measure of the osmotic pressure exerted by substances dissolved in the fluid
   a. Upon leaving the glomerulus, filtrate normally has the same osmolarity as body fluids — about 300 mOsm/L; as filtrate passes along the renal tubule, its osmolarity changes in different parts of the nephron from 1,200 mOsm/L in the descending limb of the loop of Henle to 70 mOsm/L in the collecting tubule
   b. The osmolarity of interstitial fluids in the kidney varies from 300 mOsm/L in the cortex to 1,200 mOsm/L in the medulla near the renal papillae
3. The kidneys' ability to excrete urine of variable osmolarity depends on the anatomic arrangement of the loop of Henle, vasa recta, and collecting tubules, which pass through the medulla to empty at the renal papillae
   a. These three structures are adjacent to each other in the medulla
   b. They are surrounded by interstitial fluid
4. The countercurrent mechanism concentrates urine

a. This mechanism is based on the theory of the countercurrent multiplication system
   (1) The system assumes the presence of two side-by-side tubes, each with a current flowing in opposite directions
   (2) It also assumes that the two tubes are joined at one end in a U shape
   (3) Because tubular material is transported osmotically from one tube to another across the membrane separating them, the concentration of material in the U joint is greater than that entering or leaving the tubes
b. This theory describes what occurs in the nephron
   (1) When the nephron is functioning normally, sodium is actively transported out of the solution in the proximal convoluted tubule, with water flowing passively
   (2) The solution that enters the descending limb is *isotonic* (able to bathe cells without extracting water); at this point, however, sodium from extracellular fluid enters passively, so that when the solution in the limb reaches the loop of Henle, it is highly concentrated and *hypertonic* (able to extract water from cells)
   (3) When the solution enters the ascending limb, it flows along membranes that are impermeable to water but allow active transport of chlorine and passive flow of sodium
   (4) When the solution enters the distal convoluted tubule, it is *hypotonic,* which allows additional sodium and chlorine to be pumped out actively, with water flowing passively
   (5) When the solution enters the collecting tubule, the action of ADH makes the membrane permeable to water and urea; this leaves a hypertonic solution that enters the renal pelvis as urine

B. Countercurrent mechanism function
1. Glomerular filtrate flows through the proximal tubule, which reabsorbs water and dissolved substances in equal proportions; this reabsorption reduces the filtrate volume by 80% but does not change its osmolarity
2. The filtrate flows into the descending limb of the loop of Henle, which is freely permeable to water and sodium chloride
3. As filtrate passes down the descending limb, it is exposed to the high osmolarity of the interstitial fluid in the medulla
   a. Water moves from the descending limb into the interstitial tissue by osmosis
   b. Sodium chloride diffuses into the tubular filtrate from the interstitial tissue, where the sodium chloride concentration is much higher

   c. As a result, tubular filtrate osmolarity increases as the fluid passes down the descending limb until its osmolarity is as high as that of the interstitial fluid in the medulla
4. The filtrate moves into the ascending limb of the loop of Henle
   a. This limb is relatively impermeable to water and possesses an aldosterone-regulated transport mechanism that pumps sodium out of the filtrate
   b. Chloride moves out passively with sodium; water remains in the filtrate
   c. As a result, tubular filtrate osmolarity falls as the filtrate moves through the ascending limb
5. When the filtrate reaches the distal tubule, its osmolarity has fallen to 100 mOsm/L; it continues to fall to as low as 70 mOsm/L until it enters the collecting tubule
6. ADH regulates the final urine concentration
   a. If the body has insufficient water, ADH is secreted and collecting tubule permeability increases
   b. This allows water to move out of the collecting tubule by osmosis into the hypertonic interstitial fluid, which produces concentrated urine for excretion
   c. If the body has excess water, ADH is not excreted; the collecting tubules remain impermeable to water, which produces dilute urine for excretion

♦ VIII. Renal regulation of blood pressure and volume

A. General information
1. Juxtaglomerular cells in the kidneys regulate blood pressure and blood volume by secreting renin
2. They secrete renin in response to decreased blood pressure, blood volume, or plasma sodium concentration

B. Regulation process
1. Renin interacts with a blood protein called renin substrate to yield the polypeptide angiotensin I
2. Angiotensin I is converted to angiotensin II by enzymes in endothelial cells in the lungs and other tissues
3. Angiotensin II raises blood pressure by increasing vasoconstriction and stimulating the adrenal cortex to secrete aldosterone
4. Aldosterone increases sodium and water reabsorption in the renal tubule, which increases blood volume
5. The renin-angiotensin-aldosterone system is self-regulating
   a. Blood pressure, blood volume, and sodium concentration rise in response to renin secretion

b. When these levels reach the normal range, the juxtaglomerular cells are no longer stimulated, causing renin secretion to fall

ALERT

6. When the renin-angiotensin-aldosterone system functions improperly, hypertension can result

♦ IX. Urine elimination

A. General information
1. After urine is formed in the nephrons, it passes from the collecting tubules through the calyxes of the kidney to the renal pelvis
2. From the pelvis, urine is conveyed by the ureters to the bladder
   a. Smooth-muscle contractions move urine down the ureter
   b. These peristaltic contractions occur at a rate of about 1 to 5 per minute
3. The bladder stores urine until the VOIDING REFLEX is triggered; the bladder can hold 500 to 600 ml in an adult
4. Urine elimination results from involuntary and voluntary processes
5. Urine flows from the bladder through the urethra; it is expelled from the body through the external urethral opening

B. Voiding reflex
1. The voiding reflex typically is activated when the bladder contains 300 to 400 ml of urine
2. As urine fills the bladder, it stretches the bladder walls, triggering the voiding reflex
3. Stretch receptors in the bladder walls transmit sensory impulses to the spinal cord, which stimulates parasympathetic neurons
4. The spine relays motor impulses that cause bladder wall contraction and relaxation of the external urethral sphincter; this leads to urination unless voluntary control is exerted

ALERT

   a. In neurogenic bladder, normal impulse transmission from the spinal cord to the bladder is interrupted or delayed
   b. This leads to voiding problems, such as incontinence and incomplete bladder emptying
5. Besides being transmitted to the spinal cord, sensory impulses from the bladder walls are sent to higher brain centers; they are interpreted as a sense of bladder fullness or the need to urinate
6. The brain can inhibit or stimulate the voiding reflex
   a. When urination must be delayed, the individual inhibits the reflex by contracting the external sphincter, which is composed of striated muscle and is under voluntary control
   b. When the opportunity to urinate becomes available, the individual voluntarily contracts the abdominal muscles, which raises intra-abdominal pressure and helps expel urine from the bladder

Points to remember

- The urinary system includes the kidneys, ureters, bladder, and urethra. The kidneys form urine, which is excreted by the other structures.
- In the kidneys, the nephrons perform reabsorption, secretion, and maintenance of an osmolality gradient within the interstitial fluid.
- The nephrons' tubules reabsorb and secrete various substances from glomerular filtrate, altering its composition and concentration and ultimately producing urine.
- The steroid hormone aldosterone and the pituitary hormone ADH regulate urine volume and concentration.
- The countercurrent mechanism allows the kidneys to concentrate urine to the proper osmolarity.
- The renin-angiotensin-aldosterone system regulates blood pressure and blood volume by altering sodium and water reabsorption.
- The voiding reflex triggers urine elimination, which results from involuntary and voluntary processes.

Study questions

To evaluate your understanding of this chapter, answer the following questions in the space provided. Then compare your responses with the correct answers in Appendix B, page 333.

1. Where are the renal pyramids located and what is their function? ________
____
____

2. Where do the ureters, renal blood vessels, lymphatic vessels, and nerves enter or exit the kidney? ________________________________
____
____

3. What are the major functions of the kidneys? ____________________
____
____

4. What are the main functions of the bladder? ______________________

____

____

5. Which three factors influence the glomerular filtration rate? __________

____

____

6. Which hormones regulate urine volume and concentration? How do they do this?____

____

____

7. What triggers the voiding reflex?_______________________________

____

____

CRITICAL THINKING AND APPLICATION EXERCISES

1. On a three-dimensional model, trace the flow of urine through the structures of the urinary system.
2. Draw a nephron and identify its parts.
3. Create a chart that compares the effects of glomerular filtration, tubular reabsorption, and tubular secretion.
4. Prepare a presentation on the theory and effects of the countercurrent mechanism.
5. Write a one-page paper that contrasts the effects of aldosterone and ADH on urine volume and concentration.

CHAPTER

16

Fluid, Electrolyte, and Acid-Base Balance

LEARNING OBJECTIVES

After studying this chapter, you should be able to:

- Identify the two major body fluid compartments and their contents.
- Identify the routes by which water enters and leaves the body, and explain the mechanisms of water balance.
- Differentiate among the major cations and anions.
- Compare the mechanisms of electrolyte balance.
- Define pH and describe its importance in acid-base balance.
- Explain how the buffer systems, lungs, and kidneys help maintain acid-base balance.

CHAPTER OVERVIEW

Fluid, electrolyte, and acid-base balance is essential to homeostasis, health, and well-being. However, numerous factors (such as illness, injury, surgery, and treatments) can disrupt this balance and may lead to potentially fatal changes in metabolic activity. Because most patients are at risk for a fluid, electrolyte, or acid-base imbalance, the health care professional must have current, comprehensive knowledge of the substances and their regulatory mechanisms.

♦ I. Body fluids

A. General information

1. Homeostasis depends on a complex interrelationship among fluid, electrolyte, and acid-base metabolism
2. More than 50% of the average adult's body consists of water
3. The proportion of body water varies inversely with the body's fat content because fat contains no water
   a. An obese individual has a lower percentage of water than a lean person
   b. Most women have a lower percentage of water than men because their bodies normally have a higher percentage of body fat
4. Body water contains dissolved substances (solutes) that are necessary for physiological functioning; solutes include ELECTROLYTES, glucose, amino acids, and other nutrients
5. Body fluid composition differs by compartment

B. Body fluid compartments

1. The INTRACELLULAR FLUID COMPARTMENT consists of the fluid in the body's cells
2. The *intravascular fluid compartment* consists of the fluid in blood plasma and the lymphatic system
3. The *interstitial fluid compartment* consists of fluid distributed diffusely through the loose tissue surrounding the cells
4. Intravascular and interstitial fluids are separated by a capillary endothelium that is freely permeable to water, electrolytes, and other solutes
   a. Therefore, intravascular and interstitial fluids are similar in composition
   b. The intravascular and interstitial fluid compartments commonly are grouped together in a single compartment called the EXTRACELLULAR FLUID COMPARTMENT
5. The composition of intracellular fluid (ICF) differs from that of extracellular fluid (ECF)
   a. ICF has higher concentrations of protein, potassium, magnesium, phosphate, and sulfate
   b. ICF has lower concentrations of sodium, calcium, chloride, and bicarbonate
6. Active transport helps maintain different concentrations of sodium and potassium in the ICF and ECF (for details, see Chapter 3, Cell Organization)

C. Body fluid osmolarity

1. When a semipermeable membrane separates two solutions of unequal solute concentration, water shifts by *osmosis* from the less concentrated solution to the more concentrated solution

2. The ability of the more concentrated solution to attract water is called its *osmotic activity*
3. The solution's osmotic activity depends on the number of particles dissolved in the solution
   a. Osmotic activity is unrelated to the particles' molecular weight or valence
   b. The same osmotic activity results from a solution that contains equal numbers of sodium ions (which are monovalent), calcium ions (which are divalent), or glucose molecules (which do not dissociate into ions)
   c. The osmotic pressure of a solution (pressure exerted by a solution on a semipermeable membrane) usually is measured in terms of *osmolarity*
      (1) A solution of 1 L of water that contains 1 gram molecular weight of a substance that does not dissociate in solution (such as glucose) has an osmolarity of 1 Osm/L
      (2) A solution of 1 L of water that contains 1 gram molecular weight of an electrolyte that dissociates into two ions (such as sodium chloride, NaCl) has an osmolarity of 2 Osm/L
      (3) A solution of 1 L of water that contains 1 gram molecular weight of an electrolyte that dissociates into three ions (such as calcium chloride, $CaCl_2$) has an osmolarity of 3 Osm/L
   d. Because body fluids have low concentrations of dissolved particles, their osmolarity usually is expressed in milliosmols per liter (mOsm/L)

♦ II. Fluid balance

A. General information
   1. Water is essential to normal physiological functioning
   2. The body gains and loses water daily through fluid intake and output; water enters the body via the GI tract and leaves via the skin, lungs, GI tract, and urinary tract
   3. These gains and losses must be balanced to stabilize the body's water content and to permit proper physiological functioning
   4. Two mechanisms help maintain fluid balance: thirst, which regulates water intake, and the *countercurrent mechanism,* which regulates urine concentration

B. Fluid intake
   1. Water normally enters the body from the GI tract
   2. Each day, the body derives about 1,500 ml of water from consumed liquids
   3. The body also receives 700 ml from consumption of solid foods, which may contain up to 97% water

4. Food oxidation in the body generates carbon dioxide and 250 ml of water (water of oxidation)

C. Fluid output
1. Water leaves the body through the skin (in perspiration), lungs (in exhaled air), GI tract (in feces), and urinary tract (in urine)

ALERT

2. Each day, the body loses 800 ml of water through the skin and lungs; this amount of water loss may increase dramatically with strenuous exertion, predisposing the individual to dehydration
3. Although the GI tract contents include large amounts of fluid, the colon normally absorbs almost all the water; the body loses only about 200 ml of water in feces
4. Urine excretion is the main route of water loss; output typically varies from 1,000 to 1,500 ml daily

D. Mechanisms of fluid balance
1. Two mechanisms help maintain fluid balance: thirst and the countercurrent mechanism
2. Thirst (conscious desire for water) primarily regulates fluid intake
   a. Dehydration decreases the ECF volume, which increases its sodium concentration and osmolarity
   b. When the sodium concentration reaches about 2 mEq/L above normal, it stimulates the neurons of the thirst center in the hypothalamus
   c. When the brain directs motor neurons to satisfy thirst, the individual drinks the proper amount of fluid to restore the ECF to normal
3. Through the countercurrent mechanism, the kidneys can regulate fluid output by excreting urine of greater or lesser concentration (for details, see Chapter 15, Urinary System)

ALERT

4. Interruption or dysfunction of either mechanism can lead to a fluid imbalance

♦ III. Electrolyte balance

A. General information
1. *Electrolytes* are substances that dissociate into *ions* (electrically charged particles) when dissolved in water; normal metabolism and function require sufficient quantities of each major electrolyte and proper balance among electrolytes
2. Ions may be positively charged *cations* or negatively charged *anions*
3. The ICF and ECF normally contain different concentrations of electrolytes
4. Electrolyte balance is maintained by various mechanisms

B. Electrolytes

1. Major cations include sodium (Na^+), potassium (K^+), calcium (Ca^{++}), and magnesium (Mg^{++})
2. Major anions include chloride (Cl^-), bicarbonate (HCO_3^-), and phosphate (HPO_4^-)
3. Normally, the electrical charges of the cations and anions are balanced so that body fluids are electrically neutral
4. Ion concentration is expressed in terms of the ion's *equivalent weight* (ability to combine with other ions); equivalent weight equals the ion's gram molecular weight (amount of a substance that has a weight in grams equal to its molecular weight) divided by its chemical valence (numerical expression of chemical combining capacity)
   a. Ions with the same number of equivalents in a solution have equal combining powers; their concentrations are considered equal even though their gram molecular weights are different
   b. In body fluids, ions are present in such low concentrations that they usually are expressed in milliequivalents per liter (mEq/L)
5. The ICF and ECF normally have different electrolyte compositions because their cells are permeable to different substances
   a. Sodium concentration in ICF is 10 mEq/L; in ECF, 136 to 146 mEq/L
   b. Potassium concentration in ICF is 140 mEq/L; in ECF, 3.6 to 5 mEq/L
   c. Calcium concentration in ICF is 10 mEq/L; in ECF, 4.5 to 5.8 mEq/L
   d. Magnesium concentration in ICF is 40 mEq/L; in ECF, 1.6 to 2.2 mEq/L
   e. Chloride concentration in ICF is 4 mEq/L; in ECF, 96 to 106 mEq/L
   f. Bicarbonate concentration in ICF is 10 mEq/L; in ECF, 24 to 28 mEq/L
   g. Phosphate concentration in ICF is 100 mEq/L; in ECF, 1 to 1.5 mEq/L

C. Mechanisms of electrolyte balance

1. Homeostasis depends on a complex interrelationship among water, electrolyte, and acid-base metabolism; electrolytes profoundly affect water distribution, osmolarity, and acid-base balance
2. The body uses various mechanisms to maintain electrolyte balance (for details on selected mechanisms, see Chapter 15, Urinary System)
   a. Sodium is regulated chiefly by the kidneys through the action of aldosterone
      (1) Sodium is absorbed readily from food by the small intestine and is excreted through the skin and kidneys

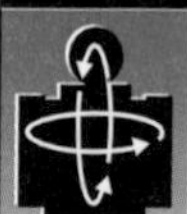

PHYSIOLOGIC PROCESS

Osmotic regulation of sodium and water

The flowchart below shows two compensatory mechanisms used to restore sodium and water balance.

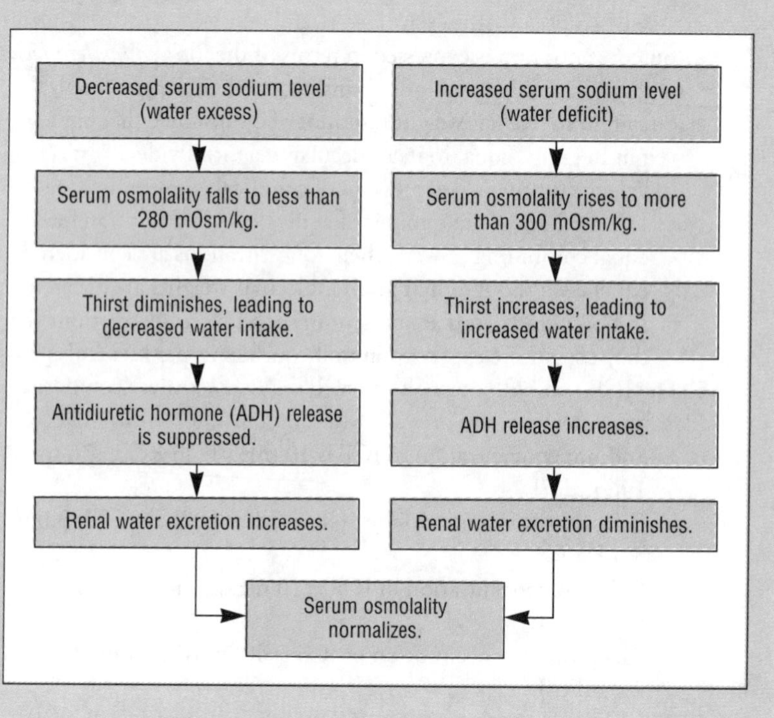

(2) Sodium and water balances are closely interrelated (see *Osmotic regulation of sodium and water*)

b. Potassium also is regulated by the kidneys through the action of aldosterone; most of it is absorbed from food in the GI tract, and the amount of potassium excreted in urine normally equals dietary potassium intake

c. Calcium in blood is in equilibrium with calcium salts in bone; calcium is regulated primarily by parathyroid hormone, which controls calcium uptake from the intestinal tract and calcium excretion by the kidneys

d. Magnesium is regulated by aldosterone, which controls renal reabsorption of magnesium; it is absorbed from the GI tract and is excreted in urine, breast milk, and saliva

e. Chloride is regulated by the kidneys; chloride ions move with sodium ions

TEACHING TIPS

Patient with an electrolyte imbalance

Be sure to include the following topics when teaching a patient with an electrolyte imbalance.

- Type and possible causes of the specific imbalance
- Signs and symptoms of the imbalance
- Diagnostic tests, such as serum electrolyte levels and electrocardiography
- Treatments, such as drugs, electrolyte replacement, and dietary supplementation
- Avoidance of foods and over-the-counter drugs that contain the electrolyte
- Medical follow-up, including diagnostic testing.

f. Bicarbonate is regulated by the kidneys, which may excrete, absorb, or form bicarbonate; it plays an important role in regulating *acid-base balance*

g. Phosphate is regulated by the kidneys; it is absorbed well from food, incorporated with calcium in bone, and regulated by parathyroid hormone along with calcium

ALERT

3. Interruption or dysfunction of any regulatory mechanism can lead to an electrolyte imbalance (for teaching tips, see *Patient with an electrolyte imbalance*)

♦ IV. Acid-base balance

A. General information

1. Acid-base balance results in a stable hydrogen ion (H^+) concentration in body fluids
2. An *acid* is a substance that dissociates in water and releases hydrogen ions
   a. A strong acid is one that dissociates virtually completely, releasing a large number of hydrogen ions
   b. A weak acid does not dissociate readily and releases fewer hydrogen ions
3. A *base* is a substance that dissociates in water and releases ions that can combine with hydrogen ions, such as hydroxyl ions (OH^-)
   a. A strong base is one that dissociates virtually completely, releasing a large number of ions
   b. A weak base does not dissociate readily and releases fewer ions
4. The hydrogen ion concentration of a fluid determines whether it is acidic or basic (alkaline)
   a. A neutral solution, such as pure water, dissociates only slightly; it contains 0.0000001 (one ten-millionth) gram molecular weight

(mol) of hydrogen ions per liter and the same amount of hydroxyl ions

b. This minute quantity may be expressed in exponential form as 10^{-7} g/L

c. More commonly, hydrogen ion concentration is expressed as pH, which is the value of the exponent without the minus sign; for example, a neutral solution that contains 10^{-7} mols of hydrogen ions per liter has a pH of 7

(1) An acidic solution contains more hydrogen ions; its pH is less than 7

(2) An alkaline solution contains fewer hydrogen ions; its pH is greater than 7

d. Because pH is an exponential expression, a change of 1 pH unit represents a tenfold change in hydrogen ion concentration; for example, a solution with a pH of 6 has ten times more hydrogen ions than one with a pH of 7

B. Sources of hydrogen ions

1. The body is an acid-producing organism
2. Protein catabolism produces several nonvolatile acids, such as sulfuric, phosphoric, and uric acid
3. Fat oxidation produces acid ketone bodies (acetoacetic acid and beta-hydroxybutyric acid)
4. Anaerobic glucose catabolism produces lactic acid
5. Intracellular metabolism creates a large quantity of carbon dioxide as a by-product; some of the carbon dioxide dissolves in body fluids to form carbonic acid

♦ V. Mechanisms of acid-base balance

A. General information

1. Buffer systems and the lungs and kidneys maintain the blood pH within a narrow range — 7.38 to 7.42 — by neutralizing and eliminating acids as rapidly as they are formed; these actions help maintain acid-base balance
2. The *sodium bicarbonate–carbonic acid buffer system* is the principal buffer in the ECF
3. The lungs affect acid-base balance by excreting carbon dioxide and regulating the carbonic acid content of the blood
4. The kidneys regulate acid-base balance by allowing tubular filtrate reabsorption of bicarbonate and by forming bicarbonate

ALERT

5. Interruption or dysfunction of a buffer system or other regulatory mechanism can lead to an acid-base imbalance

B. Buffer systems
1. Buffer systems minimize pH changes caused by excess acids or bases
2. A buffer system consists of a weak acid and a salt of that acid, or a weak base and its salt
3. The buffer system reduces the effect of a sudden change in hydrogen ion concentration by converting a strong acid or base, which normally would dissociate completely, into a weak acid or base, which releases a smaller number of free hydrogen or hydroxyl ions
4. The pH of any buffer system depends on the ratio of the two components in the buffer and not on their absolute amounts
5. The sodium bicarbonate–carbonic acid buffer system is the principal buffer in ECF
    a. This system works better in vivo than in vitro; if acid were added continuously to a fixed amount of bicarbonate-carbonic acid buffer in a beaker, eventually all of the sodium bicarbonate would be consumed by neutralizing the acid, and the buffer would lose its effectiveness because it would no longer contain bicarbonate
    b. In the body, this buffer system maintains its efficiency for two reasons
        (1) Both components of the buffer are replenished continually
        (2) The concentration of both components is regulated physiologically — sodium bicarbonate by the kidneys and carbonic acid by the lungs
    c. In the sodium bicarbonate-carbonic acid buffer system, the normal ratio of the components (20 parts sodium bicarbonate to 1 part carbonic acid) maintains a pH of 7.4
        (1) A change in the 20:1 ratio causes a corresponding change in the pH of the buffer and the body fluids it regulates
        (2) This relationship can be visualized in terms of a board on a fulcrum
            (a) Normally, one end of the board is weighted by 20 parts sodium bicarbonate, and the other end is weighted by 1 part carbonic acid
            (b) The fulcrum is positioned so the board balances at a pH of 7.4

ALERT

            (c) Changes in the ratio of sodium bicarbonate to carbonic acid will unbalance the board and shift the system to a higher or lower pH
6. The *phosphate buffer system* also helps maintain normal pH, especially in ECF
    a. The phosphate buffer uses sodium dihydrogen phosphate (NaH_2PO_4) as the acidic component and sodium monohydrogen phosphate (Na_2HPO_4) as the alkaline component

b. This buffer system is especially important in neutralizing hydrogen ions secreted by the renal tubules
7. The *protein buffer system* helps maintain normal pH; in this system, intracellular proteins function as buffers by absorbing hydrogen ions generated by the body's metabolic processes

C. Lungs
1. The lungs excrete carbon dioxide (CO_2) and regulate the carbonic acid (H_2CO_3) content of the blood
a. Carbonic acid is derived from the carbon dioxide and water (H_2O) released as a by-product of cellular metabolic activity
b. Carbon dioxide is soluble in blood plasma
(1) Some of the dissolved gas reacts with water to form carbonic acid, a weak acid that partially dissociates to form hydrogen and bicarbonate ions
(2) All three substances are in equilibrium:
$CO_2 + H_2O \leftrightarrow H_2CO_3 \leftrightarrow H^+ + HCO_3^-$
c. Carbon dioxide dissolved in plasma is in equilibrium with the carbon dioxide in the pulmonary alveoli
(1) The alveolar carbon dioxide concentration is expressed as a partial pressure (PCO_2)
(2) Consequently, an equilibrium exists between alveolar PCO_2 and the various forms of carbon dioxide in the plasma:
$PCO_2 \leftrightarrow CO_2 + H_2O \leftrightarrow H_2CO_3 \leftrightarrow H^+ + HCO_3^-$
2. The carbon dioxide content of alveolar air and the alveolar PCO_2 vary with the rate and depth of respirations
3. A change in alveolar PCO_2 causes a corresponding change in the amount of carbonic acid formed by dissolved carbon dioxide; these changes stimulate the respiratory center to alter the respiratory rate and depth
a. A rise in alveolar PCO_2 increases the blood concentration of carbon dioxide and carbonic acid, which stimulates the respiratory center to increase the rate and depth of respirations; this stimulation lowers alveolar PCO_2 and leads to a corresponding decrease in the carbonic acid and carbon dioxide concentrations in blood
b. A decrease in the rate and depth of respirations has an opposite effect, elevating the alveolar PCO_2, which leads to a corresponding increase in the carbon dioxide and carbonic acid concentrations in blood

D. Kidneys
1. The kidneys excrete various acid waste products
2. They also regulate the bicarbonate concentration in the blood in two ways
a. They allow bicarbonate reabsorption from tubular filtrate

   b. They can form additional bicarbonate to replace that used in buffering acids
3. Bicarbonate recovery and formation in the kidneys depend on hydrogen ion secretion by the renal tubules in exchange for sodium ions, which simultaneously are reabsorbed from the tubular filtrate into the circulation
4. The renal tubules secrete hydrogen ions
   a. Under the influence of the enzyme carbonic anhydrase, tubular epithelial cells form carbonic acid from carbon dioxide and water
   b. This carbonic acid rapidly dissociates into hydrogen and bicarbonate ions
   c. The hydrogen ions enter the tubular filtrate in exchange for sodium ions
   d. The bicarbonate ions enter the bloodstream along with sodium ions that have been absorbed from the filtrate
5. Bicarbonate is reabsorbed from tubular filtrate
   a. Each hydrogen ion secreted into tubular filtrate (in exchange for a sodium ion) combines with a bicarbonate ion to form carbonic acid, which rapidly dissociates into carbon dioxide and water
   b. The carbon dioxide diffuses into the tubular epithelial cell, where it can combine with more water to form more carbonic acid
   c. The leftover water molecule in the tubular filtrate is excreted in urine
   d. As each hydrogen ion moves into tubular filtrate to combine with a bicarbonate ion there, a bicarbonate ion in the tubular epithelial cell diffuses into the circulation
   e. This process is called *bicarbonate reabsorption,* even though the bicarbonate ion that enters the circulation is not the same one as in the tubular filtrate
6. To form more bicarbonate, the kidneys must secrete additional hydrogen ions in exchange for sodium ions
   a. The renal tubules cannot continue to secrete hydrogen ions unless the excess ions can be combined with other substances in the filtrate and excreted
   b. Excess hydrogen ions in the filtrate may combine with ammonia, which is produced by the renal tubules, or with phosphate salts, which are present in tubular filtrate
      (1) Ammonia (NH_3) is formed in the tubular epithelial cells by removal of the amino groups from glutamine (an amino acid derivative) and from amino acids that are delivered from the circulation to the tubular epithelial cells
         (a) Ammonia diffuses into the filtrate and combines with the secreted hydrogen ions to form ammonium ions

(NH_4^+), which are excreted in the urine with chloride and other anions
(b) Each ammonia molecule secreted eliminates one hydrogen ion in the filtrate
(c) Simultaneously, sodium ions that have been absorbed from the filtrate and exchanged for hydrogen ions enter the circulation; so does the bicarbonate formed in the tubular epithelial cells
(2) Some secreted hydrogen ions combine with Na_2HPO_4, a disodium phosphate salt in the tubular filtrate
(a) Each secreted hydrogen ion that combines with the disodium salt converts it to the monosodium salt NaH_2PO_4
(b) This reaction releases a sodium ion, which is absorbed into the circulation along with a newly formed bicarbonate ion

7. Two factors affect the rate of bicarbonate formation by the renal tubular epithelial cells: the amount of dissolved carbon dioxide in the plasma and the potassium content of the tubular cells
a. If the amount of carbon dioxide in the plasma increases, the renal tubular cells form more bicarbonate
(1) Increased plasma carbon dioxide promotes increased carbonic acid formation by the renal tubular cells
(2) Carbonic acid partially dissociates, yielding more hydrogen ions for excretion into the tubular filtrate and additional bicarbonate ions for entry into the circulation
(3) This raises the plasma bicarbonate level and decreases the plasma level of dissolved carbon dioxide toward normal
b. If the amount of carbon dioxide in the plasma decreases, the renal tubular cells form less carbonic acid
(1) Fewer hydrogen ions are formed and excreted
(2) This causes fewer bicarbonate ions to enter the circulation
(3) The plasma bicarbonate level falls correspondingly
c. The potassium content of the renal tubular cells also regulates plasma bicarbonate concentration by influencing the rate at which the renal tubules secrete hydrogen ions
(1) Tubular cell potassium content and hydrogen ion secretion are interrelated
(2) The rates at which potassium and hydrogen ions are secreted vary inversely (for details, see Chapter 15, Urinary System)
(a) If tubular secretion of potassium ions falls, hydrogen ion secretion rises
(b) If tubular secretion of potassium ions increases, hydrogen ion secretion declines

(3) Each hydrogen ion secreted into the tubular filtrate is accompanied by the addition of a bicarbonate ion to the blood plasma
   (a) Therefore, the plasma bicarbonate content rises when tubular secretion of hydrogen ions increases

ALERT

   (b) For example, if vomiting or diarrhea cause potassium depletion, then potassium secretion by the tubular epithelial cells falls, and hydrogen ion secretion rises
   (c) When body potassium is depleted, more bicarbonate enters the circulation, and the plasma bicarbonate level increases above normal

(4) The tubules excrete more potassium when the body contains excess potassium; when this occurs, fewer hydrogen ions are secreted, less bicarbonate is formed, and the plasma bicarbonate concentration decreases

POINTS TO REMEMBER

- Compared to ECF, ICF has higher concentrations of protein, potassium, magnesium, phosphate, and sulfate and lower concentrations of sodium, calcium, chloride, and bicarbonate.
- The body gains and loses water daily through fluid intake and output. Thirst regulates intake, and the countercurrent mechanism helps regulate output.
- Normally, the charges of cations (positive ions, such as sodium and potassium) and anions (negative ions, such as chloride and bicarbonate) are balanced, making body fluids electrically neutral.
- The body uses various mechanisms to maintain electrolyte balance. Many electrolytes are regulated by the kidneys and hormones.
- When acids and bases are balanced, the hydrogen ion concentration is stable and the pH is neutral (7). Acids have a pH of less than 7; bases have a higher pH.
- Buffer systems and the lungs and kidneys maintain the blood pH within a narrow range — 7.38 to 7.42 — by neutralizing and eliminating acids as rapidly as they are formed.

STUDY QUESTIONS

To evaluate your understanding of this chapter, answer the following questions in the space provided. Then compare your responses with the correct answers in Appendix B, page 333.

1. What do the intracellular and extracellular fluid compartments contain?

2. Through which organs does water enter and leave the body? ___________

3. Which mechanisms help the body achieve water balance? ___________

4. What is the difference between a cation and an anion? ___________

5. How are acids and bases similar? How do they differ? ___________

6. By which mechanisms does the body maintain acid-base balance? ___________

CRITICAL THINKING AND APPLICATION EXERCISES

1. Make a drawing that depicts the body fluid compartments.
2. Record your fluid intake and urine output for 2 days. Analyze your findings.
3. Create a chart that compares the concentrations (in mEq/L) of the major cations and anions in ICF and ECF.

4. In a one-page paper, describe the mechanisms of electrolyte balance for the major cations and anions.
5. In the laboratory, test several substances that neutralize acid. Compare their effectiveness.
6. On an illustration of the renal tubules, trace the movement of hydrogen and bicarbonate ions into and out of the renal tubule epithelial cells.

CHAPTER

17

Endocrine System

Learning objectives

After studying this chapter, you should be able to:

- Differentiate between endocrine and exocrine glands.
- Describe the general function of hormones and explain how feedback mechanisms control their levels.
- Explain how the hypothalamus controls pituitary hormone secretion.
- Compare the functions of the major pituitary hormones.
- Discuss the synthesis, secretion, and effects of thyroid hormones.
- Explain how parathyroid hormone, vitamin D, and calcitonin regulate blood calcium.
- Compare the effects of the major hormones produced by the adrenal cortex and medulla.
- Name the endocrine cells of the pancreas and the hormones that they secrete.

Chapter overview

Endocrine glands are largely responsible for maintaining the homeostasis of about 50 billion cells. These glands secrete many hormones into the bloodstream, regulating the hundreds of chemical reactions involved in growth, maturation, reproduction, metabolism, and behavior. The complexity of endocrine function contributes to the number and diversity of endocrine disorders, which can challenge your health care skills. To meet these challenges, the health care professional must be familiar with endocrine anatomy and physiology, including the functions of hormones and their effects on target cells.

♦ I. Glands and hormones

A. General information
1. The endocrine system is composed of endocrine glands, which are located throughout the body, and other structures
   a. The major endocrine glands include the *pituitary, thyroid, parathyroid,* and *adrenal glands; islets of Langerhans;* and the *ovaries* and *testes* (for details on the ovaries and testes, see Chapter 18, Reproductive System)
   b. Other structures, such as the pineal and thymus glands, are considered minor endocrine glands
2. *Endocrine glands* are ductless glands that release HORMONES directly into the blood or lymph
   a. In contrast, EXOCRINE GLANDS — sweat glands, SEBACEOUS GLANDS, mucous glands, and digestive glands — secrete their products through one or more ducts into the body's cavities or onto its surface
   b. Other tissues besides endocrine glands also produce hormones; these include the placenta and cell clusters in the walls of the GI tract, and kidneys (for details, see Chapter 18, Reproductive System; Chapter 14, Gastrointestinal System; and Chapter 15, Urinary System, respectively)

B. Functions and actions
1. The endocrine system and nervous system (sometimes collectively termed the neuroendocrine system) control all body functions
2. The endocrine system exerts its control through hormones — chemical substances that regulate the activities of specific organs
   a. Hormones control reproduction and growth; mobilize the body against stress; maintain electrolyte, water, and nutrient balance; and regulate metabolism and energy balance
   b. Once secreted by endocrine glands into the bloodstream, hormones travel to their target tissue
      (1) Specific hormone receptors within target cells or on their cell membranes determine the cell's responsiveness to a specific hormone
      (2) The number of hormone receptors in target cells varies with changes in circulating hormone levels

(a) When hormone levels are above normal, the number of receptors decreases; this compensates for the hormone excess by reducing target cell affinity for the hormone
(b) When hormone levels are below normal, the number of receptors increases; this increases target cell affinity for the hormone

c. Hormones act by altering the metabolism of specific cells in target tissue; they affect target tissue through one of two mechanisms
(1) Acting directly, hormones activate deoxyribonucleic acid (DNA) in the cells of target tissue; DNA initiates synthesis of certain protein molecules, such as enzymes, that promote metabolic activity
(2) Acting indirectly, hormones produce one or more intracellular secondary messengers that mediate the response of target tissue
(a) For example, an amino acid–based hormone produces cyclic adenosine monophosphate (cyclic AMP), an intracellular secondary messenger
(b) Cyclic AMP, in turn, activates protein kinase enzymes within the cell

3. Hormone output may be controlled directly or indirectly by feedback mechanisms
   a. Output can be regulated *directly* by the hormone level produced by a gland
   b. Output can be regulated *indirectly* by the level of a substance under hormonal control, such as glucose or sodium
4. Usually, an elevated level of hormone or hormone-regulated substance suppresses further hormone output; this arrangement is called a NEGATIVE FEEDBACK MECHANISM
5. Less commonly, a rising hormone level stimulates hormone output; this arrangement is called a *positive feedback mechanism*

C. Cyclic adenosine monophosphate and hormone function
1. Some hormones (steroid and thyroid hormones) can enter the cell and bind with intracellular hormone receptors to exert their effect
2. However, many hormones cannot enter the target cell and must bind to receptors on the cell membrane
3. Receptor binding to the cell membrane activates other enzymes to cause the desired effect in the cell
   a. Receptor binding activates the enzyme adenylate cyclase, located on the inner surface of the cell membrane
   b. This catalyzes the conversion of intracellular adenosine triphosphate (ATP) into cyclic adenosine monophosphate (AMP); this conversion continues as long as the hormone acts on the cell membrane

c. Cyclic AMP activates certain intracellular enzymes in the target cells
d. The activated enzymes perform a specific function based on target cell characteristics; for example, enzymes cause glucose liberation from glycogen in liver cells or lipid synthesis in fat cells
e. Duration of action of cyclic AMP is brief because the intracellular enzyme phosphodiesterase degrades cyclic AMP and converts it into the inactive form, AMP
f. Through this process, a hormone attached to the exterior of a cell can exert intracellular effects

♦ II. Pituitary gland

A. General information
1. The *pituitary gland,* also called the hypophysis or master gland, is located at the base of the brain in the sella turcica of the sphenoid bone
2. It receives chemical and nervous stimulation from the hypothalamus
3. The pituitary gland has two main lobes — the anterior lobe (adenohypophysis) and the posterior lobe (neurohypophysis)

B. Structure
1. The pituitary gland is a small, pea-shaped gland connected to the hypothalamus by a narrow stalk
2. The gland lies in a small depression at the base of the skull (sella turcica) just behind the optic chasm and optic nerves
3. It has an anterior lobe and a posterior lobe, which are connected by a small rudimentary intermediate lobe, which has no function in humans
   a. Releasing factors from the hypothalamus regulate hormone release from anterior lobe cells
   b. After being synthesized in the hypothalamus, posterior lobe hormones are transported by nerve axons to the posterior lobe cells, where they are stored; then they are released from the posterior lobe in response to nerve impulses transmitted from the hypothalamus down the pituitary stalk

C. Hypothalamic control
1. The hypothalamus, a portion of the diencephalon of the brain, activates, controls, and integrates various endocrine functions
2. It produces releasing and inhibiting factors (regulatory hormones) that control the anterior pituitary; these factors enter the pituitary through portal venous pathways
3. The hypothalamus also produces hormones that are stored in and secreted by the posterior pituitary
4. A negative feedback mechanism controls the release of hypothalamic substances

a. Cells in the hypothalamus regulate the level of most pituitary hormones; these cells continually monitor the levels of circulating hormones produced by target glands, such as the thyroid gland
b. When the target gland hormone level declines, the hypothalamus produces releasing factors that are carried through the portal venous pathways to the pituitary; the factors induce the release of TROPIC HORMONES that stimulate hormone production by the target gland
c. The level of the hormone produced by the target gland rises until it reaches the upper range of normal; then the elevated hormone level "shuts off" further release of releasing factors and tropic hormones

5. The mechanism maintains a relatively steady hormone output from the target gland and prevents wide fluctuations in hormone levels that might disrupt normal body functions
6. Higher cortical centers also can affect hypothalamic control of hormone release; for example, pituitary secretion may change in response to strong emotions, such as anxiety, anger, or fear (see *Mechanism of hypothalamic control*)

D. Anterior lobe hormones

1. The anterior lobe is composed of cords of epithelial cells that contain granules of stored hormone
2. Five different cell types secrete six hormones

a. Somatotropes secrete *growth hormone (GH)*, or somatotropin; GH stimulates bone and muscle growth

ALERT

(1) Hyposecretion of growth hormone in children can lead to dwarfism (abnormal underdevelopment of the body)
(2) Hypersecretion in children can result in gigantism; in adults, it leads to acromegaly (chronic disease marked by elongation and enlargement of arm, leg, jaw, and nose bones)

b. Thyrotropes secrete *thyroid-stimulating hormone (TSH)*, or thyrotropin; TSH stimulates the thyroid gland to release thyroid hormone

ALERT

(1) Hyposecretion of TSH in children results in cretinism (condition marked by hypothyroidism and arrested development); in adults, it causes myxedema (condition marked by slow speech, slow metabolism, hand and facial swelling, and coarse, edematous skin)
(2) Hypersecretion causes Graves' disease (condition marked by hyperthyroidism and thyroid enlargement)

c. Corticotropes secrete *adrenocorticotropic hormone (ACTH)*, or corticotropin; ACTH stimulates the adrenal cortex to release glucocorticoids and androgens

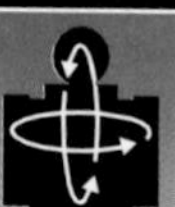

PHYSIOLOGIC PROCESS

Mechanism of hypothalamic control

Through a feedback mechanism, the hypothalamus regulates anterior pituitary hormones, which trigger hormone release by other endocrine glands, as illustrated below.

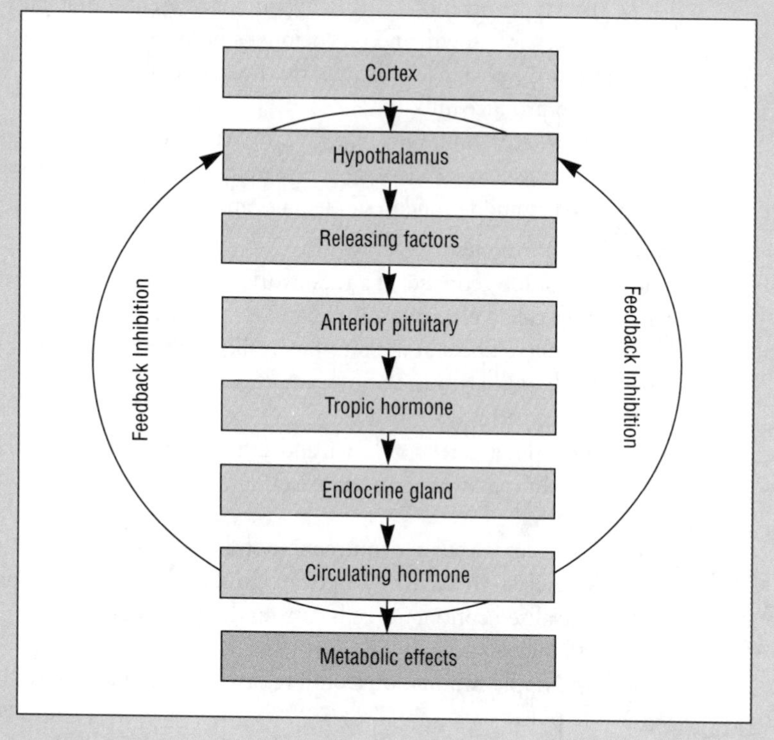

ALERT

(1) Hyposecretion of ACTH results in Addison's disease (disorder marked by increased pigmentation of skin and mucous membranes, hypotension, nausea, anorexia, and in some cases hypoglycemia)

(2) Hypersecretion results in Cushing's disease (disorder marked by fatigue, weakness, and adiposity of the face, neck, and trunk)

d. Gonadotropes secrete *follicle-stimulating hormone (FSH)* and *luteinizing hormone (LH)*

(1) FSH stimulates ovarian follicle maturation and ovarian estrogen production in females and sperm production in males

ALERT

(a) Hyposecretion inhibits sexual maturation

(b) Hypersecretion results in precocious puberty

(2) LH stimulates ovulation and ovarian production of progesterone in females and testicular production of testosterone in males

ALERT

(a) Hyposecretion results in primary or secondary hypogonadism, causing retarded growth and sexual development
(b) Hypersecretion leads to hypergonadism, resulting in excessive growth and precocious puberty

e. Mammotropes secrete *prolactin;* this hormone stimulates the breast to produce milk

ALERT

(1) Hyposecretion results in poor milk secretion
(2) Hypersecretion causes galactorrhea (persistent milk secretion) and cessation of menses in females and impotence in males

E. Posterior lobe hormones

1. The posterior lobe consists of a meshwork of nerve fibers and specialized cells called pituicytes
2. Bundles of nerve fibers in the pituitary stalk connect the posterior lobe to the hypothalamus; these structures are not linked by the portal venous pathways
3. The posterior lobe secretes oxytocin and antidiuretic hormone (ADH)

a. *Oxytocin* stimulates uterine contractions and causes MILK EJECTION from the breasts

(1) Oxytocin stimulates contraction of the pregnant uterus
(2) Milk ejection occurs when oxytocin stimulates contraction of specialized contractile cells surrounding the breast glands and ducts

(a) Nipple stimulation from breast-feeding initiates nerve impulses
(b) These impulses are transmitted to neurons in the hypothalamus, which send impulses to the posterior lobe and cause oxytocin release

b. *ADH* causes the cells of the renal and collecting tubules to become more permeable to water, altering the urine concentration (see Chapter 15, Urinary System, for more information)

(1) Osmoreceptors in the hypothalamus regulate ADH secretion by responding to osmolarity variations in the extracellular fluid (ECF)
(2) If ECF osmolarity rises above normal, hypothalamic neurons send impulses to the posterior lobe, stimulating ADH release; this causes water retention, diluting the ECF and lowering its osmolarity
(3) If ECF osmolarity falls below normal, the hypothalamus reduces ADH output from the posterior lobe; this prevents reabsorption of excess water in the tubular filtrate and caus-

es it to be excreted in the urine, concentrating the ECF and increasing its osmolarity

♦ III. Thyroid gland

A. General information
  1. One of the largest endocrine glands, the thyroid gland lies in the lower anterior neck
  2. The gland is composed of spherical follicle cells that produce the hormones *thyroxine* (T_4) and *triiodothyronine* (T_3)
  3. The gland secretes T_4, T_3, and *thyrocalcitonin;* the general term *thyroid hormone* refers to T_4 and T_3

B. Structure
  1. The thyroid gland is located in the anterior neck, overlying the inferior border of the larynx; it is fixed to the anterior surface of the upper trachea by loose connective tissue
  2. It consists of two lateral lobes — one on either side of the trachea — connected by a narrow isthmus
  3. The gland is composed of spherical thyroid follicles that contain colloid surrounded by a layer of cuboidal follicular cells; these cells synthesize the thyroid hormones T_4 and T_3
  4. Parafollicular cells, located between the follicles, secrete the hormone thyrocalcitonin (also called calcitonin)

C. Hormones
  1. T_4 and T_3 are the major metabolic hormones of the body
     a. They regulate metabolism by speeding cellular respiration
     b. T_3 has several times the biologic activity of T_4
  2. Thyrocalcitonin maintains the blood calcium level by inhibiting calcium release from bone; the calcium concentration of the fluid surrounding thyroid cells controls thyrocalcitonin secretion

D. Thyroid hormone synthesis
  1. Follicular cells actively concentrate iodine; they contain enzymes that can synthesize thyroid hormone from iodine and the amino acid tyrosine
  2. Iodine circulates in the bloodstream as iodide ions (I^-)
     a. The thyroid gland takes up these ions and oxidizes them to iodine (I_2)
     b. Iodine combines with tyrosine to form monoiodotyrosine (MIT) and diiodotyrosine
     c. Condensation of MIT and diiodotyrosine molecules yields T_3 and T_4
  3. T_3 and T_4 combine with the large protein molecule thyroglobulin and form the colloid of the thyroid follicles

TEACHING TIPS

Patient with hypothyroidism

Be sure to include the following topics when teaching a patient with hypothyroidism.
- Explanation of hypothyroidism and its causes
- Signs and symptoms of hypothyroidism
- Possible complications
- Preparation for diagnostic tests, such as laboratory tests for blood levels of thyroid hormones
- Activity restrictions
- Dietary guidelines to ensure adequate nutrition
- Importance of lifelong thyroid hormone replacement therapy
- Symptoms of hyperthyroidism (in accidental thyroid hormone overdose)

E. Thyroid hormone secretion
1. Pituitary TSH controls T_3 and T_4 output, which is regulated by a negative feedback mechanism
2. Thyroid hormone stored as colloid must be released from thyroglobulin before it can be secreted; thyroid follicular cells perform this function
   a. These cells ingest colloid by pinocytosis
   b. This causes T_3 and T_4 to split off and be secreted into the bloodstream
   c. It also degrades thyroglobulin into its component amino acids, which become part of the amino acid pool
3. Most of the thyroid hormone is metabolically inactive and circulates bound to a plasma protein called thyroid-binding globulin; only the small amount of free (unbound) hormone is metabolically active
4. Most of the secreted hormone is T_4, but much of the T_4 is converted to T_3 in the tissues where it exerts its effect

F. Metabolic effects of thyroid hormone
1. Thyroid hormone controls the rate of metabolic processes
2. It is required for normal growth and development and for development and maturation of the nervous system

ALERT

3. A thyroid hormone excess (hyperthyroidism) or deficiency (hypothyroidism) leads to a corresponding increase or decrease in metabolic processes (for teaching tips, see *Patient with hypothyroidism*)

♦ IV. Parathyroid glands

A. General information
1. The parathyroid glands are located on the thyroid gland; most people have four parathyroid glands

2. These glands secrete *parathyroid hormone* (PTH, or parahormone), the principal regulator of calcium metabolism

B. Structure

1. Four small parathyroid glands are embedded in the posterior surface of the thyroid gland
2. Pea-sized, they are the smallest endocrine glands

C. Hormones

ALERT

1. The main function of PTH is to help control the calcium level in the blood, which normally ranges from 8.5 to 10.5 mg/dl; an adequate calcium level is required for normal cardiac and skeletal muscle contraction, nerve impulse transmission, and blood coagulation
   a. Too little calcium greatly increases nerve and muscle excitability; it results from such disorders as burns, diarrhea, and vitamin D deficiency
   b. Too much calcium diminishes nerve and muscle excitability; it results from such disorders as hyperparathyroidism, vitamin D excess, prolonged immobilization, and renal or neoplastic disease
2. PTH affects the kidneys by adjusting the rate at which calcium and magnesium ions are removed from the urine
3. It also increases the movement of phosphate ions from the blood to urine for excretion
4. A reciprocal relationship exists between the calcium and phosphorus levels in the blood
   a. A decreased calcium level tends to increase the phosphorus level
   b. An increased calcium level tends to decrease the phosphorus level
5. PTH, vitamin D, and thyrocalcitonin regulate the blood calcium level
   a. PTH and vitamin D raise the blood calcium level
   b. Thyrocalcitonin lowers the blood calcium level
6. Because calcium in the blood is in equilibrium with calcium salts in bone, changes in blood calcium level eventually cause changes in the amount of calcium salts in the bone

D. Regulation of calcium metabolism

1. PTH helps regulate calcium metabolism
   a. This hormone is not stored, but is synthesized and secreted continuously
   b. The ionized calcium level in the blood regulates PTH hormone output by a negative feedback mechanism
      (1) A decrease in the ionized calcium level causes increased PTH output, which raises the blood calcium level
      (2) An increase in the ionized calcium level suppresses PTH secretion, which reduces the blood calcium level

c. PTH has three sites of action — the skeletal system, intestines, and kidneys
   (1) Its main function is to mobilize calcium from bone by promoting bone matrix breakdown and liberating calcium, which diffuses into the blood and raises the blood calcium level
   (2) In the intestines, PTH increases calcium absorption, which tends to raise the blood calcium level
   (3) In the kidneys, PTH increases calcium reabsorption by the renal tubules and promotes phosphate excretion
      (a) Increased phosphate excretion in urine lowers the phosphate concentration in blood
      (b) Because calcium and phosphate blood levels have a reciprocal relationship, the calcium level rises correspondingly

2. Vitamin D also regulates calcium metabolism
   a. This vitamin promotes calcium absorption from the intestines
   b. It is formed by a complex process from a cholesterol derivative in the skin
      (1) Ultraviolet light in sunlight converts this sterol into an intermediate compound
      (2) The liver and kidneys further metabolize the intermediate compound into the active form of vitamin D
3. Thyrocalcitonin acts as an antagonist to PTH
   a. Thyrocalcitonin is secreted in response to an increased blood calcium level
   b. It tends to lower the blood calcium level, primarily by inhibiting calcium mobilization from bone

♦ V. Adrenal glands

A. General information
1. The adrenal glands (also called suprarenal glands) are located on top of the kidneys; each consists of an outer cortex, which is enclosed in a fibrous capsule, and an inner medulla
2. These two parts of the glands secrete different hormones
   a. The adrenal cortex secretes three types of steroid hormones: glucocorticoids, mineralocorticoids, and sex hormones
   b. The adrenal medulla produces two similar hormones: norepinephrine and epinephrine

B. Structure
1. The two parts of the almond-shaped adrenal glands function as separate endocrine glands
   a. The *adrenal cortex* forms the bulk of the gland
      (1) It has three zones, or cell layers

(2) Although each zone primarily produces different hormones (called corticosteroids), the entire spectrum of corticosteroids is produced by all three zones
   (a) The zona glomerulosa, the outermost zone, secretes mineralocorticoids (such as aldosterone)
   (b) The zona fasciculata, the middle zone, secretes glucocorticoids (such as hydrocortisone, corticosterone, and cortisone)
   (c) The zona reticularis, the innermost layer, also secretes glucocorticoids and small amounts of gonadocorticoids (adrenal sex hormones); the glucocorticoids are androgens (male sex hormones) and small amounts of estrogen and progesterone (female sex hormones)

b. The *adrenal medulla* forms the inner part of the adrenal gland
   (1) It functions as part of the sympathetic nervous system
   (2) The adrenal medulla's chromaffin cells secrete the catecholamines epinephrine (adrenaline) and norepinephrine (noradrenaline)

C. Glucocorticoids
   1. The major glucocorticoid is cortisol (hydrocortisone); others include corticosterone and cortisone
   2. Cortisol and other glucocorticoids have similar actions
      a. They raise the blood glucose level by decreasing glucose metabolism and by promoting glucose formation from protein and fat (gluconeogenesis)
      b. They promote protein breakdown into amino acids, some of which are converted by the liver into glucose; this depletes tissue proteins, which are converted to glucose
   3. Glucocorticoids are secreted in response to ACTH stimulation
   4. Their output is controlled by a negative feedback mechanism in which a low glucocorticoid level stimulates ACTH secretion and a high level suppresses it

D. Mineralocorticoids
   1. Mineralocorticoids regulate electrolyte and water balance by promoting sodium ion (Na^+) absorption and potassium ion (K^+) excretion by the renal tubule (for details, see Chapter 15, Urinary System)
   2. The major mineralocorticoid is aldosterone; its secretion is regulated by more than one mechanism
      a. Although ACTH increases aldosterone secretion somewhat, the most potent stimulus is the renin-angiotensin-aldosterone system
      b. This system responds to variations in blood volume, blood pressure, and blood sodium concentration; its effect is mediated by the juxtaglomerular apparatus of the kidneys

E. Sex hormones
   1. Small amounts of estrogen, progesterone, and testosterone are produced by the adrenal glands of both sexes
   2. The amounts produced are minimal compared with the much larger quantities produced by the gonads
   3. The small amount of androgen produced by the adrenal glands appears to be responsible for the sex drive in women

F. Adrenal medulla hormones
   1. The adrenal medulla produces the hormones norepinephrine and epinephrine from a precursor amino acid called tyrosine
   2. Both hormones belong to a class of compounds called catecholamines; epinephrine differs from norepinephrine only in the presence of a methyl group (CH_3^-) attached to the amino group in the molecule
   3. During synthesis, norepinephrine is formed first; then some of it is converted to epinephrine by the addition of the methyl group
   4. Both hormones are stored in the cytoplasmic granules of adrenal medulla cells; they are released into circulation in response to nerve impulses transmitted by preganglionic fibers of the sympathetic nervous system
   5. Of the hormones produced in the adrenal medulla, norepinephrine accounts for about 20%; epinephrine accounts for the remainder
   6. Emotional stress, such as anger, fear, or anxiety, activates the sympathetic nervous system and causes the adrenal medulla to release these hormones
   7. The liberated catecholamines exert widespread effects that produce a physiological response to stress — the fight-or-flight response
      a. This response increases the heart rate and cardiac output and constricts the blood vessels
      b. It elevates the blood glucose level and mobilizes glycogen from the liver and free fatty acids from adipose tissue to provide glucose for energy
      c. This response also increases the responsiveness of the nervous system
   8. Small amounts of catecholamines are excreted unchanged in the urine, but most are inactivated by various enzymes and excreted in an inactive form
   9. Inactivation is accomplished in one of two ways
      a. A methyl group can be added to one of the hydroxyl groups in the catecholamine ring, forming a compound called a metanephrine
      b. The amino group can be removed, the terminal carbon oxidized to a carboxyl group, and a methyl group added to one of the hydroxyl groups attached to the ring; this produces vanillylmandelic acid (VMA)

♦ VI. Pancreas

A. General information
1. The *pancreas* is a triangular organ located in the hypogastric area and left upper quadrant of the abdomen
2. The pancreas has endocrine and exocrine functions
3. ACINAR CELLS make up most of the gland; they control the exocrine function of the pancreas, secreting pancreatic juice (an alkaline substance that contains digestive enzymes)
4. Scattered among the acinar cells are clusters of endocrine cells called the *islets of Langerhans,* which secrete pancreatic hormones

B. Structure
1. The head and neck of the pancreas lie in the curve of the duodenum, its body stretches horizontally behind the stomach, and its tail reaches the spleen
2. The islets of Langerhans are about one million cell clusters scattered throughout the pancreas; each islet is composed of three major cell types and three minor cell types
   a. The major types are classified as ALPHA CELLS, BETA CELLS, and gamma cells
   b. The minor types are classified as pancreatic polypeptide, D_1, and enterochromaffin cells
3. Alpha cells secrete glucagon, which raises the blood glucose level
4. Beta cells secrete insulin (the major islet hormone), which lowers the blood glucose level
5. Delta cells produce the hormone somatostatin, which suppresses insulin and glucagon release from the islets
6. Pancreatic polypeptide cells produce a hormone that stimulates GI enzyme secretion and inhibits intestinal motility
7. D_1 cells produce a hormone called vasoactive intestinal polypeptide, which increases the blood glucose level and stimulates GI secretions
8. Enterochromaffin cells synthesize serotonin

ALERT

9. Insulin is the islet cell hormone of major physiological importance; without sufficient insulin, the body develops diabetes mellitus

C. Glucagon
1. *Glucagon* is a polypeptide that helps control carbohydrate metabolism
2. The alpha cells secrete glucagon in response to hypoglycemia (decreased blood glucose level)
   a. Glucagon increases the blood glucose level by working mainly in the liver, stimulating glycogenolysis (glycogen breakdown to glucose) and gluconeogenesis (glucose synthesis from noncarbohydrate materials)

b. This process rapidly liberates glucose, increasing the blood glucose level

D. Insulin synthesis and storage
1. Within beta cells, insulin is synthesized by the endoplasmic reticulum and then transported to the Golgi apparatus
2. Next, insulin is formed into secretory granules that accumulate in the cytoplasm of the beta cells and eventually are discharged into the circulation
3. Insulin is synthesized as a large precursor peptide molecule called proinsulin, which is largely inactive
a. Chemical bonds join the two ends of the peptide chain
b. Each bond consists of a cross-bridge made of two sulfur atoms (disulfide bond); cross-linkage causes the chain to coil
4. When the proinsulin is being stored as secretory granules, a trypsinlike enzyme from Golgi apparatus membranes splits off the central part of the proinsulin coil to yield the active enzyme insulin and the connecting peptide
a. Insulin consists of two short peptide chains joined together by disulfide bonds
b. Both cleavage parts are stored in the secretory granules and secreted together into the bloodstream

E. Insulin secretion and action
1. Insulin secretion occurs in two phases
a. An initial outpouring results from the discharge of insulin stored in the cytoplasmic granules of the beta cells
b. A slower, more sustained release follows; this results from synthesis and release of additional insulin by beta cells
2. The main stimulus for insulin secretion is blood glucose elevation, which occurs after eating
3. Ingested glucose causes much more insulin to be secreted than does the same amount of intravenous glucose, because digestion triggers the release of hormones and amino acids that also stimulate insulin release
4. Several other hormones increase the blood glucose level, indirectly stimulating insulin secretion
a. Glucagon and catecholamines raise the blood glucose concentration by promoting conversion of liver glycogen into glucose
b. GH inhibits glucose use by the tissues; it promotes fat breakdown to yield free fatty acids, which are used for energy instead of glucose
c. Glucocorticoids raise the blood glucose level primarily by promoting protein breakdown into amino acids, which are converted into glucose by the liver

5. Insulin's principle action is control of carbohydrate metabolism; it also influences protein and fat metabolism
6. The chief sites of insulin action are liver cells and muscle and adipose tissue
   a. Insulin promotes the entry of glucose into the cells and enhances the use of glucose as a source of energy
   b. It promotes the storage of glucose as glycogen in muscle and liver cells; in adipose tissue, insulin enhances the conversion of glucose to triglyceride and storage of the newly formed triglyceride within fat cells
   c. Insulin also promotes the entry of amino acids into cells and stimulates protein synthesis

POINTS TO REMEMBER

- Endocrine glands release hormones directly into the blood or lymph. In most cases, hormone release is regulated by a negative feedback mechanism.
- Under hypothalamic control, the anterior lobe of the pituitary gland secretes GH, TSH, ACTH, FSH, LH, and prolactin. The posterior pituitary gland secretes ADH and oxytocin.
- Both lobes of the thyroid gland secrete T_3 and T_4, which regulate the metabolic rate, and thyrocalcitonin, which helps control calcium metabolism.
- All four parathyroid glands secrete PTH, the principle regulator of calcium metabolism.
- The adrenal cortex secretes glucocorticoids, mineralocorticoids, and sex hormones. The adrenal medulla secretes epinephrine and norepinephrine.
- In the islets of Langerhans of the pancreas, alpha cells secrete glucagon, beta cells secrete insulin, and delta cells secrete somatostatin

STUDY QUESTIONS

To evaluate your understanding of this chapter, answer the following questions in the space provided. Then compare your responses with the correct answers in Appendix B, page 334.

1. What is a hormone? ____

____

____

2. Which hormones are secreted by the anterior pituitary lobe? ___________
____
____

3. Which hormones are produced by the hypothalamus and stored in the posterior pituitary lobe? ____
____
____

4. Where are thyroid hormones synthesized and stored? _______________
____
____

5. Which substances work together to regulate calcium metabolism? _______
____
____

6. How are the adrenal medulla hormones different from the adrenal cortex hormones? ____
____
____

7. What is the chief action of insulin? _________________________
____
____

CRITICAL THINKING AND APPLICATION EXERCISES

1. In a brief presentation, compare the functions of exocrine and endocrine glands.
2. Create a poster that illustrates how hormones exert intracellular effects by binding with receptors on the exterior of cells.
3. Trace the negative feedback mechanism by which the hypothalamus controls pituitary gland secretion.
4. Write a one-page paper that describes the functions of the adrenal cortex hormones and the adrenal medulla hormones.
5. Develop of chart that compares the secretion and actions of glucagon and insulin.

CHAPTER

18

Reproductive System

Learning objectives

After studying this chapter, you should be able to:

- Describe the roles of the male and female reproductive systems.
- Identify the structures of the male reproductive system and describe their functions.
- Identify the structures of the female reproductive system and describe their functions.
- Describe the prerequisites for fertilization and the fertilization process.
- Discuss the changes that occur during the three stages of pregnancy.
- Describe the events that occur in each stage of labor.

Chapter overview

Through reproduction, parents create new individuals and pass along their genetic information to them. In this way, the reproductive system is responsible for continuation of the species. If every body system — except the reproductive system — were functioning perfectly, the individual could survive. However, the species could not. Because the reproductive system also has endocrine functions and forms an integral part of each person's self-concept, the health care professional must understand its structures and functions.

♦ I. Male reproductive system

A. General information
1. Unlike other body systems, the human reproductive system is relatively inactive until puberty
2. Although the male and female reproductive organs differ, they have a common purpose: to produce offspring
3. The role of the male reproductive system is to produce gametes (spermatozoa) and transport them to the female reproductive tract for FERTILIZATION

B. Structures
1. Structures of the male reproductive system include the penis, scrotum, testes, a duct system, and accessory organs (see *Male and female reproductive structures*)
   a. The *penis* is the copulatory organ, by which spermatozoa are placed in the female reproductive system
      (1) It consists of three cylinders of vascular erectile tissue called cavernous bodies
         (a) The upper (dorsolateral) two cylinders, the *corpora cavernosa,* are encased by dense fibrous tissue
         (b) The lower (midventral) one, the *corpus spongiosum,* encloses the urethra
      (2) Three pairs of superficial skeletal muscles attach to the bases of the cavernous bodies; contraction of these muscles compresses the urethra, which occurs during EJACULATION and urination
   b. Located posterior to the penis, the *scrotum* covers and protects the testes and spermatic cords and maintains the testes at the proper temperature for spermatozoa production
   c. The *testes,* which are located in the scrotum, are the male GONADS
      (1) They produce spermatozoa in the *seminiferous tubules*
      (2) They also produce the hormone testosterone in *Leydig's cells* (interstitial cells between the seminiferous tubules)
      (3) Gonadotropic hormones regulate testicular functions
   d. The *duct system* moves spermatozoa from the testes to outside the body
      (1) The rete testis and efferent ducts lie within each testis and drain into the epididymis, which is located on top of the testis
      (2) The duct system continues as the vas deferens, which extends to the prostate gland and joins the seminal vesicles to form the ejaculatory duct; this duct empties into the urethra

Male and female reproductive structures

Although the male and female reproductive systems share a common purpose (to produce offspring), they have vastly different structures as shown below.

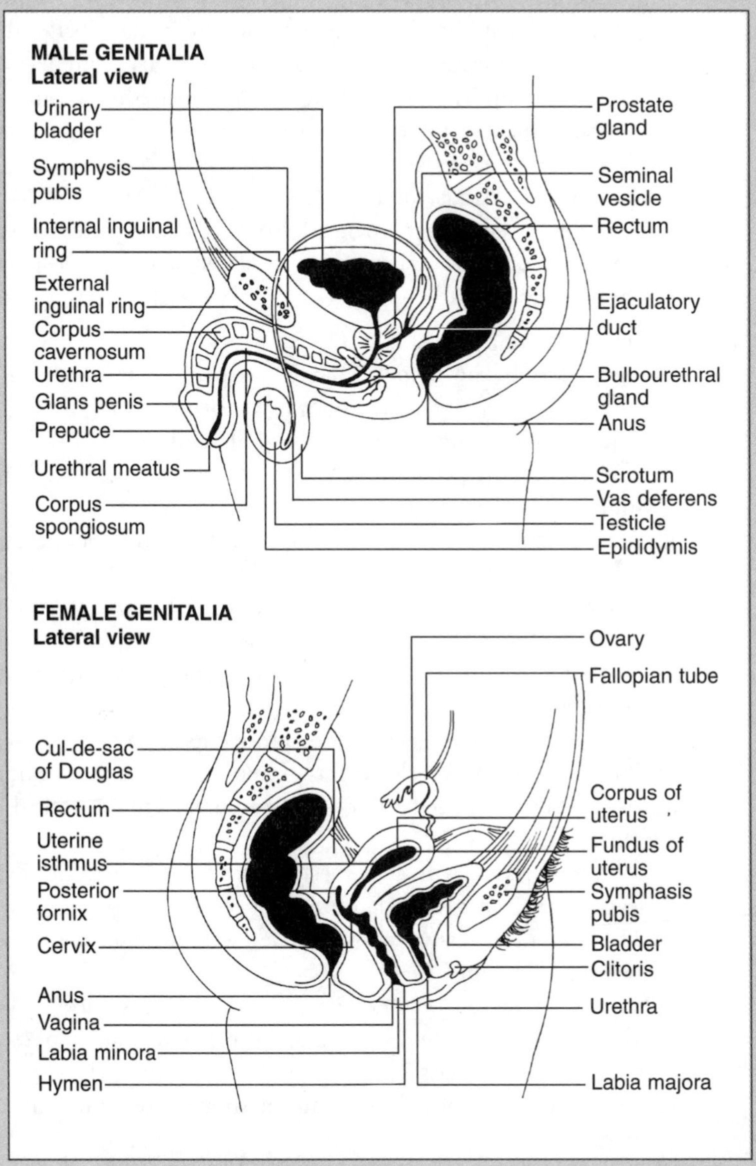

Illustrations from Cohen, S., et al. *Maternal, Neonatal, and Women's Health Nursing.* Springhouse, Pa.: Springhouse Corp., 1991.

e. The *accessory glands,* which include the seminal vesicles, prostate gland, and bulbourethral (Cowper's) glands, secrete the liquid portion of semen
   (1) The seminal vesicles merge with the vas deferens and secrete a thick alkaline fluid that nourishes spermatozoa and enhances their motility
   (2) The prostate gland surrounds the urethra and lies below the bladder; it secretes a thin alkaline fluid, which promotes sperm motility and is discharged into the urethra through small ducts that open near the orifices of the ejaculatory ducts
   (3) Cowper's glands, located below the prostate, secrete a mucoid substance that provides lubrication during intercourse

2. The male reproductive system produces semen, a mixture of spermatozoa and various fluids

C. Hormonal regulation

1. Two gonadotropic hormones regulate testicular function: *follicle-stimulating hormone (FSH)* and *luteinizing hormone (LH)*
   a. The anterior pituitary gland releases FSH and LH
   b. The hypothalamus controls FSH and LH secretion, which is continuous in males
   c. A negative feedback mechanism controls FSH and LH output; rising FSH and LH levels suppress further output of these hormones, which maintains stable gonadotropic hormone levels
2. FSH has two functions
   a. It promotes development and normal function of the seminiferous tubules
   b. FSH helps stimulate spermatozoa production
3. Inhibin suppresses FSH release; this protein (polypeptide) hormone is produced by specialized cells of the seminiferous tubules called Sertoli's cells
   a. Inhibin levels rise with active SPERMATOGENESIS; elevated inhibin levels suppress further FSH output
   b. This prevents excessive spermatogenesis and maintains normal sperm production
4. LH also promotes testosterone secretion from Leydig's cells
   a. Testosterone is responsible for sexual drive, development of secondary sex characteristics, and growth
   b. It also promotes normal spermatogenesis in the seminiferous tubules
5. Rising testosterone levels suppress further LH output, thereby maintaining a stable testosterone level
6. Spermatogenesis and testosterone production are separate functions

D. Spermatogenesis
   1. Spermatogenesis is the process of spermatozoa formation
   2. Precursor cells in the seminiferous tubules called spermatogonia contain 46 chromosomes
   3. Spermatogonia divide repeatedly by mitosis to form *primary spermatocytes*, which also contain 46 chromosomes
   4. Primary spermatocytes then undergo meiotic divisions; the number of chromosomes in the cells is reduced by half (for details on meiosis, see Chapter 3, Cell Organization)
      a. In the first meiotic division, each primary spermatocyte forms two *secondary spermatocytes* (each with 23 chromosomes)
      b. In the second meiotic division, each secondary spermatocyte forms two *spermatids* (each with 23 chromosomes), which mature into spermatozoa (with 23 chromosomes)
   5. Spermatozoa are produced continuously in the testes and seminiferous tubules; the production process takes about 2 months
   6. LH and FSH are needed to maintain normal spermatogenesis
      a. LH stimulates Leydig's cells to secrete testosterone, which is required for spermatogenesis
      b. FSH stimulates Sertoli's cells in the seminiferous tubules to secrete androgen-binding protein
         (1) This protein binds with the secreted testosterone, maintaining a high hormone level at the site of spermatogenesis
         (2) Sertoli's cells also provide nutrients to maturing spermatids, which attach themselves to these support cells

E. Spermatozoa structure and function
   1. The spermatozoon is a tadpolelike structure that consists of three parts: head, middle piece, and tail
      a. The head, which contains the chromosomes, is partially covered by a thin membranelike structure called the head cap, or acrosome; the acrosome contains enzymes that allow the spermatozoon to penetrate and fertilize the ovum
      b. The middle piece contains mitochondria with enzymes that provide the energy required to propel the spermatozoon
      c. The tail propels the sperm by flagellated movement (to and fro motion)
   2. Spermatozoa discharged in semen must undergo activation via CAPACITATION; this involves a structural change in the spermatozoon
      a. Small perforations appear in the acrosome of the spermatozoon
      b. These perforations allow the release of enzymes required for the spermatozoon to penetrate the ovum

F. Semen composition

1. Semen is a viscous secretion that consists of spermatozoa and secretions from the seminal vesicles and the prostate and Cowper's glands
   a. Seminal vesicles and prostate secretions contribute most of the semen volume; the slightly alkaline secretions provide nutrients for spermatozoa and protect them from acidic vaginal secretions
   b. Cowper's glands provide some lubricating fluid
2. The average volume of ejaculated semen is about 3 ml; the volume normally varies from 2 to 5 ml, depending on the time interval between ejaculations

ALERT

3. Normally, 1 ml of semen contains up to 100,000,000 spermatozoa
4. Although only one spermatozoon can enter the ovum to fertilize it, large numbers of spermatozoa are ejaculated to help ensure that one survives to achieve fertilization; a spermatozoa count under 20,000,000 per ml of semen usually is associated with sterility

G. Male sexual response

1. In men, SEXUAL RESPONSE consists of penile erection and semen discharge
2. The penile erectile tissue consists of three cylinders composed of a spongy meshwork of endothelium-lined blood sinuses supplied by many arterioles and drained by veins
3. The erectile tissue cylinders, surrounded by fibrous capsules, are called cavernous bodies
4. Because the arterioles that supply the erectile tissue of the cavernous bodies normally are contracted, little blood flows into the cavernous bodies, and the sinusoids are collapsed
5. Sexual excitement causes reflex dilation of the arterioles; this results from parasympathetic nerve stimulation and concomitant inhibition of sympathetic nerves, which normally constrict arterioles
   a. The cavernous bodies become engorged with blood, and the veins that drain them become compressed, causing the penis to become rigid
   b. The penis returns to the flaccid state as a result of parasympathetic nerve inhibition and sympathetic nerve stimulation; this causes the arterioles to constrict again and allows the excess blood to drain from the cavernous bodies
6. Semen discharge involves a two-phase spinal reflex, consisting of EMISSION and *ejaculation*
7. Emission refers to semen movement into the urethra
   a. Emission occurs when the sympathetic nervous system transmits efferent impulses from the lumbar spinal cord
   b. These impulses cause rhythmic contractions of the muscles near the epididymis, vas deferens, seminal vesicles, and prostate gland to expel semen into the urethra

8. Ejaculation is the pulsatile expulsion of semen from the penis; it is associated with erotic sensations called ORGASM
   a. Ejaculation occurs when efferent impulses from the sacral portion of the spinal cord cause rhythmic contractions of the muscles around the base of the penis
   b. This intermittently compresses the urethra, causing semen to be expelled from the penis in spurts
9. During emission and ejaculation, the sphincter muscle at the base of the bladder constricts, preventing semen reflux into the bladder
10. The two-phase spinal reflex occurs when impulses from the penis and genital region, other skin areas, and cerebral cortex reach a critical level of intensity

H. Developmental considerations
1. Before *puberty,* trace amounts of sex hormones produced by the gonads are sufficient to suppress production of gonadotropin-releasing hormones by the hypothalamus
2. At puberty, the hypothalamus matures and loses its extreme sensitivity to the inhibitory effect of low sex hormone levels
3. Then the hypothalamus begins to release gonadotropin-releasing hormones; these cause the release of pituitary FSH and LH, which stimulate the gonads to release sex hormones (testosterone in men, estrogen and progesterone in women)
4. Sex hormones induce sexual development and other body changes characteristic of sexual maturity; production of mature spermatozoa marks puberty in males
5. With age, testosterone secretion slowly declines; this may lead to reduced sex drive and somewhat reduced spermatogenesis

♦ II. Female reproductive system

A. General information
1. The female reproductive system includes the ovaries, fallopian tubes, uterus, vagina, external genitalia, and mammary glands (see *Male and female reproductive structures,* page 293)
2. The role of the female reproductive system is to produce gametes (ova) and nurture a developing embryo
3. The normal MENSTRUAL CYCLE prepares the endometrium to receive the fertilized ovum; if fertilization does not occur, the prepared endometrium is discarded through menstruation and a new cycle starts

B. Structures
1. The female reproductive system includes external and internal genitalia and the mammary glands

2. The external genitalia, or *vulva*, include the mons pubis, labia majora, labia minora, clitoris, and vestibule
   a. The *mons pubis* is a cushion of adipose and loose connective tissue over the symphysis pubis
   b. The *labia majora* are twin folds of adipose and connective tissue that run from the mons pubis to the perineum
   c. The *labia minora* are twin folds of connective tissue between the labia majora
   d. Similar to the penis, the *clitoris* is composed of erectile tissue; it is surrounded by mucosal folds (the prepuce of the clitoris)
   e. The *vestibule* is an oval-shaped structure surrounded by the clitoris and labia; several internal structures open into the vestibule, including the urethra, vagina, and ducts from Skene's and Bartholin's glands, which secrete lubricating substances during intercourse
3. The internal genitalia include the vagina, cervix, uterus, fallopian tubes, and ovaries
   a. The *vagina* is a fibromuscular tube that extends from the vestibule to the cervix
      (1) It serves as a passageway for menstrual flow and as the receptacle for the penis during intercourse
      (2) It also is the lower part of the birth canal
   b. The *cervix* is the narrow inferior portion of the uterus; it projects into the upper end of the vagina
   c. The *uterus*, a pear-shaped structure with a thick muscular wall, is designed to receive a fertilized ovum and support fetal development
      (1) The organ is lined by a glandular mucous membrane (endometrium)
      (2) It is held in position by bands of connective tissue called ligaments
   d. The *fallopian tubes* extend laterally from the upper corners of the uterus
      (1) These tubes transport ova from the ovaries to the uterus
      (2) The fringed (fimbriated) ends partially surround the adjacent ovaries
   e. The *ovaries* are the female gonads; they produce ova
4. The *mammary glands,* located in the breasts, are specialized accessory glands that secrete milk; each mammary gland contains 15 to 25 lobes, separated by fibrous connective tissue and fat
   a. Alveolar glands within the lobes produce milk during lactation
   b. Milk passes through excretory (lactiferous) ducts to the outside of the nipple

C. Menstrual cycle hormones
  1. Pituitary and ovarian hormones induce cyclic changes in the endometrium that are responsible for the menstrual cycle
  2. These hormones also produce less pronounced cyclic changes in the breasts, fallopian tubes, and cervical mucosa
  3. The pituitary hormones FSH and LH are secreted cyclically in women
    a. FSH stimulates the ovarian follicles to grow and secrete estrogen
    b. LH acts with FSH to promote follicle maturation
      (1) Under the influence of FSH and LH, a follicle develops and discharges its ovum; this action marks OVULATION
      (2) Then LH causes the ruptured follicle to change into a large convoluted yellow structure called the *corpus luteum,* which produces the steroid hormones estrogen and progesterone
  4. Under the influence of FSH and LH, the ovary secretes estrogen and progesterone
  5. The estrogen secreted by the ovaries exerts several effects
    a. The hormone induces sexual development at puberty, including proliferation of glandular tissue of the breasts
    b. Estrogen stimulates endometrial growth during the first half (proliferative phase) of the menstrual cycle
    c. It stimulates the glandular epithelium of the cervix to secrete a thin, alkaline mucus that facilitates spermatozoa passage into the uterus and fallopian tubes
    d. Estrogen also has general metabolic effects, such as stimulation of bone growth
  6. Progesterone, secreted by the corpus luteum, produces several effects
    a. Progesterone induces marked secretory activity in the endometrial glands during the second half (secretory phase) of the menstrual cycle, preparing the endometrium for implantation of the fertilized ovum
    b. The hormone also increases cervical mucus thickness and viscosity, making it relatively resistant to spermatozoa penetration during the postovulatory phase
    c. Progesterone also causes breast development
  7. Pituitary (gonadotropic) and ovarian hormones have a reciprocal relationship
    a. A high estrogen level inhibits FSH output, stabilizing the estrogen level; it also stimulates LH release, which increases progesterone output
    b. A high progesterone level inhibits LH output

D. Oogenesis
  1. OOGENESIS is the process of ova formation
  2. Precursors of the ova, or *oogonia,* proliferate by mitosis in the fetal ovaries before birth; they form primary oocytes (with 46 chromosomes)

3. Then a single layer of granulosa or follicular cells surrounds the oocytes, forming structures called primary follicles
   a. The primary oocytes in the primary follicles enter the prophase of the first meiotic division during fetal development, but they do not continue to divide
   b. A very large number of primary follicles form; however, less than 500 ova are released in a lifetime, and only a few of these are fertilized
4. The primary follicles remain inactive until puberty, when cyclic ovulation begins under the influence of FSH and LH
5. During each menstrual cycle, primary follicles begin to grow in the ovary, but normally only one matures and is ovulated
   a. The granulosa cells around the follicles proliferate, and a layer of noncellular material called the zona pellucida is deposited on the surface of the oocyte
   b. Fluid begins to accumulate in the layer of granulosa cells; a central fluid-filled cavity forms in the mature or graafian follicle
6. About the time the oocyte is released at ovulation, it completes its first meiotic division, giving rise to two daughter cells — a secondary oocyte and the first polar body, which are of unequal size
   a. The secondary oocyte contains half the chromosomes (23) and almost all the cytoplasm
   b. The first polar body contains the remaining 23 chromosomes but almost no cytoplasm
7. The newly formed secondary oocyte begins its second meiotic division, but it does not complete this division unless it is fertilized; completion of the second division gives rise to a mature ovum and a second polar body, each containing 23 chromosomes
   a. Whether fertilization occurs or not, the first polar body immediately undergoes a second meiotic division, giving rise to two additional haploid polar bodies (for a total of three), which degenerate
   b. The ovum can survive for about 3 days after ovulation; however, it can only be fertilized successfully for about 36 hours after ovulation
8. The ovum is swept into the fimbria of the fallopian tube by the beating of cilia that cover the tubal epithelium; it is propelled down the fallopian tube by the cilia and by peristaltic contractions of smooth muscle in the wall of the tube

ALERT

9. Ova released late in a woman's reproductive life have been arrested in prophase for up to 45 years before resuming meiosis at ovulation; this may explain the high incidence of congenital abnormalities related to abnormal chromosome separation in the offspring of older women

E. Menstrual cycle
   1. The beginning of the cycle customarily is dated from the first day of menstrual flow
   2. Ovulation occurs around the middle of the cycle, dividing it into preovulatory (follicular) and postovulatory (luteal) phases
   3. Menstrual cycle duration varies considerably among individuals; it also may vary somewhat from month to month in an individual
      a. Variations usually result from differences in the preovulatory phase duration
      b. The duration of the postovulatory phase remains relatively constant at about 14 days
   4. During the preovulatory phase, the pituitary gland begins to release FSH, which stimulates a group of ovarian follicles to grow
      a. The first follicle to respond grows more rapidly and comes to full maturity
      b. The other follicles undergo involution (atrophy)
   5. Soon after FSH output rises, LH output begins to increase; together FSH and LH promote estrogen secretion by the ovarian follicles
   6. The increasing estrogen output inhibits further FSH release and stimulates LH release
      a. LH release eventually builds to a precipitous outpouring called the LH surge, which persists for about 24 hours
      b. This surge leads to rupture of the follicle and ovulation
   7. The postovulatory phase is characterized by conversion of the ruptured follicle into a corpus luteum, which produces estrogen and progesterone
   8. The corpus luteum reaches maturity about 8 to 9 days after ovulation; then it begins to degenerate if pregnancy has not occurred
   9. Menstruation results from the decline in corpus luteum activity, which reduces estrogen and progesterone output
      a. Eventually, the levels of these two hormones no longer can maintain the endometrium
      b. Then the endometrium is shed, producing the menstrual flow
      c. Menstruation lasts about 5 days; it is associated with an average total blood loss of 50 to 150 ml
   10. As estrogen and progesterone levels fall, their inhibitory effects on FSH and LH release also decline
   11. Eventually, when estrogen and progesterone have fallen to low levels, FSH and LH are released again and a new cycle begins

F. Female sexual response
   1. The physiologic effects of sexual excitement in women are similar to those in men
   2. The parasympathetic nervous system controls the dilation of arterioles that supply the erectile tissue in the clitoris and labia minora

   a. During sexual excitement, nerve impulse transmission causes the tissues to become engorged with blood
   b. Parasympathetic impulses also cause Skene's and Bartholin's glands to produce secretions that lubricate the vagina during intercourse
3. Sensory input from nerve endings in the clitoris, labia, vaginal orifice, and perineal tissues is transmitted to the lumbar and sacral spinal cord
4. When this input reaches a critical level, a spinal reflex response occurs, characterized by rhythmic contractions of the uterus and fallopian tubes; these contractions, together with rhythmic and pulsatile contractions of the skeletal muscles around the vagina, comprise the erotic sensations called orgasm
5. Female sexual climax differs from male climax; it produces no secretions comparable to the ejaculate and is not required to achieve fertilization

G. Developmental considerations
1. The hypothalamus and pituitary gland perform the same actions to achieve puberty in women as in men; however, the release of pituitary FSH and LH stimulates the gonads to release estrogen and progesterone in women
2. These sex hormones induce sexual development and other body changes characteristic of sexual maturity, including MENARCHE in women
3. With age, women's ovarian follicles degenerate without producing mature egg cells; mature egg cell production declines until about age 45, when few follicles remain
   a. The ovaries no longer respond to FSH and LH stimulation and stop producing sex hormones
   b. When the ovaries no longer can produce sufficient hormones to stimulate cyclic changes in the endometrium, menstruation ceases; this condition is called MENOPAUSE

♦ III. Fertilization

A. General information
1. Fertilization is the union of a spermatozoon and an ovum
2. Fertilization occurs only when several basic prerequisites are met
   a. Spermatozoa must be adequate in function and number
   b. A mature ovum must be available and ready to be fertilized
   c. Spermatozoa must be transported effectively through the female reproductive tract

ALERT

3. Any structural or functional problem that interferes with these prerequisites can lead to infertility (for teaching tips, see *Patient with infertility*)

TEACHING TIPS
Patient with infertility

Be sure to include the following topics when teaching a patient who is infertile.
- Definition of infertility and its causes, such as ovulatory dysfunction, structural abnormalities, or inadequate spermatozoa production
- Diagnostic tests, such as semen analysis and laparoscopy
- Treatment with fertility drugs, which alter hormone levels
- Explanation of alternative techniques for becoming pregnant, such as in vitro fertilization and artificial insemination
- Surgery to promote fertility, such as varicolectomy and laparotomy
- Psychological counseling
- Sources of information and support

B. Spermatozoa transport
1. Spermatozoa move through the female reproductive tract by two mechanisms
   a. Spermatozoa travel several millimeters per hour by flagellar propulsion
   b. They are transported up into the uterus and fallopian tubes by rhythmic contractions of uterine muscles
2. Although several hundred million spermatozoa are deposited by a single ejaculation, many are destroyed by the acidity of vaginal secretions
3. Only the spermatozoa that enter the cervical canal, where they are protected by cervical mucus, can survive
4. The ease with which spermatozoa can penetrate cervical mucus is related to the menstrual cycle phase
   a. Early in the cycle, spermatozoa have difficulty passing through the cervix because estrogen and progesterone levels cause the mucus to thicken
   b. During midcycle, spermatozoa can pass readily through the cervix because the mucus is relatively thin
   c. Later in the cycle, spermatozoa have difficulty passing through the cervix because the mucus is much thicker
5. Once through the mucus, the spermatozoa enter the uterus
   a. Only spermatozoa (not seminal fluid) enter the uterus and fallopian tubes
   b. Uterine contractions help spermatozoa ascend into the fallopian tubes
6. Spermatozoa probably can fertilize the ovum for up to 2 days after ejaculation, although they may survive for 3 to 4 days in the reproductive tract

C. Ovum fertilization
   1. Fertilization normally occurs in the distal part of the fallopian tube; it requires intercourse to occur around the time of ovulation based on the viability of the germ cells
      a. The ovum remains viable for 24 to 36 hours
      b. The spermatozoa remain viable for 48 hours or more
   2. Before a spermatozoon can penetrate the ovum, it must disperse the granulosa cells and penetrate the zona pellucida; enzymes in its acrosome allow this penetration
   3. Once the spermatozoon has penetrated, the ovum completes its second meiotic division; the zona pellucida becomes impermeable to other spermatozoa
   4. The spermatozoon head fuses with the ovum nucleus, forming a cell nucleus with 46 chromosomes
   5. The fertilized ovum is called a ZYGOTE

♦ IV. Pregnancy

A. General information
   1. Pregnancy begins with fertilization and ends with childbirth; this time period, also called *gestation,* averages 38 weeks
      a. Various structures develop as a result of pregnancy, such as the *decidua, amniotic sac and fluid, yolk sac,* and *placenta*
      b. The zygote undergoes a complex sequence of *pre-embryonic, embryonic,* and *fetal development,* finally producing a full-term fetus
   2. Because the exact date of fertilization usually is unknown, the expected delivery date may be calculated from the beginning of the last menstrual period (LMP)
      a. The length of gestation calculated from the LMP is 40 weeks — not 38 weeks — because the first day of the LMP occurs about 2 weeks before ovulation
      b. Gestation length calculated from LMP may be expressed as 280 days, as 10 lunar (28-day) months, or as 9 calendar (31-day) months
   3. A 9-calendar-month gestation may be subdivided into three periods of 3 months, or *trimesters*
   4. Because the uterus grows throughout pregnancy, uterine size provides a rough estimate of the duration of pregnancy

B. Structural development
   1. Pregnancy changes the usual development of the *corpus luteum*
      a. When a woman becomes pregnant, placental tissue secretes large amounts of human chorionic gonadotropin (HCG), which is similar to LH and FSH
         (1) HCG prevents corpus luteum degeneration

    (2) It stimulates the corpus luteum to produce large amounts of estrogen and progesterone
  b. During the first 3 months of pregnancy, the corpus luteum serves as the main source of estrogen and progesterone; these hormones are needed during pregnancy
  c. Later in pregnancy, the placenta produces most of the hormones; although it persists, the corpus luteum is no longer needed to maintain the pregnancy
2. The *decidua* is the endometrial lining that has undergone the hormone-induced changes of pregnancy; it covers the chorionic vesicle and eventually becomes part of the placenta
  a. The decidua envelops the embryo and fetus during gestation
  b. Decidual cells secrete three substances
    (1) The hormone prolactin promotes lactation
    (2) The hormone relaxin relaxes the connective tissue of the symphysis pubis and pelvic ligaments and facilitates cervical dilation
    (3) Prostaglandin mediates several physiologic functions
3. The *amniotic sac* gradually increases in size; usually by 8 weeks' gestation, it completely surrounds the developing embryo and fuses with the chorion
  a. The fused amnion and chorion extend from the placental margins to form the fluid-filled amniotic sac, which ruptures at the time of delivery
  b. The amniotic sac and its fluid have two important functions
    (1) During gestation, they protect the fetus by creating a buoyant temperature-controlled environment
    (2) During childbirth, they form a fluid wedge that helps open the cervix
  c. Amniotic fluid source and volume vary with the gestational stage
    (1) Early in pregnancy, amniotic fluid is derived chiefly from maternal and fetal blood, and fluid from the fetal skin and respiratory tract
    (2) Later in pregnancy, fetal urine becomes the major source of amniotic fluid
    (3) Maternal and fetal blood filtration and fetal urine excretion continually add to the total amniotic fluid volume
4. The *yolk sac* forms adjacent to the endoderm of the germ disc
  a. Part of the yolk sac is incorporated in the developing embryo and forms the GI tract
  b. Another part of the yolk sac gives rise to primitive germ cells, which migrate to the developing gonads and eventually form oocytes or spermatocytes

c. The yolk sac also forms blood cells during early embryonic development
d. The yolk sac never contains yolk and has no nutritive function; it eventually undergoes atrophy and disintegrates

5. The *placenta* is a flattened, disc-shaped structure that weighs about 500 grams at delivery; from the third month of pregnancy until childbirth, it supplies nutrients to and removes wastes from the fetus
   a. The placenta forms from the chorion (and its chorionic villi) and the part of the decidua in which the villi are anchored
   b. The umbilical cord connects the fetus to the placenta; the cord contains two arteries and one vein
      (1) The arteries that carry blood from the fetus to the placenta follow a spiral course on the cord, divide on the placental surface, and send branches to the chorionic villi
      (2) Large veins on the placental surface collect blood returning from the villi; these veins join to form the single umbilical vein that enters the cord and returns blood to the fetus
   c. The placenta has two circulatory systems
      (1) The UTEROPLACENTAL CIRCULATION delivers oxygenated arterial blood from the maternal circulation to the intervillous spaces (large spaces between the chorionic villi in the placenta)
         (a) Blood spurts into the intervillous spaces from many uterine arteries that penetrate the basal part of the placenta
         (b) Blood leaves the intervillous spaces and flows back into the maternal circulation through veins that penetrate the basal part of the placenta near arteries
      (2) The FETOPLACENTAL CIRCULATION delivers oxygen-depleted blood from the fetus to the chorionic villi by the two umbilical arteries; it returns oxygenated blood to the fetus by the single umbilical vein
      (3) The proximity of the placental circulatory systems brings maternal and fetal blood into close contact; although the maternal and fetal circulations exchange oxygen, nutrients, and wastes, fetal and maternal blood do not mix
   d. The placenta produces several peptide and steroid hormones
      (1) The peptide hormone *HCG* can be detected as early as 9 days after fertilization; the level increases and peaks at about 10 weeks' gestation, then gradually declines
         (a) HCG stimulates the corpus luteum to produce the estrogen and progesterone needed to maintain the pregnancy until the placenta takes over hormone production

(b) Highly sensitive pregnancy tests can detect HCG in blood and urine even before the first missed menstrual period

(2) The level of the peptide hormone *human placental lactogen (HPL)* rises progressively throughout pregnancy

(a) HPL stimulates maternal protein and fat metabolism to ensure an adequate supply of amino acids and fatty acids for the mother and fetus

(b) It antagonizes the action of insulin, decreasing maternal glucose metabolism and making more glucose available to the fetus

(c) It also stimulates breast growth in preparation for *lactation*

(3) The steroid hormone *estrogen* increases uterine muscle irritability and contractility

(a) The placenta produces three different estrogens, which differ chiefly in the number of hydroxyl groups

(b) The placenta lacks some of the enzymes needed to complete estrogen synthesis; it requires some precursor compounds produced by the fetal adrenal glands

(c) Because neither the fetus nor the placenta can synthesize estrogens independently, estrogen production reflects the functional activity of the fetus and placenta

(4) The steroid hormone *progesterone* reduces uterine muscle irritability

(a) The placenta synthesizes this hormone from maternal cholesterol

(b) The fetus plays no part in progesterone synthesis

C. Pre-embryonic development

1. The first period of prenatal development, pre-embryonic development, begins with ovum fertilization and lasts 3 weeks
2. The zygote undergoes a series of mitotic divisions, or cleavage, as it passes through the fallopian tube
3. The first cell division is completed about 30 hours after fertilization
4. Subsequent divisions occur in rapid succession; the zygote is converted into a ball of cells called a *morula,* which reaches the uterus about 3 days after fertilization
5. Fluid accumulates in the center of the morula, forming a central cavity; the structure now is called a *blastocyst*
6. Blastocyst cells differentiate in two ways

a. A peripheral rim of cells, called the *trophoblast,* develops; the trophoblast gives rise to the fetal membranes and contributes to placenta formation

b. A discrete cell cluster in the trophoblast, called the *inner cell mass,* eventually forms the embryo

7. The blastocyst is enclosed in the zona pellucida and remains unattached to the uterus for several days
8. The zona pellucida degenerates during the week after fertilization; this allows the blastocyst to attach to the endometrium and become implanted
9. The inner cell mass becomes a flat structure, called the germ disc, which differentiates into three germ layers — the *ectoderm, mesoderm,* and *endoderm*
10. A cleft appears between the ectoderm of the germ disc and the surrounding trophoblast, forming the amniotic sac
11. The yolk sac, forms on the opposite side of the germ disc
12. A layer of connective tissue lines the enlarging blastocyst cavity and covers the amniotic and yolk sacs
    a. At this point, the cavity contains the germ disc, amniotic sac, and yolk sac and is called the chorionic sac; its wall is called a *chorion*
    b. The entire chorionic sac and embryo is called the chorionic vesicle
13. Finger-like columns of cells, called chorionic villi, extend from the chorion and anchor the chorionic vesicle to the endometrium

D. Embryonic development

1. During the embryonic period, which lasts from the fourth through the seventh week, the developing zygote begins to assume a human shape and is called an embryo

ALERT

2. This period of development is critical; all the organ systems form, and the embryo is susceptible to injury by maternal drug use and other factors, such as radiation
3. During this period, each germ layer forms specific tissues and structures
    a. The ectoderm primarily forms the external covering of the embryo and the structures that will have contact with the environment
    b. The mesoderm forms the circulatory system, muscles, supporting tissues, and most of the urinary and reproductive systems
    c. The endoderm forms the internal linings of the embryo, such as the epithelial lining of the pharynx and respiratory and GI tracts

E. Fetal development

1. During the fetal period, which extends from the eighth week until birth, the fetus becomes larger and heavier as it matures; however, it experiences no major changes in its basic structure comparable to those in the embryonic period
2. The fetus displays two unusual features during early development

a. The head is disproportionately large compared to the rest of the body; this condition changes after birth as the infant grows
b. The body lacks subcutaneous fat; it fills out shortly before birth, when fat begins to accumulate

♦ V. Labor and postpartal adaptation

A. General information
1. Childbirth (parturition), delivery of the fetus, is accomplished through labor, the process in which the fetus is expelled from the uterus by uterine contractions
a. Weak uterine contractions occur irregularly throughout pregnancy
b. When labor begins, uterine contractions become strong and regular
c. Voluntary bearing-down efforts eventually supplement the contractions and lead to expulsion of the fetus and placenta
2. Usually, the head of the fetus occupies the lowest part of the uterus; in this cephalic presentation, the fetus is delivered headfirst
3. Childbirth is divided into three stages for descriptive purposes; the duration of each stage varies with uterine size, maternal age, and the number of previous pregnancies
4. After childbirth, the infant and mother undergo adaptation

B. Onset and maintenance of labor
1. Several factors contribute to the onset of labor
a. The number of oxytocin receptors on uterine muscle fibers increases progressively during pregnancy and reaches a peak just before the onset of labor; this increase causes the uterus to become more sensitive to the effects of oxytocin
b. The uterus stretches as the pregnancy progresses, initiating nerve impulses that stimulate oxytocin secretion from the posterior pituitary lobe
c. The fetus also may play a role in initiating labor
(1) Near term, increased adrenocorticotropic hormone (ACTH) secretion by the fetal pituitary causes the fetal adrenal glands to secrete more cortisol, which diffuses into the maternal circulation through the placenta
(2) Cortisol increases oxytocin and estrogen secretion and decreases progesterone secretion
(3) These changes in hormone secretion increase uterine muscle irritability and make the uterus more sensitive to oxytocin stimulation
d. Prostaglandins also may play a role in initiating labor

(1) Decreasing progesterone leads to conversion of esterified arachidonic acid into a nonesterified form
(2) The nonesterified arachidonic acid undergoes biosynthesis to form prostaglandins, which stimulate uterine contractions

ALERT

e. If labor does not begin by 2 weeks after the due date, the woman may undergo labor induction or cesarean delivery because of the increased risk of fetal brain damage or death in a postterm delivery

2. Once labor begins, several factors maintain it
   a. Cervical dilation causes nerve impulse transmission to the central nervous system, which increases oxytocin secretion from the pituitary gland
   b. Increased oxytocin secretion serves as a positive feedback mechanism; it stimulates more uterine contractions, which further dilate the cervix and cause the pituitary to secrete more oxytocin
   c. Oxytocin also may stimulate prostaglandin formation by the decidua; prostaglandins diffuse into the uterine myometrium and enhance contractions

C. Stages of labor
1. The first stage of labor is characterized by cervical effacement (thinning) and dilation; the fetus begins to descend
   a. Before labor begins, the cervix is not dilated; by the end of the first stage, the cervix is dilated fully
   b. Uterine muscles contract actively while the cervix and the lower part of the uterus thin and dilate
   c. The amniotic sac and fluid function as a hydrostatic wedge to help dilate the cervix
   d. The first stage lasts from 6 to 24 hours in primiparous women; it is much shorter in multiparous women
2. The second stage covers the time between full cervical dilation and expulsion of the fetus
   a. Uterine contractions increase in frequency and intensity, and the amniotic sac ruptures
   b. As the flexed head of the fetus enters the pelvis, pelvic muscles force the head to rotate anteriorly and force the back of the head (occiput) under the symphysis pubis
   c. Uterine contractions force the flexed head deeper into the pelvis
   d. The resistance of the pelvic floor gradually forces the head into extension
      (1) As the head presses against the pelvic floor, the vulvar tissues stretch, and the anus dilates
      (2) At this stage, the vulvovaginal orifice usually is enlarged surgically by a small incision, called an episiotomy

e. As the head is delivered, the face passes over the perineum, and maternal tissues retract under the chin
f. The head, which had been rotated anteriorly during fetal descent, rotates back to its former position after passing through the vulvovaginal orifice
g. Usually, the head undergoes lateral (external) rotation as the anterior shoulder rotates forward to pass under the pubic arch
h. Delivery of the shoulders and the rest of the fetus follows shortly afterwards
i. This stage averages about 45 minutes in primiparous women; it may be much shorter in multiparous women

3. The third stage of labor begins immediately after childbirth and ends with expulsion of the placenta
   a. After delivery of the neonate, the uterus continues to contract intermittently and reduces in size
   b. The area of placental attachment also is reduced correspondingly; because the bulky placenta cannot decrease in size, it separates from the uterus
   c. Blood seeps into the area of placental separation
   d. As the uterus continues to contract, retroplacental blood is compressed and acts as a fluid wedge, cleaving the placenta from the uterus
   e. Usually, the edges of the placenta are the last to separate from the uterine wall; the midportion of the placenta, covered by the fetal membrane, commonly is expelled first
   f. This stage averages about 10 minutes in primiparous and multiparous women

D. Infant adjustment after birth

1. The respiratory system undergoes changes after birth
   a. The fetus depends on the mother to provide oxygen and remove carbon dioxide
   b. At delivery, the oxygen supply from the mother ceases
      (1) This causes the infant's carbon dioxide level to increase, stimulating the respiratory center in the brain
      (2) In response, the brain causes the respiratory muscles to contract, allowing the infant to draw its first breath
2. The cardiovascular system also makes several adjustments after birth
   a. At birth, flaps of heart tissue fold together, closing the foramen ovale in the fetal heart and diverting blood to the lungs for the first time
   b. When the infant's lungs start to function, heart muscle contractions close the ductus arteriosus

(1) Closure normally becomes permanent about 3 months after birth

ALERT

(2) Incomplete closure results in patent ductus arteriosus

3. The liver must undergo changes at birth to regulate bile pigment production; this may lead to physiologic jaundice a few days after birth

E. Maternal adjustment after birth

1. After childbirth, the reproductive tract requires about 6 weeks to return to its former condition; this period is called the puerperium, or postpartal period

a. The uterus rapidly decreases in size; most of the involution occurs in the first 2 weeks after delivery

b. The stretched tissues of the pelvis and vulva return to their former state more slowly

c. The cervix becomes less elastic and returns to its prepregnancy firmness

2. Postpartal vaginal discharge (lochia) persists for several weeks after childbirth

a. Lochia rubra (bloody discharge) occurs from 1 to 4 days postpartum

b. *Lochia serosa* (pink-brown, serous discharge) occurs from 5 to 7 days postpartum

c. *Lochia alba* (white, brown, or colorless discharge) occurs from 1 to 3 weeks postpartum

♦ VI. Lactation

A. General information

1. LACTATION, milk production by the breasts, is regulated by the interactions of four hormones

a. Estrogen and progesterone, which are produced by the ovaries and placenta, stimulate proliferation of breast tissue

b. Prolactin and oxytocin are produced by the pituitary and decidua

(1) Prolactin causes milk secretion after the breasts have been stimulated by estrogen and progesterone

(2) Oxytocin causes contraction of specialized cells, which help expel milk during breast-feeding

2. Breast-feeding stimulates prolactin secretion; the resulting high prolactin level causes changes in the mother's menstrual cycle

B. Hormonal initiation of lactation

1. Progesterone and estrogen levels fall sharply after childbirth when the placenta is expelled

2. Because estrogen and progesterone no longer inhibit the effects of prolactin on milk production, the mammary glands begin to secrete milk
3. Prolactin secretion also decreases after delivery unless the nipples are stimulated by breast-feeding
   a. Sensory impulses from the nipples are transmitted to the hypothalamus; this stimulates prolactin release from the anterior pituitary lobe
   b. Milk secretion continues as long as the nipples are stimulated regularly by breast-feeding; if breast-feeding is discontinued, the stimulus for prolactin release is removed and milk production stops
4. Breast-feeding also stimulates oxytocin
   a. Sensory impulses from the nipples are transmitted to the hypothalamus; this causes oxytocin release from the posterior pituitary lobe
   b. Oxytocin causes contraction of the myoepithelial cells surrounding the breast lobules
   c. This contraction causes *milk ejection* (expulsion of breast milk from the secretory lobules into larger ducts)
   d. The breast-feeding infant readily obtains milk from these ducts

C. Effects of breast-feeding on the menstrual cycle
1. The high prolactin level in a postpartal woman inhibits FSH and LH release
2. If a woman does not breast-feed her infant, prolactin output soon declines and FSH and LH production by the pituitary is no longer inhibited
   a. Cyclic release of FSH and LH soon follows
   b. Normal menstrual cycles commonly resume about 6 weeks after delivery or a few weeks after discontinuation of breast-feeding
3. If the woman breast-feeds her infant, the menstrual cycle does not resume because prolactin inhibits the cyclic release of FSH and LH necessary for ovulation; consequently, a breast-feeding woman usually does not become pregnant
4. The amount of prolactin released in response to breast-feeding gradually decreases
   a. The inhibitory effect of prolactin on FSH and LH release also declines
   b. Consequently, ovulation and the menstrual cycle may resume; pregnancy may occur after this, even though the woman continues breast-feeding

Points to remember

- The male and female reproductive systems share a common purpose: to produce offspring.
- The male reproductive system includes the scrotum, testes, duct system, accessory reproductive glands, and penis. These structures work together to produce spermatozoa and then deposit them in the female reproductive system during sexual intercourse.
- The female reproductive system includes the ovaries, fallopian tubes, uterus, vagina, external genitalia, and mammary glands. These structures work together to produce ova, allow fertilization, maintain pregnancy, perform childbirth, and feed an infant.
- Fertilization (union of a spermatozoon and an ovum) usually occurs in the distal part of the fallopian tube.
- Pregnancy, which averages 38 weeks, begins with fertilization and ends with childbirth. A full-term pregnancy allows pre-embryonic, embryonic, and fetal development.
- During labor, the fetus is expelled from the uterus by uterine contractions. Hormones, the uterus, and the fetus all play a role in initiating or maintaining labor, which is divided into three stages.
- Lactation is controlled by the interaction of the hormones estrogen, progesterone, prolactin, and oxytocin.

Study questions

To evaluate your understanding of this chapter, answer the following questions in the space provided. Then compare your responses with the correct answers in Appendix B, page 334.

1. Which structures are the male and female gonads? ____________________

____

____

2. What structures comprise the external female genitalia? ______________

____

____

3. How does the female sexual climax differ from the male sexual climax?

____

____

4. What are the basic prerequisites for fertilization? _______________

____

____

5. What are the functions of the substances secreted by the decidua? _______

____

____

6. What physiological events are associated with each stage of labor? _______

____

____

7. Which hormones control lactation? _______________________

____

____

CRITICAL THINKING AND APPLICATION EXERCISES

1. On an anatomical chart, identify the major structures of the male and female reproductive systems.
2. Create a table that compares spermatogenesis with oogenesis.
3. Using three-dimensional models, trace the flow of spermatozoa through the male reproductive system and the movement of the ovum through the female reproductive system.
4. Write a one-page paper that summarizes the growth of the fertilized ovum through the pre-embryonic, embryonic, and fetal development stages.
5. Design a poster of a pregnant uterus that traces the uteroplacental and fetoplacental circulations of the placenta.
6. Prepare a table that compares the placental hormones and their functions.

APPENDIX A

Glossary

Accommodation—adjustment of the lens of the eye to change the focal length and bring images into sharp focus on the retina

Acid—substance with excess hydrogen ions and a pH under 7

Acid-base balance—stable concentration of hydrogen ions in body fluids

Acinar cells—secretory cells surrounding a cavity, such as those in the acinar glands of the pancreas

Actin—contractile protein in muscle fibers

Active transport—movement of a substance across a cell membrane by a chemical activity that allows the cell to admit larger molecules than would otherwise be able to enter; this transport mechanism requires energy

Adenosine triphosphate—compound in muscle cells that releases energy when bonds are broken

Aerobic metabolism—energy-releasing process that requires oxygen, in which glucose is converted to pyruvate and then oxidized to yield carbon dioxide, water, and adenosine triphosphate (ATP) by mitochondrial enzymes

Agglutination—clumping

Air conduction—sound wave transmission through the tympanic membrane and auditory ossicles

Alimentary canal—gastrointestinal tract; continuous tube open at both ends, extending through the ventral cavities from the mouth to the anus

All-or-none response—response that governs muscle fiber contractions in a motor unit; a nerve impulse strong enough to stimulate contraction causes all the fibers to contract

Alpha cells—glucagon-secreting cells in the pancreatic islets

Alveoli—microscopic air sacs in the lung where air and blood exchange gases

Anabolism—synthesis of simple substances into complex ones

Anaerobic metabolism—energy-releasing process that does not require oxygen, in which glycogen and glucose are broken down into lactic acid

Anterior—ventral, or toward the front of the body; the opposite of dorsal or posterior

Apices—pointed extremities of conical structures (such as the apices of the renal pyramids)

Aponeurosis—flat sheet of connective tissue that attaches muscle to bone or soft tissue

Appendicular skeleton—division of the skeleton consisting of the pectoral and pelvic girdles and the upper and lower limbs

Arcuate arteries—arc-shaped arteries that branch from the interlobar arteries

Arrectores pilorum—tiny smooth muscles of the skin attached to hair follicles whose contraction causes the hair to stand erect

Articulation—joint; point of junction of two or more bones

Atom—unit of matter that contains a nucleus and electrons and makes up a chemical element

Axial skeleton—division of the skeleton consisting of the bones that form the longitudinal axis, including those of the skull, vertebral column, and bony thorax

Axon—extension projecting from the cell body of a neuron that conducts impulses away from the cell body

Base—substance with excess hydroxide ions and a pH above 7

Basement membrane—extracellular, filamentous material composed mainly of collagen and found between the epidermis and dermis

Beta cells—insulin-secreting cells in the pancreatic islets

Binocular vision—vision that produces a three-dimensional image, which is necessary for normal depth perception

Bone conduction—sound wave transmission through the bones of the skull

Buffer system—system that minimizes pH changes caused by excess acids or bases (alkalies)

Calyces—cup-shaped organs or cavities, such as those in the renal pelvis

Capacitation—activation process for spermatozoa that allows ovum penetration; small perforations appear in the acrosome (head cap) of the spermatozoon, allowing enzyme release

Carbohydrate—organic compound that contains carbon, hydrogen, and oxygen in a specific arrangement

Cardiac cycle—events that occur during a single systole and diastole of the atria and ventricles

Cardiac output—amount of blood ejected per minute from a ventricle, which equals the stroke volume (volume of blood ejected from a ventricle at each contraction) multiplied by the heart rate in beats per minute

Catabolism—breakdown of complex substances into simpler ones or into energy

Caudal—inferior, or toward the tail or lower part of the body

Cerebellum—section of the brain located posterior and inferior to the cerebral hemispheres, divided into two hemispheres and a middle section (vermis) and linked with the brain stem by three pairs of peduncles; regulates and coordinates all complex motor activities

Cerebrospinal fluid—plasma-like fluid, composed of secretions of the ventricles of the brain, that fills the ventricles and surrounds the brain and spinal cord

Cerebrum—largest section of the brain, divided into two hemispheres by the longitudinal fissure; performs sensory, motor, and integrative functions related to mental activities

Chemotaxis—movement toward or away from a chemical stimulus

Choroid plexus—any of the masses of capillaries in the ventricles of the brain that produce cerebrospinal fluid

Cilia—hairlike processes projecting from cells

Citric acid cycle—metabolic pathway by which a molecule of acetyl-CoA is oxidized enzymatically to yield energy

Coagulation—blood clotting

Common bile duct—duct that receives bile from the hepatic and cystic ducts and transports it to the duodenum

Complement system—collection of about 20 proteins in blood and tissue fluids that, when activated, augments the effects of antibodies

Concentration gradient—differences in the concentration of the molecules on each side of a cell membrane

Conditioned reflex—reflex that can be learned as a result of past associations; for example, salivation induced by the sight or smell of specific foods

Condyle—rounded protuberance at the end of a bone

Convergence—eye alignment so that the image of a near object falls at corresponding points of both retinas, allowing depth perception

Coronary sinus—enlarged vessel at the junction of the cardiac veins that empties blood into the right atrium

Cortex—outer layer (such as the cerebral cortex of the brain)

Countercurrent mechanism—process by which the kidneys concentrate urine

Cranial—superior, or toward the head

Cross bridges—structures formed by the binding of myosin filament heads to actin filaments; they pull actin filaments toward the center of the sarcomere, causing muscle contraction

Cross over—mixing of genetic material in meiosis; during synapsis, chromatic segments of homologous chromosomes break off and interchange

Cutaneous—pertaining to the skin (sometimes used interchangeably with dermis)

Deamination—removal of the amino group $-NH_2$ from a compound

Deep—farthest from the body surface

Dendrite—branched extension projecting from the cell body of a neuron that receives impulses and conducts them toward the neuron

Depolarization—change in resting membrane potential toward zero

Diastole—cardiac relaxation

Diffusion—movement of dissolved particles (solute) across the cell membrane from one solution to a less concentrated one

Digestion—breakdown of food into absorbable nutrients in the GI tract

Distal—farthest from the trunk, point of origin of a part, or center of the body; the opposite of proximal

Dorsal—posterior, or toward the back of the body; the opposite of anterior or ventral

Effector cells—cells capable of being stimulated to produce an effect

Ejaculation—pulsatile expulsion of semen from the penis; it is associated with the erotic sensations called orgasm

Ejection fraction—amount of blood ejected during each ventricular contraction in relation to the end-diastolic volume

Electrolyte—substance that dissociates into ions when dissolved in water and can conduct an electrical current

Electron—particle with a negative charge that orbits the nucleus in different electron shells

Electron transport system—metabolic pathway that converts products of the citric acid cycle into energy

Element—substance that cannot be broken down into smaller substances

Emission—semen movement into the urethra

End-diastolic volume—total blood volume in each ventricle before ventricular systole

Endochondral bone formation—type of ossification in which a mass of cartilage forms, is invaded by osteoblasts, and is converted into bone

End-systolic volume—blood volume that remains in a ventricle after systole

Equilibrium—sense of balance

Erythropoiesis—process of red blood cell (erythrocyte) formation

Exocrine gland—gland that releases secretions through one or more ducts that open onto an internal or external body surface

Expiratory reserve volume—amount of air that can be exhaled forcefully at the end of a normal tidal expiration (about 1,300 ml in the average adult)

Extracellular fluid compartment—intravascular fluid (in blood plasma and lymph) and interstitial fluid (in loose tissue surrounding the cells)

Facilitated diffusion—type of diffusion involving a carrier molecule in the cell membrane that picks up the diffusing substance on one side of the membrane and deposits it on the other side

Fascia—fibrous membrane covering that supports and separates skeletal muscles

Fasciculi—small bundles, such as of muscle or nerve cells

Fertilization—union of a spermatozoon and ovum

Fetoplacental circulation—circulatory system that delivers oxygen-depleted blood from the fetus to the placenta by the umbilical arteries; it returns oxygenated blood to the fetus by the umbilical vein

Fibrinolysis—blood clot dissolution

Fight-or-flight response—response to stimulation of the sympathetic nervous system; it prepares an individual to cope with stress; also called alarm response

Focal length—distance from a convex lens to its focal point

Focal point—point behind a convex lens at which parallel light rays are brought into focus

Foramen—hole in a bone for passage of vessels and nerves

Fossa—shallow depression

Functional areas—parts of the cerebral cortex related to specialized functions

Gamete—sex cell (spermatozoon or ovum)

Ganglion—collection of nerve cell bodies located outside the central nervous system

Gas exchange—process of respiration in which gases are transported between the air and capillaries in the lungs

Glabella—region above the root of the nose, between the eyebrows

Glomerulus—filtering portion of the nephron, consisting of a cluster of capillaries

Gluconeogenesis—glucose synthesis from amino acids

Glycogenesis—glycogen synthesis from glucose

Glycogenolysis—glycogen breakdown into glucose

Glycolysis—metabolic pathway that converts glucose to pyruvic acid or lactic acid and yields energy

Gonad—primary reproductive organ

Gray matter—nervous tissue that appears gray from lack of myelinated fibers

Hematocrit—measurement of the volume of red blood cells packed by centrifuge, expressed as a percentage of the total blood volume

Hematopoiesis—formation and development of blood cells from stem cells

Hemoglobin—protein-iron compound in red blood cells that carries oxygen to cells from the lungs and transports carbon dioxide from cells to the lungs

Hemostasis—arrest of bleeding by complex mechanisms that include vasoconstriction and coagulation

Homeostasis—maintenance of a stable internal environment

Heterozygous—having different alleles at a given locus on homologous chromosomes

Homozygous—having identical alleles at a given locus on homologous chromosomes

Hormone—chemical substance produced in one part of the body that regulates or initiates the activity of an organ or cells in another part; typically a steroid or amino acid derivative

Hyaline cartilage—flexible, semitransparent material composed of a basophilic, fibril-containing, interstitial substance with cavities containing chondrocytes; covers the articular surface of bones (also called chondroid cartilage)

Hydrolysis—chemical reaction in which a chemical bond is broken and the atoms of a water molecule are added across the break. Hydrogen is added to one side, and the hydroxyl group to the other side

Hydrostatic pressure—pressure that filters fluid from the blood through the capillary endothelium

Ileocecal valve—valve (sphincter muscle) located between the ileum of the small intestine and the cecum of the large intestine; permits only forward passage of intestinal contents

Immunity—ability to resist organisms or toxins that can damage tissues

Inferior—caudal, or toward the tail or lower part of the body

Inspiratory reserve volume—amount of air that can be inhaled forcefully at the end of a normal tidal inspiration (about 3,000 ml in the average adult)

Integument—covering, such as the skin and its derivatives

Intracellular fluid compartment—fluid in the body's cells

Intramembranous bone formation—type of ossification in which osteoblasts form bone without a preliminary cartilage mass

Intrapleural pressure—pressure in the pleural cavity (space between the lung and chest wall)

Intrapulmonary pressure—air pressure in the lungs

Keratinize—to become hard or horny

Lateral—away from the midline of the body

Lipids—organic compounds made of carbon, hydrogen, and water that usually is insoluble in water; fat

Lipogenesis—lipid synthesis from glucose

Long bone—bone whose length exceeds its width

Matrix—extracellular substance secreted by connective tissue that determines the specialized function of the tissue; typically includes collagen, elastic, or reticular fibers and ground substances (material occupying intercellular spaces in fibrous connective tissue, cartilage, or bone)

Medial—toward the midline of the body

Mediastinum—central region of the thoracic cavity between the lungs that contains all thoracic viscera except the lungs

Meiosis—special type of cell division in gametes, in which the daughter cells receive half the number of chromosomes of the parent cells

Menarche—onset of menses

Meninges—connective tissue membranes that enclose the brain and spinal cord; the three meninges are the dura mater, arachnoid, and pia mater

Menopause—cessation of menses, resulting from ovarian follicle depression; typically occurs around age 45

Menstrual cycle—recurring cycle in which a layer of the endometrium is shed, and then regrows, proliferates, and sheds again

Metabolism—transformation of substances into energy or materials the body can use or store; consists of the two processes anabolism and catabolism

Milk ejection—expulsion of breast milk from the secretory lobules into larger ducts of the breast

Mitochondria—cytoplasmic organelles that generate adenosine triphosphate

Mitosis—type of cell division in which the parent cell produces identical daughter cells with chromosomes duplicated from the parent; it occurs in all human cells, except gametes

Lactation—milk production and secretion

Myelin sheath—segmented, fatty wrapping around the axons of many nerve fibers

Myofibril—threadlike contractile filaments found in skeletal muscle cells

Myosin—contractile protein in muscle fibers; its interaction with actin is crucial to muscle contraction

Negative feedback mechanism—mechanism in which an elevated level of a hormone or hormone-regulated substance suppresses further hormone output

Nephron—functional and structural unit of the kidney, consisting of the renal corpuscle, loop of Henle, and renal tubule

Nucleic acid—organic compound made of nucleotides that contain pentose, a phosphate group, and a nitrogenous base

Neurilemma—thin, membranous sheath composed of Schwann cells that surrounds the segmented myelin sheaths of peripheral nerve fibers

Neuromuscular junction—motor endplate and axon terminal associated with it

Neutron—electrically neutral particle in an atom

Oogenesis—process of ova formation

Opsonization—process by which phagocytosis increases

Optic tracts—bundles of optic nerve fibers that connect the optic chiasma and the brain stem

Orgasm—climax of sexual excitement usually accompanied by seminal fluid ejaculation in the male

Osmolarity—measure of osmotic pressure exerted by a solution

Osmosis—movement of water molecules across the membrane from a dilute solution (having a high concentration of water molecules) to a concentrated one (having a lower concentration of water molecules)

Osmotic pressure—pressure exerted by a solution on a semipermeable membrane

Osteoblast—mesodermal cell that participates in bone formation

Osteoclast—large, multinucleated cell that reabsorbs the bone matrix

Ovulation—ovum release from an ovarian follicle

Oxidation—loss of electrons by a chemical compound

Pacemaker—specialized cardiac tissue (specifically, the sinoatrial node) that generates impulses that spread to other regions of the heart; sets the contraction rate of the heart

Pacinian corpuscles—encapsulated sensory nerve endings responsive to vibration and deep or heavy pressure, found in sensitive skin, subcutaneous tissue, and other specialized areas (such as the pancreas, penis, clitoris, and nipple)

Pain—sensation of discomfort or suffering caused by pain receptor stimulation

Partial pressure—pressure exerted by a single gas in a mixture of gases; it is designated by the letter "P" preceding the chemical symbol for the gas

Passive transport—movement of small molecules across the cell membrane by diffusion; this transport mechanism requires no energy

Peptide—substance derived from two or more amino acids

Periosteum—fibrous membrane that covers bones except at joint surfaces

Peripheral resistance—degree of impedance to blood flow, which may be increased by vasoconstriction

Peristalsis—movement of the contents of a tubular organ through wavelike, rhythmic muscular contractions

pH—measurement of the hydrogen ion concentration in body fluids; a pH of 7 is neutral, less than 7 is acidic, and more than 7 is basic, or alkaline

Phagocyte—cell that surrounds, engulfs, and digests harmful particles or cells

Phagocytosis—process by which specialized cells engulf and dispose of organisms, other cells, and foreign particles

Plasma—straw-colored fluid that remains after formed elements (blood cells) have been removed from the blood

Pleura—double-layered serous membrane that encloses the lungs and lines the thoracic cavity

Polarization—state of a nerve fiber not transmitting an impulse; the fiber exterior has a positive charge, the interior a negative charge

Posterior—dorsal, or toward the back of the body; the opposite of anterior or ventral

Process—prominence or projection (such as of bone)

Protein—organic compound made of carbon, hydrogen, oxygen, and nitrogen and containing amino acids

Proton—particle with a positive electrical charge in an atom

Proximal—closest to the trunk, point of origin of a part, or center of the body; the opposite of distal

Pseudostratified columnar epithelium—columnar epithelial tissue that appears to be (but is not) multilayered

Purkinje fibers—modified cardiac muscle fibers that form part of the conduction system of the heart

Pylorus—lower portion of the stomach through which stomach contents empty into the duodenum

Reduction—gain of electrons by a chemical compound

Referred pain—internal organ pain that is perceived as coming from the body surface at a site distant from the organ

Reflex—automatic or involuntary action in response to a stimulus, usually mediated through the spinal cord

Reflex arc—chain of sensory, connecting, and motor neurons that produces a reflex when stimulated

Refraction—bending of light rays as they pass from one medium to another of different density

Refractive index—measurement of the refractive power of a medium; the greater the refractive index, the more the light rays are bent as they pass through the medium

Refractory period—brief period after nerve impulse transmission during which the nerve fiber is unresponsive and cannot transmit another impulse

Renal plexus—network of autonomic nerve fibers branching from the celiac plexus and accompanying the renal artery to the kidney; innervates the kidneys and ureters

Renin-angiotensin-aldosterone mechanism—self-regulating mechanism that helps control blood pressure, blood volume, and sodium plasma concentration

Residual volume—amount of air left after the lungs expel the expiatory reserve volume (about 1,200 ml in the average adult)

Resorption—bone breakdown, which normally equals bone formation during adulthood

Respiratory center—control center in the brain stem that regulates the rate and depth of respiration

Resting membrane potential—voltage difference between the interior and exterior of a nerve fiber

Retroperitoneally—behind the peritoneum or outside the peritoneal cavity

Reuptake—absorption of a neurotransmitter into the synaptic vesicles of the axon terminals that originally released it

Sagittal plane—vertical plane through the longitudinal axis of the trunk that divides the body into right and left regions

Salt—substance that ionizes into anions and cations, but not into H^+ or OH^- ions

Saltatory conduction—type of conduction in myelinated nerves in which the depolarization wave jumps between gaps in the myelin sheath rather than moving progressively along the fiber, as in unmyelinated nerves

Sarcomere—smallest contractile unit of myofibrils in skeletal muscle

Sebaceous gland—simple alveolar gland that secretes oil (sebum)

Secretory coil—coiled secretory duct found in certain glands

Serosa—serous membrane, such as the peritoneum, pleura, or pericardium

Serum—watery fluid that remains after coagulating elements (clotting factors) have been removed from the plasma

Sexual response—penile erection and semen discharge (in men) or erection of the clitoris and labia minora without ejaculation of secretions (in women)

Sinoatrial node—specialized cardiac tissue that sets the rate of cardiac contraction; also called the pacemaker of the heart

Sinus rhythm—normal cardiac rhythm, originating in the sinoatrial node

Sodium-potassium pump—active transport mechanism that transports potassium ions through the cell membrane and simultaneously transports sodium ions out

Spermatogenesis—process of spermatozoa formation

Starling's law—the amount of stretching of cardiac muscle fiber helps regulate stroke volume

Stratum germinativum—growth layer of the epidermis; collective term for the stratum basale and stratum spinosum

Striated—marked by streaks (striae), such as striated muscle

Stroke volume—volume of blood ejected from a single ventricle with each contraction

Superficial—toward or at the body surface

Superior—cranial, or toward the head

Suture—fibrous joint in which the opposed surfaces are closely joined; an immovable articulation

Synapse—small gap between two neurons or between a neuron and an effect or organ

Synovial fluid—viscid fluid that lubricates the joint

Systole—cardiac contraction

Tendon—strong, flexible, fibrous band of connective tissue that attaches muscle to bone and other parts

Tidal volume—amount of air inhaled in one breath (about 500 ml in the average adult)

Transamination—exchange of an amino group in an amino acid for a keto group in a keto acid, through the action of transaminase enzymes

Tropic hormone—substance that stimulates hormone production by a target gland

Tubercle—small, rounded process

Tuberosity—elevation or protuberance; a broad, large process

Uteroplacental circulation—circulatory system that delivers oxygenated arterial blood from the maternal circulation to the placenta by the uterine arteries; it returns blood to maternal circulation by veins near the arteries

Ventilation—process of respiration in which air moves in and out of the lungs

Ventral—anterior, or toward the front of the body; the opposite of dorsal

Visceral peritoneum—serous membrane that covers the external surfaces of most abdominal organs (also called perimetrium)

Vital capacity—maximum amount of air that can be moved in and out of the lungs by maximum inspiration and maximum expiration (about 4,800 ml in the average adult)

Voiding reflex—involuntary reflex that causes the urge to urinate when the bladder contains 300 to 400 ml of urine; it is under a high degree of voluntary control

White matter—nervous tissue that appears white from myelinated sheaths surrounding nerve fibers

Zygote—fertilized ovum

APPENDIX B

Answers to Study Questions

CHAPTER 1

1. The functions of a body part (physiology) reflect its structure (anatomy). This relationship is called the complementarity of structure and function.
2. In increasing order of complexity, the levels of structural organization are: the chemical level, cellular level, tissue level, organ level, systems level, and organismic level.
3. Anatomical features are demarcated by dividing the body into planes, cavities, and regions.
4. The dorsal cavity includes the brain and spinal cord. The ventral cavity includes the lungs, heart (with large vessels), trachea, esophagus, thymus, lymph nodes, portions of other vessels and nerves, stomach, intestines, spleen, liver, bladder, rectum, and some reproductive organs.

CHAPTER 2

1. Carbon, hydrogen, nitrogen, and oxygen comprise 96% of the human body, by weight. Calcium and phosphorus account for 2.5% of the body weight.
2. An atom with unpaired electrons in its outer electron shell can participate in chemical reactions. All atoms try to achieve stability by emptying their outermost electron shell or by filling it as much as possible. To do this, atoms must accept, release, or share electrons with other atoms.
3. An ionic bond forms when valence electrons are transferred from one atom to another. A covalent bond forms when atoms share pairs of valence electrons.
4. Water acts as a solvent, suspension medium, and lubricant; enters into chemical reactions; helps the body maintain homeostasis; and keeps the body cool through perspiration.
5. Dehydration synthesis converts monosaccharides into more complex carbohydrates and water. Hydrolysis breaks down complex carbohydrates into monosaccharides by adding water.
6. DNA has a double-helix structure, contains deoxyribose, and consists of arginine, cytosine, guanine, and thymine. RNA has a single-chain structure, contains ribose, and substitutes uracil for the base thymine.

CHAPTER 3

1. Although most cells are specialized, they all have these four major components: cell membrane, cytosol, organelles, and inclusions.
2. Mitochondria contain enzymes that oxidize food nutrients. This oxidation produces ATP, which

provides the energy for many cellular activities.

3. Active transport methods, such as endocytosis, require energy; passive transport methods, such as diffusion and osmosis, do not.
4. A dominant gene is expressed in the heterozygous state. A recessive gene is expressed only in the homozygous state.
5. DNA's primary function is to carry the genetic information in living cells.
6. Ribosomal RNA (rRNA) is used to make ribosome in the endoplasmic reticulum. Messenger RNA (mRNA) specifies the amino acid arrangement for making proteins at the ribosomes. Transfer RNA (tRNA) carries specific amino acids during protein synthesis.
7. The four phases of cell division are prophase, metaphase, anaphase, and telophase.

CHAPTER 4

1. The three layers of epithelial tissue are the simple epithelium, stratified epithelium, and pseudostratified epithelium.
2. The connective tissue matrix is composed of collagenous, elastic, and reticular fibers.
3. Striated muscle tissue is attached to the bones. Cardiac muscle tissue forms the heart wall. Smooth-muscle tissue is found in the GI, respiratory, and genitourinary tracts; arrectores pilorum; nipples and scrotum; and ciliary body and iris of the eye.
4. Neurons generate and conduct nerve impulses. Neuroglia insulate and protect neurons.

CHAPTER 5

1. The two fused layers of the skin are the epidermis and dermis.
2. When blood is needed by other parts of the body, the skin shunts its blood to the general circulation.
3. The epidermis contains keratinocytes, melanocytes, Merkel's cells, and Langerhans' cells.
4. The dermis contains fibroblasts, macrophages, mast cells, and white blood cells.
5. Under sympathetic nervous system control, sudoriferous glands secrete sweat through a duct on the body's surface.
6. The skin regulates body temperature by a negative feedback mechanism, which affects sweat glands and blood vessels in response to environmental temperature changes.

CHAPTER 6

1. The two types of bone tissue are compact tissue, which is dense and smooth, and cancellous tissue, which has a spongy or latticelike structure.
2. Based on shape, bones may be classified as long, short, flat, or irregular.
3. Cartilage supports and shapes various body structures and cushions the bones.
4. The axial skeleton forms the body's vertical axis (skull, vertebrae, and bony thorax). The ap-

pendicular skeleton includes all the bones that hang off the axial skeleton (shoulder and pelvic girdles and upper and lower limbs).

5. Synarthroses allow little or no movement; amphiarthroses allow slight movement; and diarthrosis allow free movement.

CHAPTER 7

1. Muscle excitability is the property that allows a muscle to receive and respond to a stimulus.
2. Skeletal and cardiac muscle tissues are striated.
3. Cardiac and smooth muscle tissues are under involuntary control.
4. Actin and myosin are the principle proteins involved in muscle contractions.
5. Smooth muscle may be single-unit or multi-unit tissue.
6. The name of a skeletal muscle may come from its location, action, size, shape, point of attachment, number of divisions, or direction of fibers.
7. The all-or-none response governs skeletal muscle fiber contraction. If an impulse is strong enough to stimulate a contraction, all the fibers in the motor unit contract. If not, none of them contracts.
8. Cross bridges form during skeletal muscle contraction, when myosin heads bind to actin filaments. Cross bridges pull the actin filaments toward the center of the sarcomere, which causes muscle fiber shortening.

CHAPTER 8

1. The endocrine system works with the nervous system to maintain homeostasis.
2. The brain and spinal cord are the major components of the CNS
3. Neurons have more specialized functions than neuroglia. Also, they conduct impulses, but cannot reproduce; neuroglia cannot conduct impulses, but can reproduce.
4. The major regions of the brain are the cerebrum, diencephalon, cerebellum, and brain stem.
5. The autonomic and somatic nervous systems are both parts of the PNS.
6. A simple reflex arc requires sensory, connecting, and motor neurons.

CHAPTER 9

1. Receptors for the special senses are found in complex organs in a relatively small area of the body. Receptors for the general senses are found throughout the body.
2. When light waves hit the retina, they stimulate an impulse that is conveyed to the brain, where it is interpreted as a visual image.
3. Near vision allows viewing of objects closer than 20′ (6.1 m) from the eye, which requires accommodation, pupillary constriction, and eye convergence. Binocular vision (single vision with two eyes) permits depth or distance perception and creates a larger field of vision. It relies on convergence and transmission of two slightly different images to

the brain, where they are synthesized (fused) into a single image.

4. The external ear collects sound; the middle ear conducts it. The inner ear transmits sound waves and maintains equilibrium.
5. Differences in the loudness result from variations in hair cell stimulation. Loud sounds stimulate more hair cells, which generate more impulses than soft sounds.
6. The sense of smell must be functioning properly in order for taste perception to occur.
7. Pain impulses are transmitted by myelinated and unmyelinated nerve fibers via the same transmission route as the other general senses. Different types of pain result from stimulation of different areas.

CHAPTER 10

1. The right side of the heart acts as a pulmonary pump; the left side, as a systemic pump.
2. When the atria contract, blood flows into the relaxed ventricles. When the atria relax, the ventricles contract, ejecting the blood into the arteries. At the same time, venous blood flows into the relaxed atria. After expelling blood, the ventricles relax in preparation for the next cardiac cycle.
3. The SA node is the heart's pacemaker. It is located in the posterior wall of the right atrium near the opening of the superior vena cava.
4. Arteries carry blood away from the heart; veins transport blood to the heart. Veins are larger than arteries, but arteries have thicker walls. Unlike arteries, veins have one-way valves. Mean arterial pressure remains around 100 mm Hg; venous pressure, less than 15 mm Hg.
5. Systolic pressure measures the force of ventricular contraction. Diastolic pressure measures peripheral resistance caused by arteriolar vasoconstriction.

CHAPTER 11

1. Blood delivers oxygen and nutrients to body cells; transports wastes away from the cells; transports hormones to target tissues; maintains body temperature; maintains acid-base balance; maintains adequate fluid volume; helps prevent blood loss through hemostasis; and helps prevent infection.
2. Granulocytes (neutrophils, eosinophils, and basophils) contain cytoplasmic granules. Agranulocytes (lymphocytes and monocytes) lack these granules.
3. Hematopoiesis produces seven types of blood cells from one stem cell.
4. A compound in RBCs, hemoglobin carries oxygen from the lungs to the cells and transports carbon dioxide from cells to the lungs. Iron is an essential component of hemoglobin.
5. WBCs participate in inflammatory and immune responses, defending the body against viruses, bacteria, and other foreign particles
6. Platelets aggregate and adhere to the injury site, release vasocon-

strictors and a phospholipid that initiates coagulation, and form a plug in small capillary breaks.
7. The ABO and Rh blood groups are both based on the presence of antigens of the surface of RBCs.

CHAPTER 12

1. The major lymph tissues are the lymph nodes, spleen, and thymus.
2. Lymph conveys foreign substances to the lymph nodes (where lymphocytes act on them), helps maintain the osmotic pressure of interstitial fluid, and transports nutrients absorbed from the digestive tract.
3. Both types begin development in the bone marrow. T lymphocytes finish it in the thymus; B lymphocytes, in the bone marrow.
4. The body maintains nonspecific resistance through factors in the skin and mucous membranes, antimicrobial substances, phagocytosis, inflammation, and fever.
5. The body obtains acquired immunity after exposure to a foreign substance causes antibody formation or lymphatic activation.
6. In cell-mediated immunity, cytotoxic T cells directly kill organisms or other invading cells. Helper T cells interact with other T and B lymphocytes to enhance the immune response. Suppressor T cells prevent the other T cells from causing excessive immune reactions and severe tissue damage.
7. The cause of an allergic response is reexposure to a sensitizing antigen. Effects can range from allergic symptoms, such as sneezing, stuffy nose, and itchy eyes, to life-threatening anaphylaxis.

CHAPTER 13

1. The upper airways include the nose, pharynx, and larynx. The lower airways include the trachea and bronchi.
2. Gas exchange takes place in the alveoli.
3. The lungs remain expanded in the pleural cavity because the intrapleural pressure is less than the intrapulmonary pressure.
4. The inspiratory reserve volume is the amount of air (3,000 ml) than an adult can forcefully inhale after a normal inspiration. The expiratory reserve volume is the amount of air (1,300 ml) than an adult can forcefully exhale after a normal inspiration.
5. During diffusion, gases move from an area with a high partial pressure of the gas to one with a low partial pressure.
6. Carbon dioxide travels to the lungs dissolved in plasma, combined with hemoglobin, and combined with water as carbonic acid and its component ions.
7. The respiratory center is primarily regulated by arterial P_{CO_2}.

CHAPTER 14

1. The GI system ingests, digests, and absorbs food.
2. The large intestine's main function is to absorb water and eliminate digestive waste products.

3. Accessory organs include gastrin glands, intestinal glands, the liver, gallbladder, and pancreas. Most of them produce or store secretions needed for the digestion.
4. Enzymes hydrolyze nutrients in the GI tract.
5. Anabolism and catabolism are both metabolic processes. Anabolism allows the synthesis of complex substances; catabolism allows their breakdown.
6. Unlike the citric acid cycle and electron transport system, glycolysis requires no oxygen.
7. Keto acid–acetyl CoA conversion causes excess amino acids to be converted into fat.
8. Glucagon and epinephrine both promote glycogenolysis, gluconeogenesis, and lipolysis.

CHAPTER 15

1. The renal pyramids are located in the renal medulla. These triangular, striated wedges discharge urine from their apices into the renal pelvis, which forms the upper end of the ureters.
2. The ureters, renal blood vessels, lymphatic vessels, and nerves enter or exit the kidneys through the hilus.
3. The kidneys dispose of wastes and excess ions in the form of urine; filter blood, regulating its volume and chemical makeup; maintain fluid, electrolyte, and acid-base balances; produce several hormones and enzymes; and convert vitamin D to a more active form.
4. The bladder stores urine and works with the urethra to eliminate urine.
5. The glomerular filtration rate depends on glomerular capillary permeability, blood pressure, and effective filtration rate.
6. Aldosterone regulates the rate of sodium reabsorption from the tubules. Antidiuretic hormone controls water reabsorption from the collecting tubules. These actions regulate urine volume and concentration.
7. Stretching of the bladder walls by accumulated urine triggers the voiding reflex.

CHAPTER 16

1. The intracellular fluid compartment includes fluid in the body's cells. The extracellular fluid compartment contains the intravascular and interstitial fluid compartments.
2. Water enters the body via the GI tract. It leaves via the skin, lungs, GI tract, and urinary tract.
3. Thirst and the countercurrent mechanism help the body achieve water balance.
4. A cation is a positively charged ion; an anion is a negatively charged ion.
5. Acids and bases both dissociate in water and help maintain a stable hydrogen ion concentration in body fluids. However, acids release hydrogen ions; whereas bases release ions that combine with hydrogen ions.
6. The body maintains acid-base balance by buffer systems and the lungs and kidneys.

CHAPTER 17

1. A hormone is a chemical substance that regulates the activities of specific organs by affecting target cells.
2. The anterior pituitary lobe secretes growth hormone, thyroid-stimulating hormone, adrenocorticotropic hormone, follicle-stimulating hormone, luteinizing hormone, and prolactin.
3. The hypothalamus produces antidiuretic hormone and oxytocin, which are stored in the posterior pituitary lobe.
4. Thyroid hormones are synthesized and stored in follicular cells in the thyroid gland.
5. Calcium metabolism is regulated by parathyroid hormone, vitamin D, and thyrocalcitonin.
6. The adrenal medulla produces steroid hormones; the adrenal cortex produces catecholamines.
7. Insulin chiefly controls carbohydrate metabolism.

CHAPTER 18

1. The male gonads are the testes; the female gonads are the ovaries.
2. The external female genitalia include the mons pubis, labia majora, labia minora, clitoris, and vestibule.
3. Unlike the male sexual climax, the female climax produces no secretions similar to ejaculate and is not required to achieve fertilization.
4. Fertilization requires sufficient spermatozoa, a mature ovum, and effective spermatozoa transport through the female reproductive tract.
5. Prolactin promotes lactation. Relaxin relaxes the connective tissue and pelvic ligaments and promotes cervical dilation. Prostaglandin mediates several physiological functions.
6. The first stage of labor is associated with cervical effacement and dilation and the beginning of fetal descent. The second stage covers the time between full cervical dilation and fetal expulsion. This third stage begins immediately after childbirth and ends with delivery of the placenta.
7. Estrogen, progesterone, prolactin, and oxytocin control lactation.

Selected References

Berkow, R., ed. *Merck Manual of Diagnosis and Therapy,* 16th ed. Rahway, N.J.: Merck & Co., Inc., 1992.

Crowley, L.V., and Abrams, C. *Applied Science Review: Physiology.* Springhouse, Pa.: Springhouse Corp., 1993.

Guyton, A.C., and Hall, J.E. *Textbook of Medical Physiology,* 9th ed. Philadelphia: W.B. Saunders Co., 1995.

Johnston, C. *Applied Science Review: Anatomy.* Springhouse, Pa.: Springhouse Corp., 1993.

Marieb, E.N. *Human Anatomy and Physiology,* 2nd ed. Reading, Mass.: Addison-Wesley Publishing Co., 1992.

Patrick, M.L., et al. *Medical Surgical Nursing: Pathophysiological Concepts,* 4th ed. Philadelphia: J.B. Lippincott Co., 1994.

Porth, C. *Pathophysiology*, 4th ed. Philadelphia: J.B. Lippincott Co., 1994.

Seeley, R.R., et al. *Essentials of Anatomy and Physiology,* 2nd ed. St. Louis: Mosby-Year Book, Inc., 1994.

Sheldon, H. *Boyd's Introduction to the Study of Disease,* 11th ed. Baltimore: Williams & Wilkins Co., 1992.

Spence, A., and Mason, E.B. *Human Anatomy and Physiology,* 4th ed. St. Paul, Minn.: West Publishing Co., 1992.

Tortora, G.J., and Grabowski, S.R. *Principles of Anatomy and Physiology,* 7th ed. New York: HarperCollins College Publishers, 1993.

Vander, A.J., et al. *Human Physiology: The Mechanisms of Body Function,* 6th ed. New York: McGraw-Hill Book Co., 1993.

Van De Graaff, K.M. *Human Anatomy.* Dubuque, Iowa: Wm. C. Brown Publishers, 1995.

Index

i refers to an illustration; t refers to a table

i refers to an illustration; t refers to a table

D

E

i refers to an illustration; t refers to a table

i refers to an illustration; t refers to a table

i refers to an illustration; t refers to a table

i refers to an illustration; t refers to a table

i refers to an illustration; t refers to a table

i refers to an illustration; t refers to a table

i refers to an illustration; t refers to a table

About the StudySmart Disk

StudySmart Disk lets you:

- review subject areas of your choice and learn the rationales for the correct answers
- take tests of varying lengths on subjects of your choice
- print the results of your tests to gauge your progress over time.

Recommended system requirements
486 IBM-compatible personal computer (386 minimum)
Windows® 3.1 or greater (Windows® 95/98 compatible)
High-density 3½″ floppy drive
8 MB RAM (4 MB minimum)
S-VGA monitor (VGA minimum)
2 MB of available space on hard drive

Installing and running the program

- Start Windows®.
- In Program Manager, choose Run from File menu.
- Insert disk, type a:\setup.exe (where a: is the letter of your floppy drive), and click OK.

For Windows® 95/98 Installation

- Start Windows.
- Select Start button and then Run.
- Insert disk, type a:\setup.exe (where a: is the letter of your floppy drive), and click OK.

For technical support, call 215-628-7744 Monday through Friday, 9 a.m. to 6 p.m. Eastern Standard Time.

The clinical information and tools in the StudySmart Disk are based on research and consultation with nursing, medical, and legal authorities. To the best of our knowledge, the program reflects currently accepted practice; nevertheless, it can't be considered absolute or universal. For individual application, all recommendations must be considered in light of the patient's clinical condition and, before administration of new or infrequently used drugs, in light of the latest package-insert information. The authors and publisher disclaim responsibility for any adverse effects resulting directly or indirectly from the suggested procedures, from any undetected errors, or from the reader's misunderstanding of the program.

Springhouse Corporation warrants to the user that the program media on which the software is recorded shall be free from defects in materials and workmanship for a period of ninety (90) days from the date of the user's purchase. Springhouse Corporation's liability shall be limited to correction or replacement of defective media.

This book cannot be returned for credit or refund if the vinyl disk holder has been opened, broken, or otherwise tampered with.